Contemporary Neuropsychiatry

Contemporary Neuropsychiatry:

Implications from Cognitive Neuroscience

Edited by

Drozdstoy Stoyanov

Cambridge Scholars Publishing

Contemporary Neuropsychiatry:
Implications from Cognitive Neuroscience

Edited by Drozdstoy Stoyanov

This book first published 2023

Cambridge Scholars Publishing

Lady Stephenson Library, Newcastle upon Tyne, NE6 2PA, UK

British Library Cataloguing in Publication Data
A catalogue record for this book is available from the British Library

ISBN (10): 1-5275-9455-6
ISBN (13): 978-1-5275-9455-5

TABLE OF CONTENTS

PREFACE

Contemporary neuropsychiatry is largely informed by the methods and sources of cognitive neuroscience and phenomenology.

This book attempts to consolidate some of the recent developments in the field.

The first part covers topics from phenomenology and clinical psychopathology.

Phenomenology and neurobiology of well-being set the stage in the opening chapter to formulate a comprehensive understanding of the limits of mental health and the premises of psychopathology. This fundamental chapter is delivered by David Foreman.

Phenomenological discourse is adopted in further investigation of the embodied attention by Francesca Brencio.

Formal thought disorder is explored by Dornelles and Telles-Correia in view of its pathogenetic mechanisms. Depression is reviewed from the perspective of developmental neuro-psychology in the next chapter by Matanova and Kostova.

Okan Caliyurt focuses on the meeting of descriptive psychopathology, inherited from the XX century tradition with post-modern trends in artificial intelligence approaches to construction of psychiatric diagnosis and treatment.

The second part includes topics explaining the mechanisms of mental disorders.

Chronobiological factors are largely underestimated as explanatory models in psychiatry. The contribution of Nadejda Madjirova is a tour-de-force introduction to this field and represents her legacy generated for decades of intensive research commitment.

Neurogenesis, more specifically stress-related alterations in hippocampus are presented in the chapter to follow by Peshev and Milanova.

Cerebellar mechanisms, ataxia and movement regulation are implicated in most of the mental disorders. The work of Haralanova and associates summarizes an effort to link neurological methods to psychiatry, with an emphasis on the potential application of original quantitative methods for evaluation of the movement pattern disorders in schizophrenia.

Finally, Basli and Bounaas present innovative treatment strategies in Alzheimer's disease, driven by the advances of molecular neuroscience.

This book is produced by an international group of established scholars with the intention to serve as state-of-the-art update about applications of neuroscience, cognitive science and phenomenology in the transition of psychiatry from a hybrid proto-science to a medical discipline.

It is dedicated to the loving memory of our colleague Prof. Dr Nadejda P. Madjirova (1945-2021), who authored one of the chapters in it.

Plovdiv
October 27th 2022
Drozdstoy Stoyanov

CHAPTER ONE

WELL-BEING THEORY: USING THE FREE ENERGY PRINCIPLE AND ACTIVE INFERENCE TO CONNECT PHENOMENOLOGY AND PSYCHOPATHOLOGY TO BIOLOGY THROUGH WELL-BEING

DAVID FOREMAN
KING'S COLLEGE & ROYAL COLLEGE OF PSYCHIATRISTS, LONDON

Abstract

Explaining the relationship between biology and subjectivity is challenging. Well-Being Theory uses the Free Energy Principle and Active Inference Model to formally connect objective biology to subjective phenomenology and psychopathology through well-being. The first section introduces the concepts of Markov blankets as necessary for an organism's survival. Generative modelling of informational free energy up to a bound is necessary for the organism to maintain adaptation to its environment without breaching its Markov blanket. Well-being becomes an organism's subjective measure of free energy, extending from simple to hierarchical organisms such as us, and is shown to be equivalent to ordinary measures of well-being, such as health-related quality of life. However, we must redefine our concept of our everyday selves as a set of nested environments, with upper and lower scale boundaries defined by embodiments of information-theoretic estimations. The second section shows how the embodiment of well-being across scale creates the unscalable subjective dimensions of our minds, while we can deduce both ordinary and pathological psychological phenomena from the necessary properties of our generative models. Well-Being Theory can thus be a useful tool for modelling general principles of phenomenology and psychopathology in terms of plausible biology, thus replacing the biopsychosocial model, which is shown to be inadequate to model well-being across scale.

Keywords: well-being; phenomenology; free energy principle

Introduction

It is current orthodoxy that the domains of genetics, neurobiology, economics, and sociocultural factors all contribute to disturbances in our mental health, expressed as psychopathology. However, our theories about how this happens are extremely vague. The face validity of concepts such as the biopsychosocial model have not been matched by advances in construct or predictive validity (e.g., Ghaemi, 2011), and quantification remains elusive.

Enormous strides have been made in methodology, reflected in large and increasing numbers of valuable, insightful publications. However, the practical obstacles to a purely empirical search strategy for finding efficient causes are insuperable. For example, in psychiatric genetics & genomics, sample sizes are now tens of thousands and still inadequate for complex interactions (e.g., Sullivan et al., 2018). In neuroimaging, the small sample sizes that the cost of the technologies impose, together with the number of investigator-sensitive parameters each methodology possesses, have generated a literature full of noise (Botvinik-Nezer et al., 2020; Marek et al., 2020, 2022). At the other end of the scale, indubitable societal influences on mental health, such as poverty, are also noisy, being only weakly predictive of mental health difficulties at the individual level (Das, Do, Friedman, McKenzie, & Scott, 2007; Ridley, Rao, Schilbach, & Patel, 2020). Practically, this means that advances in mental health therapy remain largely serendipitous, while biological and sociocultural psychopathologists propose competing potential explanations that are necessarily incomplete.

This failure may reflect the "curse of dimensionality" (Spruyt, 2014) that challenges artificial intelligence and machine learning (AI/ML): here, the dimensions arise from the progress of empirical research in discovering ever more parameters—with their associated errors in measurement—to be considered. These difficulties are compounded as the parameters have different scales, affecting how the errors in their measurement can be managed in respect of each other. In AI/ML, the solution is some form of weighting, where previous experience is abstracted to produce a set of rules which guide the search for the best solutions. Theories about mental health could provide such weighting in determining research choices, but currently, those available are either highly localised, frequently compete, or, if high-level, are vague, and the relationship between different theories remains undefined.

The introduction of Research Domain Criteria (RDoC) (NIMH, 2016) attempted to provide an empirically based framework that would scale sufficiently for cross-domain research. However, Patrick and Hajcak (2016) observed that further progress would depend upon developing

> "... a systematic measurement-oriented approach to clarifying relations between psychological phenomena and physiological variables in the service of understanding clinical problems." (Patrick & Hajcak, 2016)

In short, RDoC will fail without some measure-related theory to link those parameters. Unfortunately, Carcone & Ruocco (2017) found that research using the RDoC paradigm tended to sit within specific RDoC domains rather than form bridges between them and empirical attempts to link to other measurements struggle (Funkhouser et al., 2021). Within biology, successful theories are scalable; Darwinian evolution's random mutation and selection are good examples. In contrast, psychopathology, which dominates our attempts to understand mental disorders, is extremely resistant to scaling, as it is based on mapping humans 'subjectivities using principles derived from Husserl's phenomenology (Jaspers, 1963). Viewing well-being as psychopathology's inverse can resolve these scaling difficulties as it is not limited to subjectivity, and treating it as "model evidence" for free energy minimisation allows its embodiment within a scalable theory of biological cognition, called here the Free Energy Principle (FEP) (Kirchhoff, Parr, Palacios, Friston, & Kiverstein, 2018) which may give an account of the genesis of well-being and psychopathology (Corcoran & Hohwy, 2017; Miller, Rietveld, & Kiverstein, 2021). Here, the approach is used to develop an embodied general theory of phenomenology to help empirical research link biology with subjectivity.

Imagining a Biological Organism from the Perspective of Well-Being

Imagine an organism O living in an environment $\boldsymbol{E}$. We are interested in how O can persist in $\boldsymbol{E}$, given that only a subset of $\boldsymbol{E}$, E, will permit this, and $\boldsymbol{E}$ is subject to random variation. We consider two points of view. There is the observer's perspective, but also the perspective of the organism itself, and the two will not always coincide, e.g., when O makes a mistake. Formulae reflecting an observer's point of view will be written in black, but those from the organism's point of view in red to aid clarity. Table 1 provides a list of symbols.

Symbol	Interpretation
Red, Black	Organism's (subjective) perspective observer's (objective) perspective
O	Biological organism
$\mathbb{O}$	Observer
$\boldsymbol{E}$	General specifier of environment
E	Subset of environment which can sustain the organism
V	Generic random variable
$\subset$	Subset
$\sqcup$	Disjoint union
$\perp$	Conditional independence
$\backslash$	Disjoint sets
V_O	Environmental variable values that support the organism
$V_{\mathbb{O}}$	Environmental variable set of an arbitrary observer
$D_{KL}(X \parallel Y)$	Kullback-Liebler divergence (between X and Y)
$\boldsymbol{S}$	Entropy
$\mathbb{S}$	Relative Informational Free Energy between X and Y
$\mapsto$	X maps to Y
δ	Modifier indicating a small increment or variation to a max/min value.

Symbol	Interpretation
$ForF$	Objective or Subjective Well-being
$\mathcal{L}, \mathcal{L}$	Laplace transformation
s	The frequency parameter of the Laplace transformation
C	Constant of integration
$\mathfrak{S} or \mathfrak{S}$	Surprisal (satisficing is $-\mathfrak{S}$)
m	Model used to generate predictions (generative model)
Θ	Parameters of generative model
p, q	Generic probability distributions
iid	Variable(s) drawn from identical & identically distributed populations
R, R	The organism's biology, understood from its own perspective
L	Lagrangian
T	Total kinetic energy in a system
V	Total potential energy in a system
S	Action in a Lagrangian system
U	Economic utility
$\succ$	Succeeds (also with reference to scale)
W	Embodied subjective well-being
Ψ, Ψ	O's communication, command and control system (C3)
ψ	That part of C3 phenomenologically represented as "mind"
$\hat{F}, \hat{\mathbb{S}}$	Imputed well-being or relative informational free energy

Symbol	Interpretation
$\mathcal{F}$	Subjective embodiment of $\mathcal{L}$; dimension of phenomenological space
$\tilde{\mathcal{F}}$	Psychopathological dimension

Table 1: List of Symbols (in order of use)

The Markov Blanket

Defining $\boldsymbol{E}$ as generally as possible, we can say that it is a set of random variables $\{V_1 \ldots V_n\}$. An organism may be present, but, as observers, we do not yet know. We guess that $O \subset \boldsymbol{E}$, as we assume O will include at most $\{V_{a\geq 1} \ldots V_{b<n}\}$, for any O will need some separable environment. We also note that $O \sqcup \boldsymbol{E}$ so it can sustain itself in its environment and not dissolve. A Markov blanket $O \perp \boldsymbol{E} \backslash V_O | V_O$ can enable this for O, as it defines a boundary between O and $\boldsymbol{E}$. It means that we, or O, can deduce its existence from observing V_O. It follows that $V_O = E$. We should note that if either we or O do not observe V_O (E) we will not conclude an organism is present, and O must be able to self-identity, as otherwise it will be destroyed when it meets values of $\{V_1 \ldots V_n\}$ that are not compatible with its continued existence. In symbols, this is $O \sqcup \boldsymbol{E} | E \subseteq V_{\mathbb{O}}$. Observers have Markov blankets, too. We shall see that $E \subseteq E$.

Deriving Well-Being from Informational Free Energy

The problem of how O can do this without breaching its Markov blanket (and so invite dissolution) is solved by invoking the Free Energy Principle (FEP). In general, informational free energy is defined as $\boldsymbol{S}(Q|\{X_i\}) = -K \sum_i p_i \, log \, p_i$, where $\boldsymbol{S}$ is entropy, Q the quantity being considered, $\{X_i\}$ is a set of variables and p_i their probability distributions. Free energy is high when there are many equivalently possible outcomes; it decreases as the number of possibilities falls.

Provided it has some prior information, O can make a reasonably informed guess about what is out there without breaching its Markov blanket. In our notation, this is E. If the guess is correct, all is well, so it needs to know how different its guess is from what is *really* out there. Then, it can adapt. The Kullback-Liebler divergence between predictions E and reality E $D_{KL}(E \parallel E)$ will capture this, which is also the relative informational free energy of that difference, $\mathbb{S}$ (Buckley, Kim, McGregor, & Seth, 2017). The asymmetry of D_{KL} makes space for subjectivity, implicit in E. For O, The difference in terms of free energy is $\mathbb{S}(O \sqcup \boldsymbol{E}|E) = -K \sum_O p_O \ln p_O$.

However, our organism still must get from E to E without breaking its Markov blanket, as what it needs to survive is $\mathbb{S}(O \sqcup \boldsymbol{E}|E) = -K \sum_O p_O \ln p_O$. It can do this by acting as if E were true, monitoring its consequential experiences (which are subjective) and plugging them into a loss function, something that reaches a minimum (or equivalent maximum) when $\boldsymbol{E} = E$. This is equivalent to trying to minimise $\mathbb{S}$ through its actions, symbolised as $\lim_{\mathbb{S}\to 0} f\colon \nabla\mathbb{S} \mapsto \nabla\mathbb{S}$; the red indicates that O needs to map the real gradient change into subjectivity to act upon it. O needs time $t + \delta t$ to enact its prediction, so the quantity of interest to O is actually $\lim_{\mathbb{S}\to 0} \int \mathbb{S}dt \sim \lim_{\mathbb{S}\to 0} \int \mathbb{S}dt|O$. A Laplace transform can estimate this as an expected value for a probability distribution (here shown for the gradient $\nabla\mathbb{S}$)

$$\mathcal{L}\{f\colon \nabla\mathbb{S}(t)\} = \int_0^\infty e^{-st} f\colon \nabla\mathbb{S}(t)dt$$

This maximises O's model evidence for its prediction E, getting its predictions E into an *objective* comparison with $\boldsymbol{E}$ so that it can get to $\mathbb{S}$. If we think of O's behaviour as modelling its predictions, we can understand that this quantity is the total change in evidence for its world model (hence "model evidence" above) following its action. This model is frequently called a "generative model" as it generates the evidence the organism relies on to decide its next actions. We will denote it as m; note that while it exists objectively, there is no need for O to be aware of more enough to enable appropriate actions, so $E \subseteq E$.

This model evidence is F or F, depending on the point of view. For the time being, let us assume O is getting it right, so $F = F$. If O has leached every possible benefit from its environment by its action, then $F = 1$, but with no environmental support $F = 0$, and O dies. It now makes sense to call this model evidence "well-being" but note that "well-being" inverts the value of $\mathbb{S}$: well-being F is maximised when $\mathbb{S}$ is minimised.

Surprisal

Compare a beloved goldfish in its aquarium with a mackerel being grilled for tea. In terms of our model, we can hope, for the goldfish, that $F \approx F \approx 1$. For the grilling mackerel, it is clear $F = 0$, but F simply does not exist, as there is no longer a functioning mackerel to model it. As the illustration shows, organisms can only minimise $\mathbb{S}$ up to some bound; what lies beyond that is called "surprisal." Surprisal is why severe burns may be less painful than minor ones: with pain and temperature receptors gone, we can no longer model what has happened to us. Mathematically, surprisal is $\mathfrak{S} = -log(prob\boldsymbol{E} = E)$ so it grows as the environment becomes more hostile, but it can never be incorporated into F, as that refers to *model* evidence, and surprisal, by this definition, cannot be modelled.

Limits to modelling

There are more limits to O than E. Implicit in minimising $\mathbb{S}$ is O updating itself accurately in the light of new information. This involves the prior information O has, the structure of the model m it uses, and the parameters Θ in that model, which define the dependencies between the model's variables. The number of variables in $\boldsymbol{E}$ is typically enormous, and the parameters of all possible interactions $\Theta \sim {}^{\boldsymbol{E}!}/_{E!\,(\boldsymbol{E} - E)!}\,|O$ potentially much larger still, so $\int \Theta$, necessary to determine $\mathbb{S}$, is intractable. However, we have seen O only needs to model up to a boundary, which permits a variational approach to updating. The Laplace approximation to a Gaussian distribution enables an approximate factorisation of the distribution of interest $q(E, \Theta) \approx q_E(E)q_\Theta(\Theta)$. If E is iid, all E can be treated as mutually independent, while $N(\Theta_E) = N(E)$. The price paid is ignoring how fluctuations in E require fluctuations in Θ to accurately model $q(E, \Theta)$. Laplace's approximation also greatly simplifies finding integrals—here $q_E(E)$—by allowing variation distant from a global maximum to be ignored. This lets a (computationally tractable) variational Bayesian approach find $-\mathbb{S} = F$ (Buckley et al., 2017), but the maximum F identified may not be global. So, these approximations and assumptions also contribute to surprisal. As this surprisal reflects computational limits rather than environmental incompatibility, it is subjective & denoted as $\mathfrak{S}$. Despite being subjective, it is still outside F. It is usually (imprecisely) referred to by its negative, i.e., what we can comprehend given our cognitive limits—satisficing, denoted as $-\mathfrak{S}$.

Scaling Well-Being

Organisms function at several scales. We, for example, are composed of organs, which are composed of cells, which have their own organelles, each with its individual biochemistry. Well-being must be expressed across all those scales, and each level must make its separate contribution to total well-being F, independently and interactively. The generative model m is therefore hierarchical. From the above, we can write

$$F = \lim_{\mathbb{S} \to min} \left(\prod_{1}^{m} F_i \to 1 \right)$$

For any individual level

$$F_i = E_i R_i F_{i-1}$$

To understand the new term R, consider the relevant Laplace transform $\mathcal{L}_i\{f \colon \nabla\mathbb{S}_i(t)\} = \int_0^\infty e^{-st_i} f \colon \nabla\mathbb{S}_i(t)dt$. Remember that $\lim_{\mathbb{S} \to min} \sim F|O$ and F is being measured at its maximal, steady state. R_i is, therefore, the integral of e^{-st_i} with respect to time, $e^{-st_i}/s + C$. $1/_s$ is not level specific, so it may be applied recursively across all levels. The constant of integration, C, can be interpreted as representing all the unknown structures and processes O uses to generate e^{-st_i}, allowing C to be proportionally scaled as 1. R will also behave as a normalising constant, as the probability for F at steady state is also (approximately) 1. Therefore, it represents the organism's biology from the organism's perspective and sets its upper and lower scale boundaries. Beyond the upper boundary lies the organism's environment, and beneath the lower is the chemistry from which the organism arises. We can think of these boundaries as phase transitions in how informational free energy is embodied across scale.

A problem estimating well-being arises at the lower boundary $m = 1$, as $F_i = F_0$ does not exist, stopping evaluation of F_1 and thus the whole system.

Recalling $R_i = e^{-st_i}/s + C$ and taking logs, we can write (assuming $C = 1$ as above)

$$\lim_{F\to 1}\left(\sum_{1}^{m} \log E_i + \log F_{i-1} - st_i - \log s \to 0\right)$$

For $m = 1$, we can write $\lim_{F\to 1}(\log E_1 = st_1 - \log s)$. So, not only may an organism estimate well-being even at its lowest level from its biology, but organisms without internal hierarchy are possible, too, while s is a frequency parameter, so it can coordinate levels in m across temporal and spatial scales.

Environment, Individual Identity, and Action

Our consideration of how we need to measure our well-being, especially across scale, leads us to a novel interpretation of what it means to be ourselves. We are not material individuals in an environment, but a nested set of environments, structured and coordinated by some shared rules, which also define the everyday boundary between ourselves and our world, and a less familiar boundary with the small-scale world of biochemistry. Each nested environment, while following the recursive rules expressed in s and embodied in C, functions to a different timescale t_i. The ability to process information to ensure survival is not just a function of our nervous system but is a fundamental property of any living system, so implies similar nesting of our subjectivity, which is no longer coterminous with our awareness.

All this sounds strange and alien, but we have an everyday illustration available in our own blood. At our scale, it looks like a thickish liquid that comes in various shades of red and brownish purple. Put a drop under a microscope, and we see a liquid environment containing white and red blood cells. Some of the former seem to have, at the very least, more awareness than the latter, displaying what looks like purposeful intention as they engulf bacteria. Drilling down further, we see sets of chemical reactions organised by a micro-architecture that seems purposefully arranged. While it is easy to observe the difference in timescale here—e.g., macrophages engulfing bacteria takes seconds to minutes, but a successful immune response may take days to complete—more is needed to understand how it happens.

From a purely physical perspective, an organism, like its environment, is just a bunch of stuff moving around. So, like all other stuff in our universe, a mechanical model may describe its behaviour, and the Lagrangian one is helpful here. Especially, its "principle of least action" is a thermodynamic equivalent to the loss function discussed above, which enables the descent/ascent (equivalent here) of *informational* gradients to be accurately embodied by *thermodynamic* ones.

The basic Lagrangian formalism is very simple, with a numerical summary of the total dynamics of a system, called the Lagrangian (L) being the difference between the system's total kinetic energy (T) and potential energy (V); $L = T - V$. As T includes velocity and therefore implies motion, V can be conceived as a gradient (slope or potential) in any space (or field) necessary for motion (or its equivalent, e.g., current) to occur. If the beginning and end of the motion are points in time, the path between them is called an action (S). There are many possible paths connecting two time points. The path of least action is the most direct one. We can thus conceive of O's continued existence as an action and its environment as a kind of landscape, where it needs to find the most direct route to each and every future point that best sustains its existence. We can formalise this path as $S = \int_{t_1}^{t_2} L dt$, where $\delta L = 0$. O finds it through embodying the equivalent informational gradient— $\underset{F \to 1}{min}(\mathbb{S} \approx \mathbb{S}) \equiv (\delta L \to 0)$ —as discussed above. When, like us, O is hierarchical, $S = \prod_m S_i$, with each integral nested up to m. So, superordinate integrals, being integrals of integrals with respect to time, will define longer timescales. If we now focus on the kinetic energy T associated with each action S, the longer timescales of superordinate actions will make them seem like gradients V to their subordinate components. So hierarchical development allows more sophisticated actions by letting O manipulate both T and V at multiple scales, using its objective biology R.

Rhythm, Control, and the Non-Equilibrium Steady State

Organisms are one example of Non-Equilibrium Steady States (NESS), systems that maintain themselves by constant correction, though remaining far from their environmental equilibrium. If we think about the Lagrangian associated with that, it will need to follow a closed route, which, extended in time, will form a sinusoidal path as it drifts away from and then moves back towards optimal conditions to maintain the NESS. Breathing is one example. Embodying s provides adjustable frequency parameters to deliver this. In reality, δL represents random perturbations, not a regular rhythm. However, as the Fourier transform demonstrates, any irregular waveform can be represented by a superposition of enough regular ones, and in hierarchical organisms, m's nested levels can provide these (Rue, Martino, & Chopin, 2009).

Empirical Assessment of Well-Being

In everyday language, "well-being" denotes individuals flourishing (or not) in their environments. As defined by our model, embodied well-being represents us as the uppermost level in the nested environments of O. Let us denote this level as I (for individuals) and its associated well-being as F_I. There must be an F_{I-1}, which fits our understanding of "health" as it estimates the well-being of those nested environments that, together and connected by R, make up our bodies.

From the arguments above, F estimates the usable fraction (E) of $\boldsymbol{E}$ available to O, so it describes a utility U. In health economics, the health-related version is Health-Related Quality of Life (HRQOL), which is measured by differences in health-state preference, with a presumption that health will be preferred. It may be directly estimated by evaluating how much loss would be equivalent to a particular suboptimal health state, which is also $\max_{\boldsymbol{S}}(\boldsymbol{S}(Q|\{X_{loss}, X_{health-state}\}) = -K\sum_i p_i \ln p_i) = -F_{max}$ as there is, at estimation, no information to allow preference of one over the other. This utility is scaled to 1 being perfect health and 0 death (Payakachat, Murawski, & Summers, 2009). We can therefore state $F_{I-1} \propto U_{HRQOL}$, as they are derived equivalently. Defining well-being as embodied model evidence has turned out to include everyday health-related well-being, which latter requires no reinterpretation.

HRQOL is not considered qualitatively distinct from any other utility considered in economics (Payakachat et al., 2009). We also have an everyday word for the set of affordances we need to survive as individuals; they constitute our welfare. If we accept that HRQOL is what we understand as "being healthy" in everyday language (which implicitly sets $m = I$), we can therefore say $Well - being \sim (Welfare \times Health)|R$, or, forgetting R as everyday language is wont to do $Well - being = Welfare \times Health$. In its complete form, we can express this as previously

$$\lim_{F \to max} \left(\prod_{Health}^{Welfare} E_{Welfare} R F_{Health} \to 1 \right)$$

We can see that our model does not undermine or redefine our current measures of well-being. Instead, it clarifies the otherwise vague concepts, such as "welfare", "health", or "utility", which underpin them, in terms of our necessary biology.

From Well-Being to Psychopathology

Death, Disease and Disadvantage

It is essential to check if our imagined model can cope with these if it is to include psychopathology. From the above, we can write, from the perspective of an observer only

$$F_{death} = U_E = 0$$

As O is dead, there is no perspective to create R. We can say that the environment provides no utility to our dead O, but we cannot observe E either, because the organism's conditional independence from its environment is gone—the dead mackerel cannot resist being grilled. The multiplication rules say that any $U_{E_i} = 0$ is sufficient to determine death. An everyday example is $U_{E_{I-1}} = 0$, which is the same as saying $HRQOL = 0$. Death can therefore be defined as an instance of a level-specific environment (or more) being unable to provide sufficient utility to $\prod_1^m O_i = O$, which matches everyday experience.

It makes sense to say that disease is something intermediate between life and death, as modelled by HRQOL. Our model can cope with this, by setting at least one $U_{E_i} \ll 1$. Impaired welfare, or disadvantage, now becomes a special case of disease, where $U_{E_i} = U_{E_{I+1}}$, the external environment to O. It is "special" because, being outside R, our ability to regulate V (the gradients in our environment) can only be achieved by actions expressed through T_I. From this, we may draw the unsurprising conclusion that there is no clear boundary between ordinary ($U_E < 1$) and impaired ($U_E \ll 1$) health or well-being. Our model is consistent with our ordinary intuitions about these. However, there is a caveat, discussed next.

The Biopsychosocial Model Fails for Well-Being

The biopsychosocial model remains the most popular way to understand mental health. Because m_i is associated with a unique U_{E_i}, $F_{death} = U_E = 0$ can test whether a proposed level m_i is valid. The model can be formalised as

$$F_I \sim \left(\prod_{1}^{I+1} m_i \, , m = \{m_{social} \succ m_{psychological} \succ m_{physical}\} \right) |R$$

The physical level precedes, so is nested within the psychological, which is nested within the social level. We situate our identity in the middle layer. The biopsychosocial model makes no distinction between subjective and objective perspectives, so we treat it as objective (from the observer's perspective). From this, we deduce a set of objective level-specific environmental utilities $\{U_{E_{physical}}, U_{E_{psychological}}, U_{E_{social}}\}$. We do not have to consider ordering, as any product including a zero will result in death, so disagreements over the order of nesting make no difference. Setting $U_{E_{physical}} = 0$ will lead to death, as that is HRQOL. However, coma or anaesthesia set $U_{E_{psychological}} = 0$, without death being in any way inevitable. So, it seems that $m_{psychological}$ is not a valid level in our model. Instead, we might want to say $m_{psychological} \subset m_i$, though we cannot yet say what the whole of m_i encompasses. A similar problem arises with and $U_{E_{social}} = 0$ though the latter is beyond this chapter's scope. We consider alternatives to $m_{psychological}$ next.

Imagining a Biologically Valid Psychology

The Dimensions of Subjectivity

We have already seen that subjectivity is the inevitable consequence of O needing to traverse its environment while maintaining its Markov blanket. We have acknowledged that F is information-theoretic, so it needs embodiment. We define our assessment of our well-being as $\{W\}$ as there are many ways that we can monitor our well-being. A helpful analogy is to think of a tool. If we liken F_i to a ruler, then W_i is the ruler we happen to own, with all its virtues and flaws. We can state $\{W\} = \{\mathcal{F}Fe\}$, where $\mathcal{F}$

denotes the transformation our measurement tools perform, so is the subjective embodiment of $\mathcal{L}$, and e is the error they introduce. As $F = \prod_1^m F_i$, we will need at least m subjective scales W_i to evaluate F. By substitution, we can say $W_i = \mathcal{F}_i F_i e_i$ as each W_i is likely to need a different transformative function and, therefore, will have a different error. We can therefore write, for a simple 2-level case, such as welfare and health, and substituting utilities for "objective" well-being to improve clarity

$$W = \prod_{Health}^{Welfare} W_i = \{W_{Welfare}, W_{Health}\} = \prod_{Health}^{Welfare} \mathcal{F}_i U_i\, e_i$$

We may scale W between 0 and 1, but $\max_{F \to 1} W < F$ because of e_i, and $\mathcal{F}_i$ is not recursive: the rules that embody R could, and indeed need to, produce many different forms of $\mathcal{F}$. This is consistent with our intuition—we use different vocabularies to discuss each, and our subjective awareness of our health is quite different from our welfare. This is despite measuring level-specific utilities U_i, which are simply components of the total utility U_E that O needs to survive. While this is "error" in terms of measuring U_E it is not mistaken, as it needs to match the E_i it is monitoring. For example, we cannot use our ruler to measure the distance between stars, but using a telescope instead gives output that is qualitatively distinct from that of the ruler, despite referring to the same metric of length.

We can now write, again substituting utilities

$$\begin{aligned} W_I &\sim (\mathcal{F}_{Welfare} U_{Welfare} e_{Welfare})(\mathcal{F}_{Health} U_{Health} e_{Health}) | R \\ &= \mathcal{F}_{Welfare} \mathcal{F}_{Health} \left(U_{Welfare} e_{Welfare} U_{Health} e_{Health} \right) | R \end{aligned}$$

The qualitative differences necessary to measure utility across our nested environments have created a multidimensional (in this case, the two dimensions are $\mathcal{F}_{Welfare}\mathcal{F}_{Health}$) space within which the total utility, and hence well-being, can be measured. Notice, as discussed above, that the multidimensionality of W_I encodes the transformation introduced by $\{\mathcal{F}_i\}$, so does not apply to U_I. Recall that monitoring our well-being is to shape our behaviour appropriately. We generalise $\mathcal{F}_{Welfare}\mathcal{F}_{Health}$ to $\prod_1^m \mathcal{F}_i$, as we might well be monitoring more levels of which we are not subjectively aware. $\prod_1^M \mathcal{F}_i$ is, therefore, a space in which well-being can be represented subjectively: Ψ. This gives us $W \sim U\Psi \prod_1^m e_i \,|R$ Think back to our ruler and telescope analogy. The distances they measure comprise U, encoded as F (remember, obtaining utility U from environment E is why organisms need to measure F in the first place). The difference in processing needed to obtain each measurement generates the qualitative differences that set the dimensions of Ψ, while the total within-measurement error is $\prod_1^m e_i$.

The subjective space Ψ we have just outlined is a superset of what is usually considered "psychological" in the biopsychosocial model. This becomes clearer if we consider that this definition of subjectivity extends to things that we would not typically attach subjectivity to, due to scaling. Consider a white blood cell. In its environment, it faces the same task of self-evidencing as we do in ours, and, as we have seen, subjectivity to some degree is an inevitable consequence of Active Inference to maintain a NESS Markov blanket. While this may feel odd, it fits with modern philosophical developments in intentionality (van Hateren, 2020). A helpful analogy is that of "Communication, Command and Control" (C3) in military and cybernetic studies. We can think of the Central Nervous System (CNS) as just one part of a more extensive C3 system, perhaps including endocrine, metabolic, and immune control systems. If we consider $m_{\Psi\equiv\Psi}$, it is evident that depriving that level of what it needs ($U_{\Psi\equiv\Psi} \rightarrow 0$) will result in death, as organised function will be lost, leading to failure to maintain O's Markov blankets. So, while $O_{psychological}$ is not a valid level in our model, O_Ψ is.

The Properties of Psychological Subjectivity

Let us concentrate on well-being estimates we evaluate psychologically. First, we define $\psi \subset \Psi$ to represent this subset, making ψ everyday subjectivity. We can already deduce some properties of ψ.

1. The fabric of ψ is dimensional.
2. The whole of ψ—both dimensions and the objects they constitute—is subject to updating, so it will change with time.
3. The data that ψ encodes is composited, with both a predictive component generated subjectively, and an error component generated comparatively.
4. All evaluations will include a preference dimension that will reflect their utility.

This sets out the formal properties of ψ, including ascribing a common nature to its contents. Note that O_ψ is no longer commensurate with other levels of O due to $\{\mathcal{F}\}$ so it cannot scale to them. Such a space is apt for phenomenology and fits our conception and experience of "mind".

Defining the Contents of Mind

W estimates F, but we have not yet discussed how that is achieved, beyond specifying some function $\mathcal{F}$. As $F = -\mathbb{S} \approx -\mathbb{S}$, all our estimates are (minimised) predicted differences. However, maximising well-being may entail either approaching or avoiding some state of affairs, and these will be instantiated differently. Imagine O is confronted by a dangerous fire. Putting the fire out and running away from it both minimise $\mathbb{S} = D_{KL}(E \parallel E)$ but the first modifies this through acting on $\boldsymbol{E}$ and the second through acting on O. However, internal sensory information is generated in anticipation of experience and can be detected through interoception (Barrett & Simmons, 2015), which imputes a potential E, not a real E. Empirical demonstration of this has been achieved for hunger and thirst (Livneh et al., 2020). This difference is $\hat{F} = -\hat{\mathbb{S}}$, the circumflex indicating the estimated prediction error has arisen entirely from O, without E. Consider "Willingness To Pay" (WTP) an amount of money for a particular good: two items with the same WTP would be considered to contribute equally to well-being. This technique is used to evaluate HRQOL, for example, as discussed above. However, in HRQOL estimation, WTP is often to avoid a sickness, disability, or similar. If the person has experienced the illness, witnessed it, or even read a description, it is probably safe to assume $\mathbb{S} = \hat{\mathbb{S}}$ and this presumption underlies much WTP usage in practice as a tool to evaluate consumer preference for new goods (e.g., Taylor & Armour, 2002). But, without external input from E, $\hat{\mathbb{S}}$ can go wrong, as the story below illustrates.

> A man was seen covering his garden with rolled-up newspaper. When his neighbours asked him why he replied, "It's to keep the tigers away." Puzzled, his neighbours assured him there were no tigers where they lived. "That's right," he replied, "It's really effective."

We may see how this arises in Ψ by considering $\{W\} = \{\mathcal{F}Ue\}$. Our man and his neighbours have similar well-being estimates $\{W\}$; both were quite content in their lives until the conversation in the story. Similarly, there is no appreciable difference in $\{e\}$; all agree on the absence of tigers and the presence of a garden covered with rolled-up newspaper. To explain the difference, we must presume that our man additionally possesses some functions $\{\mathcal{F}_{Man}\}$ to allow him to deduce a necessary and sufficient connection between his behaviour and the local absence of tigers. We also need to distinguish the different classes of evaluation discussed above. For $F = -\mathbb{S}$ the term "direct" emphasises that it has been evaluated with direct reference to E. For $\hat{F} = -\hat{\mathbb{S}}$ the term "imputed" implies E has been predicted from interoceptive anticipation, so distinguishing a current situation we predict from some postulated state we seek.

The Roots of Emotional and Imaginary Thinking

Let us assume $\{W_i\}$ generates a set of estimators $\{\omega_j\}$. The use of Greek lowercase reminds us that we will experience these estimators within Ψ, and we assume $i \leq j$. Some of these estimators will be of $\hat{\mathbb{S}}$, where the action minimises *imputed* free energy. Subjectively, W will scale to unity, as we have seen above. We can therefore write $\{\omega_j\} = \{\omega_{j-k}, 1 - \omega_k\}$, where $\{\omega_{j-k}\}$ are direct estimators, and $\{1 - \omega_k\}$ are imputed estimators. However, this leaves the unsatisfactory position that sometimes we estimate directly and sometimes by imputation, without explaining how this can happen or how we can tell which is which.

The goal of either estimation is to identify the utilities $\{U_E\}$ we need from our environment. Put another way, the environmental variables providing those utilities $\{V_O\} = E$ are salient to us, and to evaluate them, we must express preferences. From this perspective, O is behaving as an investor in its environment; it is betting its predictions against what its environment will afford, e.g., oxygen when it respires or nourishment when it eats. Economists observe that these preferences can arise either from rational deduction or emotional state, which they call "sentiment", and its separate existence as a subjective predictor of value may be reliably deduced (e.g., Ryu, Kim, & Yang, 2017). The equivalent term in psychology is "valence" (cf. Shuman, Sander, & Scherer, 2013). Active Inference can successfully model valence, at least in silico (Hesp et al., 2019). A full discussion of that model is inappropriate here, but the functions which deliver valence are bounded within specific hierarchical levels, while Shuman et al. (2013) attribute a hierarchical structure to valence itself, according to its level of complexity. From our principle that levels in O are represented as dimensions in Ψ, evaluations via sentiment will be represented by a different order of dimensions to cognitive evaluations. As Hesp et al. (2019) and Ryu et al. (2017) point out, valence/sentiment is expressed as confidence in belief. At the neurocognitive level, this is the precision of the predictive model generated; at the economic level, it is expressed by several functions of the volume and share closing prices with respect to time. We notice that at either level, valence/sentiment can generate values for $\hat{\mathbb{S}}$ though, of course, that value may be mistaken. I suggest that the imputed estimators $\{1 - \omega_k\}$ provide the *affective* dimensions of our subjectivity, which we typically experience differently from subjectivity's cognitive components. This is consistent with empirical work on the relationship between emotion and interoception. For example, the absence of the ability to express emotion, alexithymia, has been related to interoceptive failure (Murphy, 2017). Interoception also links emotion, time (which we have discussed above), and music, which are mutually related to normal and psychopathological states (Droit-Volet, 2013; Juslin & Sloboda, 2013; Vicario, Nitsche, Salehinejad, Avanzino, & Martino, 2020).

We are conscious of at least some of ψ. Emotion is conscious sentiment or affect, whose creation we have discussed above. Being conscious of at least some subjective predictions without engagement with error-correction from sensation also allows for a class of *imaginary* objects in our subjectivity. Unlike emotions, they are unconnected with sense-data or proxies, so no prediction of $\hat{\mathbb{S}}$ will be made, i.e., they do not imply action. We may deduce four classes of construction in our subjectivities.

a) Dimensions. These encode the estimators of our level-specific environments.
b) "Real" objects. These arise from imaginary objects composited with sense data.
c) "Imaginary" objects. These are predictions resulting from our generative models, which have not been composited.
d) Emotions. These are estimates of the utility of potential states created by imputation.

In short, we have been able to deduce the familiar contents of our everyday subjectivity from applying FEP to well-being.

From Errors in Self-Evidencing to Psychopathology

Let us return to our man and his unorthodox approach to tiger prevention. It follows from the above that our psychopathological interest centres on $\{\mathcal{F}_{Man}\}$. We assume, of course, that he is wrong, so $\{\mathcal{F}_{Man}\} = False$. This lets us imagine a superset of faulty functions generating false dimensions $\{\tilde{\mathcal{F}}_{Man}\} \subset \{\tilde{\mathcal{F}}\}$. Can $\{\tilde{\mathcal{F}}\}$ account for the psychopathology we observe in reality?

Consider a single errant function $\tilde{\mathcal{F}}_i$. Psychopathology refers to some aspect of subjectivity that is not part of our shared reality. So, it follows that it will be informed by (at least) one incorrectly imputed estimator $\tilde{\omega}_{k=i}$. The effort wasted generating this imposes a net loss to U_{E_O}, so psychopathology will always reduce F and be harmful. In our imaginary example, our man has spent useless time, money, and effort accumulating and spreading rolled-up newspaper around his garden, so incurring, at the very least, an opportunity cost. Were his neighbours unable to persuade him otherwise, it would be reasonable for us to assert that he is deluded. The difficulty we face is that we have defined imputed evaluations as emotions, and delusions are not understood as such. However, this objection can be overcome.

Knowledge is classically defined as "justified true belief". We need to be clear that the man's mistake is believing there is a causal connection between paper (presence) and tiger (absence). His justification is plausible, just incredibly unlikely compared to the alternative: it is the plausibility that adds the humour. The falsity is because the man's level of belief has been set at "certainty", and certainty is an emotion. So, delusions are inappropriate compositions with certainty. We can predict a subclassification depending on whether the composition was with real, imaginary, or emotional objects, and this can be found. Delusional perceptions are typically "two-limbed"; an actual occurrence leads to a delusional deduction, e.g., personal messages are perceived in public radio messages. There are emotional delusions of love (de Clerambault's Syndrome) or jealousy (Othello Syndrome). Paranoid delusions create purely imaginary webs of conspiracy. As they share a common misattribution of certainty, it is no surprise that they can co-occur. Objectively, FEP manages this well. We have seen above that emotion sets the precision associated with the predictions arising from FEP's generative models. Inappropriate certainty could either arise from over-precise predictions or impaired error correction—the latter is implicit in inappropriate composition. Paulus et al. (2019) both describe supporting evidence and explain how, once established, such errors do not automatically correct themselves.

The idea of inappropriate composition can be extended to explain hallucinations. The classic definition of a "sensory perception occurring without external stimulus" strongly suggests an imputation being inappropriately applied to an imaginary prediction. Schizophrenia is the obvious empirical model for hallucinations and delusions, as both psychopathological phenomena are found in it, and there is empirical support. The insula coordinates cognitive, emotional and somatosensory processing. Sheffield et al. (2020) describe reduced differentiation in resting-state functional connectivity within the insula in a large sample of schizophrenic patients, which is consistent with a hypothesis of increased error in composition.

While not an exhaustive list of all psychopathology, hallucinations and delusions are the prototypical exemplars of disordered perception and disordered beliefs, which covers much. In this model, both can be explained as the product of mistaken compositions of imputed error correction and subjective predictions in the ongoing process of self-evidencing by Active Inference at specific levels of biological organisation. I have not explicitly discussed the psychopathology of emotion, but I have already referenced relevant accounts framed within FEP (e.g., Paulus et al., 2019) and my account of well-being is no more than a subjective application of this theory. Therefore, it seems likely that the mechanism of inappropriate composition (by either presence or absence) will generalise across psychopathology.

Psychopathology, Surprisal and Satisficing

Astute readers may have noticed that the discussion of psychology above did not mention surprisal. This is because our psychology is a subjective expression of model evidence, and surprisal lies outside this. However, we can now understand psychopathology as a level-specific, deleterious change in our ability to generate accurate model evidence, and so signals an unwelcome increase in surprisal. All the complexities just described are to optimise $\mathcal{O}$' s path of least action $S = \int_{t_i}^{t_2} L dt, \delta L = 0$ to maintain its integrity, and so survive. The effect of psychopathology is to reduce fit or increase bias, so that $\mathbb{S} = \delta L > 0$. Because surprisal is also level-specific, the same surprisal may be represented as either $\mathfrak{S}$ (when V is an environmental property relative to level m_i), or $\mathfrak{S}$ (when the limit is computational). Recalling that psychopathology reflects a space $\{\tilde{\mathcal{F}}\}$ enables us to distinguish it from both $\mathfrak{S}$, e.g., a sound that destroys our ears cannot be heard & $-\mathfrak{S}$, which is evidenced through phenomena such as optical illusions. Objectively, $f\colon \left\{\tilde{\mathcal{F}}\right\} \mapsto \mathfrak{S} + \delta\mathfrak{S}$, so increasing the risk of both disability and death. This makes psychopathology qualitatively distinct from psychology, not in terms of its content, but in its forms, as described by Jaspers (1963).

Conclusions

It has been said that the greatest creation of the human brain is the real world. However, the world it builds for us is to aid our survival, and our awareness of it is only a means to that end, so it is not surprising to find that ideas based on our subjectivities alone, such as classical psychopathology, can be misleading. The biopsychosocial model has turned out to be, quite literally, a figment of our imaginations, as the separate orders it proposes result from necessary but illusory encoding of levels of biological organisation. Apparently obvious distinctions, such as those between "thought", "emotion", "reality", and "imagination" are anything but, and psychopathology signals when the processes which construct them break down. Our individual identities and environments are matters of perspective, while our "constitution" is an embodiment of information theory applied to survival. We are to our kidneys what our world is to us, while the social science of Macro-Economics stops at our households, as we do at our genetics, and we could, theoretically, also exist in any computer which could re-create all our Markov blankets in silico. We have even found that we may have over-privileged our brains as commanders of our lives, and other C3 systems need to be included in our understanding. However, with those corrections made, we have also found it possible to explicitly link our biological processes and the subjectivity we recognise in both its normal and pathological expressions. Further work elucidating that link will be challenging, but at least it need be mysterious no longer.

References

Barrett, L. F., & Simmons, W. K. (2015). Interoceptive predictions in the brain. *Nature Reviews Neuroscience*, *16*(7), 419–429. https://doi.org/10.1038/nrn3950

Botvinik-Nezer, R., Holzmeister, F., Camerer, C. F., Dreber, A., Huber, J., Johannesson, M., … Schonberg, T. (2020). Variability in the analysis of a single neuroimaging dataset by many teams. *Nature*, 1–7. https://doi.org/10.1038/s41586-020-2314-9

Buckley, C. L., Kim, C. S., McGregor, S., & Seth, A. K. (2017). The free energy principle for action and perception: A mathematical review. *Journal of Mathematical Psychology*, *81*, 55–79. https://doi.org/10.1016/j.jmp.2017.09.004

Carcone, D., & Ruocco, A. C. (2017). Six Years of Research on the National Institute of Mental Health's Research Domain Criteria (RDoC) Initiative: A Systematic Review. *Frontiers in Cellular Neuroscience*, *11*. https://doi.org/10.3389/fncel.2017.00046

Corcoran, A. W., & Hohwy, J. (2017). *Allostasis, interoception, and the free energy principle: Feeling our way forward*.

Das, J., Do, Q.-T., Friedman, J., McKenzie, D., & Scott, K. (2007). Mental health and poverty in developing countries: Revisiting the relationship. *Social Science & Medicine*, *65*(3), 467–480. https://doi.org/10.1016/j.socscimed.2007.02.037

Droit-Volet, S. (2013). Time perception, emotions and mood disorders. *Journal of Physiology-Paris*, *107*(4), 255–264. https://doi.org/10.1016/j.jphysparis.2013.03.005

Funkhouser, C. J., Correa, K. A., Letkiewicz, A. M., Cozza, E. M., Estabrook, R., & Shankman, S. A. (2021). Evaluating the criterion validity of hierarchical psychopathology dimensions across models: Familial aggregation and associations with research domain criteria (sub)constructs. *Journal of Abnormal Psychology*, *130*(6), 575–586. https://doi.org/10.1037/abn0000687

Ghaemi, S. N. (2011). The biopsychosocial model in psychiatry: A critique. *American Journal of Psychiatry*, *121*, 451–457.

Hesp, C., Smith, R., Parr, T., Allen, M., Friston, K., & Ramstead, M. (2019). *Deeply Felt Affect: The Emergence of Valence in Deep Active Inference*. https://doi.org/10.31234/osf.io/62pfd

Jaspers, K. (1963). *General Psychopathogy* (J. Hoenig, Ed.). Manchester: Manchester University Press.

Juslin, P. N., & Sloboda, J. A. (2013). Music and Emotion. In *The Psychology of Music* (pp. 583–645). Elsevier. https://doi.org/10.1016/B978-0-12-381460-9.00015-8

Kirchhoff, M., Parr, T., Palacios, E., Friston, K., & Kiverstein, J. (2018). The Markov blankets of life: Autonomy, active inference and the free energy principle. *Journal of The Royal Society Interface*, *15*(138), 20170792.

Livneh, Y., Sugden, A. U., Madara, J. C., Essner, R. A., Flores, V. I., Sugden, L. A., … Andermann, M. L. (2020). Estimation of Current and Future Physiological States in Insular Cortex. *Neuron*. https://doi.org/10.1016/j.neuron.2019.12.027

Marek, S., Tervo-Clemmens, B., Calabro, F. J., Montez, D. F., Kay, B. P., Hatoum, A. S., … Dosenbach, N. U. F. (2020). Towards Reproducible Brain-Wide Association Studies. *BioRxiv*, 2020.08.21.257758. https://doi.org/10.1101/2020.08.21.257758

Marek, S., Tervo-Clemmens, B., Calabro, F. J., Montez, D. F., Kay, B. P., Hatoum, A. S., … Dosenbach, N. U. F. (2022). Reproducible brain-wide association studies require thousands of individuals. *Nature*, *603*(7902), 654–660. https://doi.org/10.1038/s41586-022-04492-9

Miller, M., Rietveld, E., & Kiverstein, J. (2021, July 6). The Predictive Dynamics of Happiness and Well-Being [Preprint]. Retrieved 17 February 2022, from http://philsci-archive.pitt.edu/19282/

Murphy, J. (2017, November 20). Alexithymia is associated with a multidomain, multidimensional failure of interoception: Evidence from novel tests. https://doi.org/10.1037/xge0000366

NIMH. (2016). Research Domain Criteria (RDoC). Retrieved 20 August 2016, from http://www.nimh.nih.gov/research-priorities/rdoc/index.shtml

Patrick, C. J., & Hajcak, G. (2016). RDoC: Translating promise into progress. *Psychophysiology*, *53*(3), 415–424. https://doi.org/10.1111/psyp.12612

Paulus, M. P., Feinstein, J. S., & Khalsa, S. S. (2019). An Active Inference Approach to Interoceptive Psychopathology. *Annual Review of Clinical Psychology*, *15*(1), 97–122. https://doi.org/10.1146/annurev-clinpsy-050718-095617

Payakachat, N., Murawski, M. M., & Summers, K. H. (2009). Health utility and economic analysis: Theoretical and practical issues. *Expert Review of Pharmacoeconomics & Outcomes Research*, *9*(4), 289–292. https://doi.org/10.1586/erp.09.36

Ridley, M., Rao, G., Schilbach, F., & Patel, V. (2020). *Poverty, Depression, and Anxiety: Causal Evidence and Mechanisms* (No. w27157; p. w27157). Cambridge, MA: National Bureau of Economic Research. https://doi.org/10.3386/w27157

Rue, H., Martino, S., & Chopin, N. (2009). Approximate Bayesian inference for latent Gaussian models by using integrated nested Laplace approximations. *Journal of the Royal Statistical Society: Series B (Statistical Methodology)*, *71*(2), 319–392. https://doi.org/10.1111/j.1467-9868.2008.00700.x

Ryu, D., Kim, H., & Yang, H. (2017). Investor sentiment, trading behavior and stock returns. *Applied Economics Letters*, *24*(12), 826–830. https://doi.org/10.1080/13504851.2016.1231890

Sheffield, J. M., Rogers, B. P., Blackford, J. U., Heckers, S., & Woodward, N. D. (2020). Insula functional connectivity in schizophrenia. *Schizophrenia Research*.

Shuman, V., Sander, D., & Scherer, K. R. (2013). Levels of Valence. *Frontiers in Psychology*, *4*. https://doi.org/10.3389/fpsyg.2013.00261

Spruyt, V. (2014, April 16). The Curse of Dimensionality in Classification. Retrieved 16 October 2017, from Computer vision for dummies website: http://www.visiondummy.com/2014/04/curse-dimensionality-affect-classification/

Sullivan, P. F., Agrawal, A., Bulik, C. M., Andreassen, O. A., Børglum, A. D., Breen, G., … O'Donovan, M. C. (2018). Psychiatric Genomics: An Update and an Agenda. *The American Journal of Psychiatry*, *175*(1), 15–27. https://doi.org/10.1176/appi.ajp.2017.17030283

Taylor, S. J., & Armour, C. L. (2002). Acceptability of willingness to pay techniques to consumers. *Health Expectations: An International Journal of Public Participation in Health Care and Health Policy*, *5*(4), 341–356. https://doi.org/10.1046/j.1369-6513.2002.00201.x

van Hateren, J. H. (2020). Constructing a Naturalistic Theory of Intentionality. *Philosophia*. https://doi.org/10.1007/s11406-020-00255-w

Vicario, C. M., Nitsche, M. A., Salehinejad, M. A., Avanzino, L., & Martino, G. (2020). Time Processing, Interoception, and Insula Activation: A Mini-Review on Clinical Disorders. *Frontiers in Psychology*, *11*. https://doi.org/10.3389/fpsyg.2020.01893

CHAPTER TWO

EMBODIED ATTENTION: A PHENOMENOLOGICAL HYPOTHESIS

FRANCESCA BRENCIO
UNIVERSITY OF SEVILLE, SPAIN &ROYAL COLLEGE OF PSYCHIATRISTS, LONDON

Abstract

The significance of phenomenology for neuroscience has not yet been fully recognised. While it had a widespread application in psychology and psychiatry, it is mainly ignored or overlooked in neuroscience. Through this contribution I aim to provide an account of attention from a phenomenological perspective, the aim of which is to offer a *qualitative* interpretation of this phenomenon. I argue that we can talk about embodied attention as an ongoing process linked to the temporal structure of bodily intentionality and kinaesthetic abilities of the body. This account of embodied attention is able to enrich the neuroscientific view on attention, and to offer a phenomenological insights of attention disorders. This chapter is divided into three main sections: in the first section, I focus on the issue of attention from the perspective of cognitive psychology and neuroscience, underlying how attention is regarded as a mental event from the first perspective, and as a function of brain activity in the second one. In both cases, the body as a source of attention is excluded and attention seems to be confined to a mentalistic view on our experience, typical of a disembodied mind. In the second section, by drawing on the resources of classical phenomenological literature, I aim to discuss an account of embodied attention as an ongoing process linked to the temporal structure of bodily intentionality and kinaesthetic activities. In the third section, using the paradigm of circular causality (Fuchs 2018, 2020) I aim to show how neural processes at the core of the neurophysiological accounts of attention may be described as dispositional patterns that participate in dynamic sensorimotor cycles involving the whole organism–environment system in the form of resonance between the brain, body, and environment.

Keywords: embodied attention; phenomenology; psychopathology

What is attention?

The concept of attention as central to human performance extends back to the start of experimental psychology and it is a subject of investigation of different disciplines, such as neuroscience, psychology, psychiatry, philosophy, and even contemplative studies. Generally speaking, attention is a phenomenon mainly overlapping with others, such as perception, cognition, awareness, and consciousness, and its boundaries are difficult to define.

Attention is a broad term referring to many different mechanisms. It might encompass the ability to select, shift, and thereby focus on something, on gestures, or behaviour. The common term "paying attention" implies that attention is a unitary phenomenon; however, it is a multifaceted construct supported by multiple brain networks. There are different types of attention, such as sustained attention, alternating attention, selective attention, focused attention, limited attention, open attention, or body-centred mindfulness in contemplative studies.

The function of attention seems to be to select some aspects of stimulus input. The ability to focus one's attention on important environmental stimuli while ignoring irrelevant ones is fundamental to human cognition and intellectual function. Attention is inextricably linked to perception, learning, memory, and executive function interacting with other brain functions through interconnected neural networks. In our ordinary and daily activities, there are many forms of attention involved in any simultaneous task: i.e., while you are looking outside the window, visual attention, auditory attention, and bodily attention are all involved. Is the attention that we use in vision the same that we use in audition? While it is difficult to do two visual or two auditory tasks concurrently, it is not necessarily difficult to combine an auditory and a visual task. There is also a passive and an active element to attention: while the former is initiated in a bottom-up direction by external stimuli, the latter is controlled in a top-down direction by the individual's goals or expectations (Oyebode, 2019).

Attention should not be confused with consciousness: although they are related processes (to be explicitly conscious of something implies that I have paid attention to it), findings show that attention and consciousness can operate independently. In fact, while the function of attention seems to be selection, the function of consciousness is the summarisation and integration of all of the information available to think, to speak, to make decisions, to plan, and so on. Attention is also intimately related to memory. Perhaps you experienced the situation in which you did not pay attention to someone's words because you were scrolling through your Facebook profile. If we want to be sure that someone remembers what we are telling them, we ask them to pay attention.

When we talk about "attention" it might sound as if it is a "thing" or a causal agent that "does something". William James (1890) pointed out this question when he asked: "Is attention a resultant or a force?" Johnston and Dark (1986) looked at theories of selective attention and divided them into cause theories and effect theories, a general distinction between theories that view attention as a causal mechanism and those that view it as a natural consequence of other processes.

A substantial contribution in the definition of this phenomenon was provided by Donald Broadbent with his book entitled *Perception and Communication* (published in 1958). Focusing on the nature of information transmission between the sensory system and the central nervous system, he argued that, although the sensory system provides vast amounts of information to the central nervous system, only a small fraction of that information is available to awareness or results in voluntary responses. Broadbent attributed this reduction or "filtering" of information to limited capacity in the communication channel between sensory inputs and awareness. This filtering of information was defined by James as "selective interest", and more recently as selective attention.

Anne Treisman, who was one of the most important contributors to the development of theories of attention in cognitive psychology, stated in her paper *Selective Attention in Man* that

> Fifty years ago, psychologists thought of attention as "the focalisation of consciousness" or "the increased clearness of a particular idea". But these and other definitions in terms of mental faculties or subjective experience proved sterile for empirical research and ended in a series of inconclusive controversies. Recently interest in this problem has revived (1964, p.12).

When attention research began in the 1950s, cognitive psychology did not even have a name. It was in the mid-1950s that attention started to be investigated through the contribution of brain studies and neurophysiology:

> From the 1950s until recently, experimental research on attention has mainly been concerned with attention as the momentary focus of perception and action. The common motif is that attention is limited and that perceptual access to the world is therefore far from optimal. [...] In recent research, the paradigm shifted towards more temporally extended processes in their connection with the bodily constitution and kinaesthetic abilities of the perceiving subject (Wehrle & Breyer 2016, p. 43).

Posner (1993) divides works on attention into three phases: Initially, in the 1950s and 1960s, research centred on human performance and on the concept of "the human as a single channel processor". In the 1970s and early 1980s the field of study had become "cognition" and research was mostly concerned with looking for and studying internal representations, automatic and controlled processes, and strategies for focusing and dividing attention. By the mid-1980s "cognitive neuroscience" psychologists were taking account of biology, neuropsychological patients, and computing. Posner (1990) believed that if we think of attention as a system of several brain networks, the concept is valid.

In neuroscience, one classic brain-based model of attention includes three components: alerting, orienting, and executive networks (Posner et al., 2014; Petersen & Posner, 2012; Posner, 1980, 2011):

(a) the alerting network is indexed by quickened response times following a general warning signal or by changes in arousal throughout a prolonged task. It relies on the brainstem and right-hemisphere systems to regulate the extent to which resources should be mobilised to react to salient events in the environment in a non-selective manner.
(b) The orienting network, which recruits frontal and parietal brain regions, supports the ability to direct attention toward a specific stimulus feature or spatial location (Corbetta et al. 2008). Orienting can consist of voluntary responses toward relevant stimuli or involuntary responses toward irrelevant stimuli (Corbetta et al. 2008).
(c) Finally, the executive network is implicated in target detection; this system mobilises limited-capacity brain resources to bring stimuli to awareness and monitor conflict. It is thought to rely on the midline

anterior cingulate cortex and lateral frontal cortex (Petersen & Posner, 2012).

During a cognitively demanding task, these systems ideally allow a person to focus attention on the task without being constantly distracted (Hoyer et al. 2021). According to neuroscience, the executive control functions (ECF) of the brain broadly encompass a set of cognitive skills that are responsible for the planning, initiation, sequencing, and monitoring of complex, goal-directed behaviours, such as shifting attentional focus, inhibiting dominant response tendencies, and updating working memory contents (Royall et al., 2002; Cohen, 2014).

The development of sophisticated techniques such as positron emission tomography (PET) and functional magnetic resonance imaging (FMRI) now allow researchers to observe brain activity during cognitive tasks that involve varieties of attention. Information about the different brain areas involved in different tasks is increasing on an almost daily basis and the challenge is to interpret and understand the implications of these data for theories of attention. The brain has numerous networks that feed information back and forth and because modern neuroimaging methods allow researchers to observe the brain in action, it is becoming possible to see how these networks are activated in different "attentional" tasks. It is evident that different tasks recruit different brain areas and different networks.

In cognitive psychology, attention is primarily considered as a mental activity. In his *Principles of Psychology*, William James wrote that attention "is the taking possession by the mind, in clear and vivid form, of one out of what seem several simultaneously possible objects or trains of thought. Focalisation, concentration, of consciousness are of its essence. It implies withdrawal from some things in order to deal effectively with others, and is a condition which has a real opposite in the confused, dazed, scatter-brained state." (James, 2007, 404-405). According to James, attention improves performance in relation to the attended stimulus: it allows a person to perceive, discriminate, remember, and react better than if attention were not engaged. He stated that attention also could be active or passive. Passive attention is reflexive and effortless and elicited by novel, intense, or motivating stimuli (i.e., the aroma of bread in the oven). These mechanisms appear to operate outside of conscious awareness and, when activated, result in distraction from other activities or thoughts. Active attention, in contrast, is intentional and effortful and directed by task demands. Active attention is limited in capacity and tends to decay over time without continual effort.

The prevalence of James' account is at the core of the spotlight metaphor (Cave & Bichot 1999): according to this, attention is like a spotlight that illuminates certain sensory data or certain parts of the field of awareness (or experience).

This cognitivistic account of attention is criticised by the French phenomenologist Maurice Merleau-Ponty. In his *Phenomenology of Perception* he considers this interpretation of attention in light of two mistakes: the first is what he terms the presupposition of constancy—a consequence of an empiricist approach— i.e., the presupposition that things must already be 'there' in the world, things capable of capturing the gaze, and as such, my attention; the second mistake is that attention is seen only in quantity and not in quality. Nevertheless, Merleau-Ponty demonstrates that attention creates the form of my experience by providing meaning to it. Accordingly, attention can also be conceived as a quality attribute (1981, p. 26-28).

Another phenomenological source that we can take into consideration to enrich our understanding of attention is the work of Aaron Gurwitsch, a student of Husserl. According to Gurwitsch (1964, 1966, 1985), attention may be considered as dynamic tension of transformations of content, involving dimensional organisation principles (Gestalt-coherence of the theme, unity by relevance of the thematic context, co-presence of the margin) and transformation principles (serial-shifting, context-shifting, enlargement, elucidation, synthesis, singling out, restructuration, etc.).

The phenomenological background: bodily intentionality, protention, attention

As we have seen, in all the previous accounts on attention, the body is excluded as a source of attention, confining the various attentional phenomena to a mentalistic view typical of a disembodied mind. None of these perspectives considers the role of the body, as a medium for each experience we have. Through perception, in fact, our body can master our attention. When we talk about perception, we do not refer merely to the sole elements of sensation: this would reduce perception to a form of empiricism or sensualism. It is precisely in the attempt to overcome the dualism typical of these views that phenomenology may be a useful resource[1].

Conceived by Edmund Husserl as a method of inquiry and understanding of one's lived experience, phenomenology describes the basic structures inherent in conscious experience, such as embodiment, spatiality, temporality, intentionality, and intersubjectivity and to analyse their possible deviations and derailments. Phenomenology offers reliable descriptions of the structures of conscious lived experiences by following how they are experienced – the so-called first-person perspective (1P) (Moran 2019)— without the imposition of external explanatory frameworks. Phenomenology has a wide application in psychology and psychiatry (Brencio 2022, 2021, 2019). In recent years, phenomenology's stress on the embodied character of experience in the context of a lifeworld has majorly impacted cognitive science (Gallagher & Schmicking 2010; Gallagher & Zahavi 2008) as well as psychopathology. As recently stressed in "The Lancet Psychiatry", "phenomenology might suggest ways to approach the challenges faced by patients and professionals" (Boice 2021).

In order to understand how and why it is possible to talk about embodied attention, we must clarify two fundamental concepts at the core of this account, bodily intentionality and protention, to see how they are linked with the issue of the attention. Intentionality has been one of the major themes in Edmund Husserl's thinking (Husserl 1982, p. 187) since the publication of *Logical Investigations*. He analyses intentionality based on three central ideas: intentional act, intentional object, and intentional content. The intentional act is a particular kind of mental experience (such as perceiving, believing, evaluating, remembering, etc.) that can be distinguished from the intentional object toward which the act is directed. The intentional content may be defined as the meaning of the experience: intentional content makes consciousness intentional, furnishing the act with its directedness (Zahavi 2003, p. 22). Intentionality is the peculiar feature of our consciousness, irreducible to existing objects, but also characterises our fantasies, predictions, memories, judgments, etc. What is needed for intentionality to occur is the existence of an experience with the appropriate internal structure of object-directedness: this is its inner characteristic.

While examining the different levels of intentionality, Husserl stresses the central function of our lived body for primordial orientation in spatial,

---

[1] Fundamental studies on attention from a phenomenological perspective are Waldenfels 2004; Bégout 2007; Breyer 2011; Depraz 2014; D'Angelo 2020.

temporal, and personal terms. The body is given to intuition in a kind of 'quality', in a 'location', which has dimensional modifications. The body is both the subject and the object of intentionality: as a lived body (*Leib*), it experiences things; as an object body (*Körper*), it is experienced as a thing. For Husserl, the body links one's insertion or being-in-the-world: the body is the *Nullpunkt* (zero point) from which the perceived world is organized. Everything is oriented in relation to the lived body, which is key in the localisation of kinaesthetic and tactile sensations (Husserl 1989, pp. 151-152) and in the experience of lived time.

Embodied Attention

Maurice Merlau-Ponty took a substantial step towards bodily localisation: he developed the notion of bodily intentionality. Bodily intentionality rests on perception and action as the primary ways of interaction with the world (1981, p. 238). According to him, classical theories with consciousness at the centre of their explanations inadequately explain two phenomena: (a) the quality of our perceptual experience and (b) how our ability to move, to function, and to relate to our body breaks down in pathological cases. Perception requires the perceiver being 'in the middle' of a situation, inhabiting a spatio-temporal world. This requires a body (1981, p. 311). A disembodied mind could not enter into the objective physical world and be a part of it, nor would a mind simply dwell in a body (1981, pp. 88-89, p. 124). Our bodily experience of movement provides us with a way to access the world and the object, called 'praktognosia', which must be recognised as primary to our consciousness (1981, pp. 140-141).

How can the body be intentional? This form of intentionality, derived from the primacy of perception and action, marks a break from the traditional concept of intentionality because this form grants the latent self-knowledge that the body possesses (1981, 233-235). Another key component for understanding bodily intentionality is operative intentionality, outlined by Husserl. Merleau-Ponty distinguishes between intentionality of act (such as our judgements and our position taking) and operative intentionality (*fungierende Intentionalität*), "which produces the natural and anti-predicative unity of the world and of our life" (1981, XVIII). Operative intentionality corresponds to the structural coupling of organism and environment produced by functional cycles of sensorimotor interaction (Fuchs 2020, 4).

How is it possible to link attention to bodily intentionality? It is possible through temporality: bodily intentionality is always temporally determined. The concrete realisation of lived time is primarily achieved pre-reflectively through the lived body. Embodiment and temporality are strictly connected: lived (or implicit) time is possible as a "function of the lived body, opened up by its potentiality and capability" (Fuchs 2005, 196). In *The Phenomenology of internal time-consciousness*, Edmund Husserl distinguishes among three different layers of temporality: the objective time of the appearing objects; the subjective, immanent, or pre-empirical time of the acts, and appearances; and the absolute, pre-phenomenal flow of time constituting consciousness (Zahavi 2010, p. 324). Consequently, subjective time constitutes the ever-present undercurrent of our experience (Fuchs 2013a), and it is based on the transcendental synthesis of three moments: the first one is the presentation or the primal impression (*Urimpression*), narrowly directed toward the strictly circumscribed now-phase of the object (Zahavi 2010, p. 321); the second, the 'retention', provides us with a retained awareness of what we just experienced; and the third, the 'protention', which, in a more-or-less indefinite way, intends the phase of the object about to occur thereby providing a future-oriented temporal context for the primal impression (Zahavi 2010, p. 321). Together, these three moments constitute 'inner time consciousness', a field of experiencing, a dimension of manifestation that encompasses all three temporal modes (Zahavi 2010, p. 324). This threefold structure is present synchronically as a unified whole. The relations between protention, primal impression, and retention are not relations among items located within the temporal flow; rather, these relations constitute the flow (Zahavi 2010, p. 323). It is called inner time-consciousness because it belongs to the innermost structure of the experience itself (Zahavi 2010, p. 334).

To capture the basic structure of intentionality and embodied mental life through purposeful action, Merleau-Ponty coined the expression "intentional arc" (Fuchs 2007, p. 230). The intentional arc, conceived as the bodily mediated directedness of our attention and activity toward its goal, has a temporal structure based on the threefold structure of presentation, retention, and protention. The intentional arch shows how mental events succeed in retaining the previous events and anticipating the future ones. In other words, consciousness spreads out by its double-faced attention of retention and protention (Fuchs 2007, p. 231). The intentional arc denotes how consciousness is built up by its retentional-protentional structure. Lived time is also based on another element: the dynamic and affective dimension of lived time, also called conation (Fuchs 2013a). Conation works as the root for spontaneity, affective directedness, attention, and the pursuit of goals that are key aspects of psychic life. This "energetic" momentum is central for the experience of temporality, and when changes occur in basic motivational states, this basic drive changes accordingly. It is precisely through the joint combination of subjective temporality and the affective-conative tension that the temporal structure of intentionality may be related to the lived body, for its drives and protentions essentially open it; moreover, the lived body contributes to temporality through its habitual structure, or through body memory (Fuchs 2012).

If we consider all these elements, we can say that attention is an active concentration of the "protentional cone" (Fuchs 2007), which restricts the forward-directed protentions or anticipations, and fades out inappropriate or irrelevant protentions and stimuli. This "energetic" momentum is central for the experience of temporality, and when changes occur in basic motivational states, this basic drive changes accordingly. It is precisely through the joint combination of subjective temporality and the affective-conative tension that the temporal structure of intentionality may be related to the lived body, for its drives and protentions essentially open it; moreover, the lived body contributes to temporality through its habitual structure, or through body memory (Fuchs 2012).

Following these approaches, I argue that we can distinguish among different layers of attention and the first one is not mental nor cerebral, rather embodied: it is the body that shapes my experience and guides my attention through its kinaesthetic ability. Being conceived of as an ongoing act, embodiment manifests a circular structure regarding the cycles of homeostatic self-regulation between the brain and body, and the sensorimotor cycles between the brain, body, and environment (Fuchs 2020). This shows a strict coherence with the primary social perception issue through which we always experience others as embodied subjects. In our experience of others, we do not simply see their face, eyes, body, and gestures, but we sense all these things through our body, through a mutual bodily resonance typical of second-person interactions (Fuchs 2013b).

This bodily resonance plays a peculiar role in the phenomenon of joint attention, a behaviour in which two or more people focus on an object or event to interact with each other. Joint attention involves sharing a common focus on something with someone else. It requires the ability to gain, maintain, and shift attention and may be gained by using eye contact, gestures (i.e., pointing, following, etc.), and/or vocalisations, including spoken words. Early joint attention skills may include a child reaching out to be picked up by an adult or looking at the same object with another person. There are two ways joint attention can occur: (a) the child initiates the shared attention; (b) the child responds to someone else's efforts to gain joint attention. Joint attention crucially implies an interaffective component: infants' responsiveness to others' embodied affects is demonstrated through affective synchrony, affect attunement, bodily resonance, and intercorporality. These embodied interactions are at the core of intersubjectivity and show the role of embodied attention in the development of social perspectives.

A fundamental resource to accomplish the goals this research intends to achieve is the enactive account of intersubjectivity. From this perspective, intersubjectivity can be defined from the angle of the interaction process, which includes bodily resonance, affect, attunement, coordination of gestures, facial and vocal expression, and many others (Fuchs & De Jaegher 2009, 466). Enactive intersubjectivity is based on a complex and rich constellation of assumptions, i.e., intersubjectivity relies heavily on embodiment in a rich sense of the word. The bodily experiences of interacting are the grounds for understanding each other and of understanding the world together. The embodiment contains precisely our immediate apprehension of others: the immediate, enactive form of subjectivity and intersubjectivity are closely intertwined (Fuchs & De Jaegher H., 2009). This requires dynamic coupling and coordination among the agents. The frame within which this happens is that of a "mutual circulation between cognitive science and phenomenology in which subjectivity and experience play the vital role that they also have in the everyday doings of living, sentient, sense-making beings" (De Jaegher, et al. 2017, p. 494).

In light of phenomenology's unique contributions, one may argue that current enactive theories of intersubjectivity and embodied mind combined with the paradigm of the circular causality (Fuchs 2018, 2020), may offer the theoretical resources to draw a framework for embodied attention conceived as a circular process that links bottom-up and top-down influences, showing that neurobiological mechanisms underpin the link between the embodied mind and the disorganisation of intersubjectivity. The circular causality model works at two levels: on a vertical level, explaining relations within the organism; and on a horizontal level, explaining the interrelation between the subject and the environment. This model calls into question the neuroscientific consideration of the brain as

> a constructor, asking how the neuronal machinery produces the experienced world and the experiencing subject. Consciousness thus appears not as the

> relation of a living being to the world, but becomes an internal representation of the external world inside the head. In this conception, the brain is considered as a system in itself, in opposition to the remainder of the body as well as to the surrounding world. The body remains a physiological carrier mechanism for the brain, which supposedly even as a bodiless brain- in- a-vat could bring forth consciousness, as a "cosmos inside the head (Fuchs 2018, p.67).

Organism and environment develop and adjust themselves in a mutual relation. The discovery of neuroplasticity (i.e., the effects that subjective and intersubjective experiences, for example, in psychotherapeutic processes, have on the neural structure), has shown that "causes" and "meanings" (as that which is explainable and as that which is understandable) are only comprehensible when considered as being in constant interplay with each other (Fuchs 2014). On this basis, one may suggest that disorders of attention are connected to the fragmentation of bodily intentionality.

As already pointed out by Gallagher in *How the body shapes the mind*, in much of our everyday experience, and most of the time, our attention is directed away from the body, toward the environment, or toward some project we are undertaking; for example, when I am solving a difficult mathematical problem, am I also and at the same time aware of the position of my legs or even of my grip on the pencil? There are things so automatic that I don't need to be aware of them (2005, p. 27). This perceptual attention is trained and entrained by my projects to such an extent that the body's mode of being in the perceiving act is more than to be perceived.

When we talk about bodily self-awareness (Gallagher 2003), bodily attention and embodied attention, we are dealing with different kinds of intentionality: bodily self-awareness is not object perception, and I can be attentive to (or un-attentionally aware of) my own body; bodily attention defines a certain kind of attentional experience (Wehrle & Breyer 2016) especially in cases where kinaesthetic activities are particularly prominent (such as playing soccer, dancing, etc.); embodied attention is a circular process that links bottom-up and top-down influences. The role of kinaesthetic consciousness, not just as a conscious-of movement, but as a consciousness capable of motility, is linked both with protention primarily derived from bodily conation (Fuchs 2013a), and to body memory— what we anticipate in protention is mainly a result of embodied habits. This embodied attention is also trained by sensorimotor cycles which are performed in a focused way and are frequently repeated, thus enabling smooth, attentive performance (Fuchs 2020).

Conclusive remarks

The phenomenological hypothesis of embodied attention has many consequences at different levels: in pedagogy, psychology, psychiatry, and neuroscience. It invites us to dismantle our cultural attitude to think about the relationship between mind and brain in a reductionistic approach, mainly based on a neurocentric view, in favour of an ecological approach to the human being in its totality.

The accent of the role of embodiment also in relation to the attentional phenomena recalls the centrality of the role of our bodily existence. Bodily resonance acts as the medium of both our affective engagement in a situation (Fuchs 2016, p. 16) and of our attention. Emotions shape our attention and its layers and, at the same time, affect the way in which we can be focused on a task. If I am anxious for an expected outcome, for example, I will experience a certain difficulty in maintaining my attention at a high level; if I am happy to work on something new, this will modify accordingly my attention. How affective life shapes our attention is particularly evident on the phenomenon of joint attention in which bodily resonance plays a peculiar role.

One may argue that a diminution of bodily activity may impact the kinaesthetic ability of the body, affecting both bodily intentionality and embodied attention. This seems to be supported by recent findings on ADHD (Donovan et al. 2019), for example, which confirm a disorganisation of embodied attention on two levels: a kinaesthetic one (recovering the notion of operative intentionality and sensorimotor cycle) and a temporal one (disorganisation of the selective protention). In fact, a reduction of exposure to the environment, also conceived as a reduction of bodily experiences, may increase the exposure to attention disorders. As underlined by Donovan et al. (2019), increasing a child's lifetime exposure to country life might provide a certain protection against attention disorders. This correlation between ADHD and a low level of outdoor activities seems to corroborate the hypothesis of embodied attention: outdoor activities can help advance embodied attention capacity through sensorimotor cycles between the brain, body, and environment. Therefore, "neural processes should be described as dispositional patterns that participate in dynamic sensorimotor cycles involving the whole organism–environment system"

(Fuchs 2020, p. 6), in the form of resonance between the brain, body, and environment.

At the core of this philosophical exploration of attention there is the hope to contribute to the interdisciplinary dialogue between phenomenology and neuroscience in order to enrich our understanding of those phenomena which characterise human being as an embodied, living subject.

References

Bégout, B. (2007) "Husserl and the Phenomenology of Attention". In: Boi L., Kerszberg P., Patras F. (eds) Rediscovering Phenomenology. Phaenomenologica, vol 182. Springer, Dordrecht, pp. 13-32, https://doi.org/10.1007/978-1-4020-5881-3_1

Brencio F. (2022), (Dis)Embodied encounters. Deciphering intersubjectivity in the context of drugs' prescription, in P. A. Gargiulo, H. L. Mesones Arroyo (eds.), Psychiatry and Neuroscience Update. From Translational Research to Drug Addictions and Psychoses, Volume V, Springer, (Forthcoming in December)

Brencio F., P. Morand, L. Wilhelm, C. Sabourdy, P. R. Bauer (2021a), Intersubjectivity and social perception in epilepsy, in "Phenomenology and Mind", 21, 2021, pp. 88-99, DOI 10.17454/pam-2107

Brencio F. (2019), Befindlichkeit: Disposition, in G. Stanghellini, A. Raballo, M. Broome, A. V. Fernandez, P. Fusar-Poli, and R. Rosfort (eds.), The Oxford Handbook of Phenomenological Psychopathology, Oxford University Press, Oxford 2019, 344-353, DOI: 10.1093/oxfordhb/9780198803157.013.39

Breyer, T. (2011). Attentionalität Und Intentionalität. Grundzüge Einer Phänomenologisch-Kognitionswissenschaftlichen Theorie Der Aufmerksamkeit. München: Wilhelm Fink Verlag.

Broadbent, D. (1958) Perception and Communication. Oxford: Pergamon Press.

Boice, N., "The things themselves". In The Lancet Psychiatry, March 2021, DOI: https://doi.org/10.1016/S2215-0366(21)00033-X

Cave & Bichot (1999), "Visuospatial attention: Beyond a spotlight model". In Psychonomy Bulletin and Review, 6(2), pp. 204–223.

Cohen, R. A. (2014), The Neuropsychology of Attention. New York: Springer, pp. 60-62, 81-82.

Corbetta, M., Patel, G., & Shulman, G. L. (2008). "The reorienting system of the human brain: From environment to theory of mind". In Neuron, 58(3), 306-324.

D'Angelo, D. (2020) "The phenomenology of embodied attention". In Phenomenology and the Cognitive Sciences, 19, pp. 961–978.

De Jaegher, H. Pieper B., Clénin D., Fuchs, T. (2017), "Grasping intersubjectivity: an invitation to embody social interaction research". In Phenomenology and the Cognitive Sciences (2017) 16.

Depraz, N. (2014). Attention et vigilance. A la croisée de la phénoménologie et des sciences cognitives, Paris: Puf.

Donovan, G. H., Michael, Y. L., Gatziolis, D., Mannetje, A., Douwe, J., (2019) "Association between exposure to the natural environment, rurality, and attention-deficit hyperactivity disorder in children in New Zealand: a linkage study". In Lancet Planet Health 2019, 3: e226–34.

Fuchs, T. (2005) "Implicit and explicit temporality". In Philosophy, Psychiatry & Psychology 12: 195-198.

Fuchs, T. (2007) "The temporal structure of intentionality and its disturbance in schizophrenia". In Psychopathology 40: 229-235.

Fuchs, T., De Jaegher, (2009) "Enactive intersubjectivity: Participatory sense-making and mutual incorporation". In Phenomelogy and Cognitive Sciences 8, 465–486, DOI 10.1007/s11097-009-9136-4

Fuchs, T. (2012) The phenomenology of body memory. In: Koch, S., Fuchs, T., Summa, M., Müller, C. (eds) Body Memory, Metaphor and Movement, pp. 9-22. John Benjamins, Amsterdam.

Fuchs T. (2013a) "Temporality and Psychopathology." Phenomenology and the Cognitive Sciences 12: 75–104.

Fuchs, T. (2013b) "The self in schizophrenia: Jaspers, Schneider and beyond". In: T. Fuchs, G. Stanghellini (2013) (Hrsg.) One Century of Karl Jaspers 'General Psychopathology', Oxford University Press, Oxford, 245-257.

Fuchs, T., Koch, S. (2014) "Embodied affectivity: on moving and being moved". In Frontiers in Psychology. Psychology for Clinical Settings 5: Article 508, 1-12. DOI: 10.3389/fpsyg.2014.00508

Fuchs, T. (2016), Intercorporeality and Interaffectivity, in C. Meyer, J. Streeck & S. Jordan (eds.) (2016) Intercorporeality: Emerging Socialities in Interaction, Oxford University Press, Oxford.

Fuchs, T. (2018), "The cyclical time of the body and its relation to linear time". In Journal of Consciousness Studies, 25, No. 7–8, 2018, pp. 47–65.

Fuchs, T (2020) "The Circularity of the Embodied Mind". In Front. Psychol. 11: 1707. doi: 10.3389/fpsyg.2020.01707.

Gallagher, S. (2003). "Bodily self-awareness and object perception". In Theoria et Historia Scientiarum, 7(1), 53–68.

Gallagher S. (2005), How the Body Shapes the Mind, Oxford: Oxford University Press.

Gallagher, S., Zahavi, D. (2008). The Phenomenological Mind: An Introduction to Philosophy of Mind and Cognitive Science. London: Routledge.

Gallagher, S., & D. Schmicking (Eds.) (2010), Handbook of phenomenology and the cognitive sciences, Dordrecht: Springer,

Gurwitsch, A. (1964). The Field of Consciousness. Pittsburgh: Duquesne University Press.

Gurwitsch, A. (1966). Studies in Phenomenology and Psychology. Evanston, IL: Northwestern University Press.

Gurwitsch, A. (1985). In: L. Embree (ed), Marginal Consciousness. Athens, Ohio: Ohio University Press.

James, W. (2007) The Principles of Psychology, Harvard: Harvard University Press, Voll. II.

Johnston, W. A., & Dark, V. J. (1986). Selective attention. Annual Review of Psychology, 37, 43–75. https://doi.org/10.1146/annurev.ps.37.020186.000355

Hoyer, R. S., E. Pakulak, A. Bidet-Caulet, C.M. Karns (2021) "The development of attention and distractibility in preschool children from higher and lower socioeconomic status backgrounds". In bioRxiv.438161; doi: https://doi.org/10.1101/2021.04.06.438161

Husserl, E. (1982) Husserliana 3, Ideas Pertaining to a Pure Phenomenology and to a Phenomenological Philosophy. First Book. Trans. Fred Kersten. The Hague: Martinus Nijhoff.

Husserl, E. (1989) Husserliana 4. Ideas Pertaining to a Pure Phenomenology and to a Phenomenological Philosophy. Second Book. Trans. Richard Rojcewicz and Andre Schuwer. Dordrecht: Kluwer Academic Publishers.

Husserl, E. (1991) Husserliana 10. On the Phenomenology of the Consciousness of Internal Time (1893-1917). Trans. John Barnett Brough. Dordrecht: Kluwer Academic Publishers.

Moran D. (2019), "The phenomenological approach". In G. Stanghellini et al. The Oxford Handbook of Phenomenological Psychopathology, Oxford: Oxford University Press, 205-215.

Merleau-Ponty M. (1981), Phenomenology of Perception, New York: Routledge.

Oyebode, F. (2019). "Consciousness and its disorders". In G. Stanghellini et. al. The Oxford Handbook of Phenomenological Psychopathology, Oxford: Oxford University Press, 417-430.

O'Donnell BF. (2002). Forms of attention and attentional disorders. Semin Speech Lang. 2002 May;23(2):99-106. doi: 10.1055/s-2002-24986. PMID: 11951170.

O'Regan, J. K., Noe, A. (2001). A sensorimotor account of vision and visual consciousness. Behavioral and Brain Science, 24(5), 939–1031.

Petersen, S. E., & Posner, M. I. (2012). „The Attention System of the Human Brain: 20 Years After". In Annual review of neuroscience, 35, 73-89, https://doi.org/10.1146/annurev-neuro-062111-150525

Posner M. I. (1980) "Orienting of Attention". In Quarterly Journal of Experimental Psychology. 32(1):3-25. doi:10.1080/00335558008248231

Posner, M., & Petersen, S. (1990). "The Attention System of the Human Brain". In Annual review of neuroscience, 13, 25-42. https://doi.org/10.1146/annurev.ne.13.030190.000325

Posner, M. I. (2011). Cognitive neurosciences of attention. New York: Guildford Press.

Posner, M. I., Rothbart, M. K., Sheese, B. E., & Voelker, P. (2014). "Developing Attention: Behavioral and Brain Mechanisms". In Advances in neuroscience (Hindawi), 2014, 405094. https://doi.org/10.1155/2014/405094.

Royall, D. R., et al. (2002). "Executive Control Function: A Review of Its Promise and Challenges for Clinical Research". In J Neuropsychiatry Clin Neurosci 14:4, Fall 2002, pp. 337-405

Styles, A. (2006). The Psychology of Attention. New York: Taylor & Francis

Treisman, A. (1964) Selective Attention in man, British Medical Bulletin, Volume 20, Issue 1, January 1964, Pages 12–16, https://doi.org/10.1093/oxfordjournals.bmb.a070274

Waldenfels, B. (2004). Phänomenologie der Aufmerksamkeit. Suhrkamp: Frankfurt am Main.

Wehrle, M., & Breyer, T. (2016). Horizonal extensions of attention: A phenomenological study of the contextuality and habituality of experience. Journal of Phenomenological Psychology, 47, 41–61.

Yu, C., & Smith, L. B. (2012). Embodied attention and word learning in toddlers. Cognition, 125(2), 244–262.

Zahavi, D. (2003) Husserl's Phenomenology, Stanford University Press.

Zahavi, D. (2010a). "Inner (time-)consciousness". In D. Lohmar, & I. Yamaguchi (Eds.), On Time - New Contributions to the Husserlian Phenomenology of Time, Dordrecht: Springer, 319-339.

CHAPTER THREE

ARTIFICIAL INTELLIGENCE AGAINST DESCRIPTIVE PSYCHIATRY IN THE DIAGNOSIS AND MONITORING OF NEUROPSYCHIATRIC DISORDERS

OKAN CALIYURT
TRAKIA UNIVERSITY, TURKEY

Abstract

Descriptive psychiatry is the branch of psychiatry that deals with the description and classification of mental disorders. It is concerned with the clinical, phenomenological and nosological aspects of mental disorders. While descriptive psychiatry is useful in providing a common language for clinicians to communicate about mental disorders, it has significant limitations when it comes to making a psychiatric diagnosis. Diagnosis requires a more comprehensive understanding of the aetiology, course, and prognosis of a disorder, which is beyond the scope of descriptive psychiatry. It has not yet been possible to develop a diagnostic system based on biological markers or the aetiology of mental disorders that will allow for an objective diagnosis.

The use of artificial intelligence in medicine is becoming increasingly common, with applications ranging from diagnosis and follow-up, to treatment and prediction. Applications of artificial intelligence inevitably show up in psychiatry as well. By utilising a range of data, artificial intelligence techniques like machine learning, computer vision, and natural language processing can be employed in the diagnosis of various psychiatric disorders. The development of artificial intelligence applications to replace diagnostic tools like the DSM is still in its early stages. However, there is a lot of potential for artificial intelligence to improve diagnostic systems. For example, AI could make diagnostic systems more objective and measurable.

AI can also minimise the need for human labour, cut costs, and speed up the diagnostic process. In conclusion, artificial intelligence in psychiatry has the potential to be a far more objective way of diagnosing psychiatric disorders than descriptive psychiatry. In the future, it is anticipated that AI will help psychiatry make better diagnoses. It appears that artificial intelligence will improve already-existing descriptive systems like DSM rather than doing it automatically on its own.

Keywords: Artificial intelligence, machine learning, diagnosis, psychiatry, computer vision, natural language processing

Introduction

Our daily lives are increasingly influenced by artificial intelligence (AI) and its subfields, like machine learning. Their importance for the future of human society can be compared to that of the industrial revolution. AI means that a computer, or a machine containing a computer, can act intelligently as if it were a human. AI enables machines to behave according to the environment and external stimuli. It is a topic that has received a lot of attention in recent years. The main reasons for this are, the digital data required for artificial intelligence to reach a sufficient level, the development of computer hardware capable of processing this data, and the introduction of more successful artificial intelligence algorithms.

AI has developed over the past few years and can now be found in various areas of life. More and more industries are adopting AI and as expected, the field of medicine has inevitably started to become one of the application areas of AI. Recently, AI techniques have made a huge impact in healthcare, sparking an ongoing debate about whether AI doctors may someday replace human physicians. This is unlikely to occur in the foreseeable future, but AI can assist physicians to make better clinical decisions or even replace human judgment in certain functional areas of healthcare (e.g., radiology). The increasing availability of healthcare data and the rapid development of big data analytic methods have made possible the recent successful applications of AI in healthcare. Guided by relevant clinical questions, powerful AI techniques can unlock clinically relevant information hidden in the massive amounts of data, which in turn, can assist clinical decision-making.

The use of artificial intelligence in medicine

AI is one of the hottest topics in both the technology and medical industries today, and it is not difficult to see why: the potential applications of AI in medicine are vast and could completely transform the healthcare landscape as we know it. By improving diagnosis and treatment to reduce costs and enhance patient care, AI has the potential to change the face of healthcare. AI is already being used in many ways in medicine, from diagnosing diseases to developing new treatments. The advantages of AI have been extensively discussed in medical literature. With sophisticated algorithms, AI can 'learn' features from a large volume of healthcare data, and then use the obtained insights to assist clinical practice. It can also be equipped with learning and self-correcting abilities to improve its accuracy based on feedback. An AI system can assist physicians by providing up-to-date medical information from journals, textbooks, and clinical practices to inform proper patient care. In addition, an AI system can help to reduce the diagnostic and therapeutic errors that are inevitable in human clinical practice. Moreover, an AI system extracts useful information from a large patient population to assist in making real-time inferences for health risk alerts and health outcome predictions (Ahuja, 2019).

One particular strength of AI-based systems is their ability to gather and analyse mountains of data and draw conclusions from their analysis. This can help in predicting disease, which is a challenging task for human physicians in the best of cases. AI can assist the physician in assessing cancer risk or assessing the risk factors of heart attacks as compared to strokes. In the future, physicians could then help their patients pre-empt these conditions with a long-term plan of patient care. All these changes are poised to improve the practice of medicine in the future. This will stem from making medical practice more accurate, more comprehensive, and possibly less expensive over time by preventing diseases and reducing harmful side effects and unnecessary tests based on patient profiles. This is good news for all concerned: patients, their families, and healthcare providers.

Artificial intelligence is successful in general medicine in terms of perception ability. Medical doctors can use this ability to evaluate the symptoms and signs of diseases, or they can detect an abnormal finding on a radiological image in this way. However, artificial intelligence is still far from replacing the problem-solving, critical decision-making, or operational capabilities of medical doctors.

Computer vision, natural language processing (NLP), and machine learning are sub-branches of artificial intelligence and are used in diagnostic applications in general medicine. These artificial intelligence applications in the field of general medicine have started to be used in diagnostic applications in areas such as radiology, pathology, and dermatology (Hosny et al., 2018, Niazi et al., 2019, Young et al., 2020). Computer vision is the process of using computers to interpret and understand digital images. This technology is used in a variety of fields, including medical diagnosis, autonomous vehicles, and security systems. Computer vision is an interdisciplinary field that combines elements of computer science, engineering, and mathematics. Computer vision is increasingly used in general medicine in areas such as cancer and tumour detection, medical image analysis, and diagnostic evaluation. The ability of computers to process and interpret images is rapidly improving, and this is leading to better and faster diagnosis of diseases (Esteva et al., 2021). Additionally, computer vision can be used to create 3D models of organs, which can be used for educational purposes or to plan surgeries (Olveres et al., 2021). NLP is a field of computer science and artificial intelligence that deals with the interaction between computer and human (natural) languages. In NLP, computers are trained to understand and generate human language. NLP is used in a variety of applications, such as machine translation, speech recognition, and text classification. NLP can be used in general medicine in areas such as evaluating medical notes, transferring handwritten medical records to a digital form, and understanding patients' expressions directly (Savova et al., 2019).

> Machine learning is a field of computer science that uses statistical techniques to give computers the ability to "learn" (i.e., progressively improve performance on a specific task) with data, without being explicitly programmed. The focus of machine learning is to develop algorithms that can automatically improve given more data.

Machine learning is a powerful tool that can be used to improve diagnostic processes in general medicine. By using large datasets, machine learning algorithms can be trained to identify patterns that may be indicative of disease. Additionally, machine learning can be used to develop predictive models that can help doctors better understand a patient's prognosis. One of the advantages of using machine learning in diagnostic processes is that it can help overcome the limitations of human cognitive abilities. For example, human beings are often unable to identify patterns in data that are too complex or too large. However, machine learning algorithms can be designed to identify these patterns (Awaysheh et al., 2019). In general medicine, supervised learning is frequently used as a machine learning method. Using very large amounts of data, supervised machine learning may be more successful at performing pattern analysis than humans. Supervised learning algorithms can be used to make a diagnosis based on a patient's medical history or to predict the likelihood of a certain medical condition. Additionally, supervised learning can be used to interpret medical images and find patterns that may be indicative of disease (de Bruijne, 2016).

The use of artificial intelligence in psychiatry

Psychiatry is a branch of medicine in which the human factor is of the utmost importance. In comparison to other medical specialties, the therapeutic alliance during psychiatric evaluation and treatment is a crucial component and enables an empathetic doctor-patient interaction. Human abilities such as empathy or common sense are needed in this doctor-patient relationship. Because these abilities are not available in machines, many may think that the use of AI in the field of psychiatry will be quite limited compared to other medical fields. By analysing patterns in an extensive range of data, AI can highlight subtle relationships. However, in recent years, it has become increasingly clear that machines and AI can also use data other than electronic hospital and neuroimaging records, or images used in computer vision applications. In other words, the data obtained by psychiatrists through psychiatric interviews can now be digitised and used in AI applications. Consequently, data used in the diagnosis of psychiatric disorders such as emotions, behaviour patterns, speech styles, and content have become available to AI (Haines et al., 2019). This means machines can acquire human abilities and begin to exceed their limits.

While descriptive psychiatry has several serious problems, it remains the standard form of mental health diagnosis. This is because the underlying aetiology of psychiatric disorders and the mechanics of how the brain works are simply not understood enough to support a more causal diagnostic system. In addition to the heterogeneous nature of psychiatric disorders and the different causes of the same condition, the fact that descriptive systems do not take environmental and psychological factors into account creates a separate problem area. For these reasons, it is not possible today to make a psychiatric diagnosis with the use of artificial intelligence alone. On the other hand, the descriptive system-created diagnostic categories and the signs and symptoms associated with the diagnoses can both be used by AI. With tools such as AI, machine learning, NLP, or computer vision, these signs and symptoms can be detected more objectively and more precisely. This will allow for a quicker and more efficient automated application of the descriptive mental diagnosis method (Blease et al., 2020). The use of AI in psychiatry is the approach of using some computerised and algorithmic techniques, such as machine learning, for psychiatric diagnosis, follow-up, treatment, and prevention. Psychiatry has utilised subjective and inaccurate evaluations for years. Patient self-reports and clinical observations lead to flawed conclusions, and many treatment methods do not produce desired results. AI can aid in the mental health field and has already started to change how we think about treatment options, medication side effects, and diagnosis. It provides a level of consistency in the psychiatric evaluation process that was impossible with traditional paper and pencil assessment tools, among other benefits (Fakhoury, 2019).

Brain imaging tools are highly successful data sources in the use of AI for the diagnosis of schizophrenia. It has been shown that fMRI and PET images can successfully differentiate schizophrenia patients from the controls with Artificial Neural Network-based machine learning methods (Bose et al., 2008, Jafri and Calhoun, 2006). Similarly, another area that can be used as a data source in AI applications is possibly brain atlases. To determine four MRI parameters, including regional grey matter volume, regional homogeneity, the amplitude of low-frequency fluctuation, and degree centrality, the authors collected MRI data from patients with first-episode schizophrenia, chronic schizophrenia patients, and healthy controls. According to their findings, the groupwise whole-brain atlas with numerous regions of interest performed better than the other two brain atlases (Zang et al., 2021). In another study, MRI data and machine learning in major depressive disorder were investigated. Their findings indicated that dynamic functional connectivity is superior to static functional connectivity and offers a valid quantitative tool for the diagnosis of severe depressive disorder. The authors claimed that their findings may contribute to a better understanding of the neurological underpinnings of major depressive disorder as well as to a more precise diagnosis and early treatment of this condition (Yan et al., 2020). Brain scans can be used to diagnose dementia in people with extremely early-stage disease. The algorithms are capable of a very high success rate, which is far better than current techniques that rely on the assessments of medical professionals. This suggests that brain scans could be utilised as an objective method for the early identification of Alzheimer's disease (Popuri et al., 2020).

Unipolar and bipolar depression were compared with machine learning using a higher order functional connectivity network, it was seen that there were different divergent and convergent neural substrates, and it was concluded that these are different mental disorders. This result is remarkable in understanding the inadequacy of the DSM-based diagnostic system and revealing the importance of artificial intelligence. Although there are differences between unipolar and bipolar depression in areas such as onset, course, and treatment; the clinical presentation and symptoms are the same in both disorders in the descriptive psychiatric approach. As a result, AI applications will help the correct classification of such psychiatric disorders, and lead to the correct diagnosis and treatment (Zhang et al., 2022).

An alternative that can be used in psychiatric diagnosis as an AI application is the use of digitalisation of physiological changes. These signs and symptoms are physiological measurements that are not included in diagnostic systems such as DSM or ICD. Specific physiological changes occur in many psychiatric disorders, although most of them are not pathological enough to make a diagnosis of a physical disease. However, the data can be used successfully in the diagnosis or follow-up of psychiatric disorders. In fact, with the 24/7 detection and follow-up of these symptoms, improvement or worsening of psychiatric disorders can be monitored (Momeni et al., 2019, Saboo et al., 2019).

Changes in movement, speech, gait, and changes in their speed often occur in affective disorders (Boettcher et al., 2020, Delic et al., 2019). Some specific behaviours occur in obsessive-compulsive disorder, ADHD or autistic disorder. Similarly, autonomic hyperactivity, increase in heart rate, prominence of facial capillaries, and arousal findings related to anxiety can be detected with the help of various sensors. One study investigated the link between mobile phone keyboard activity and mood disruption in patients with bipolar disorder. As a result, among these individuals, the results showed a correlation between the keyboard activity and the changes in usage patterns. (Zulueta et al., 2018). In a study, researchers provided the subjects with mobile phones that passively collected keystroke metadata. Mood states in in bipolar disorder appear to correlate with specific changes in mobile phone usage. The creation of these models provides evidence for the feasibility of using passively collected keyboard metadata to detect and monitor mood disturbances (Zulueta et al., 2018). It is possible to determine the heart rate remotely without any physical contact with the patient. Remote photoplethysmography uses a camera to collect reflected light from the skin and analyse it to obtain heart rate. The heartbeat variability can be used for measuring mental workload or for detecting emotions such as anger and sadness (Wang et al., 2018). In a related study, it was shown that panic disorder and other anxiety disorders can be distinguished from each other by using the heart rate variability parameter through machine learning (Na et al., 2021).

Apart from the standard diagnosis approach based on signs and symptoms, artificial intelligence applications show the capacity to diagnose or screen for psychiatric disorders using a wide spectrum of data. A recent study analysed posts from social media platforms focusing on schizophrenia along with non-mental health-related posts for comparison purposes. Afterward, linguistic features were used in conjunction with subject headings for machine learning methods that classified with a 96% success rate for separating the two groups. The authors showed that their machine learning study using social media texts can be effectively used as a tool for detecting signs of schizophrenia (Bae et al., 2021). Sentiment analysis is a natural language processing technique that can be used to determine if data is positive, negative, or neutral. When applied to social media, sentiment analysis can be used as a tool for screening and following up on mental disorders. In this way, large-scale data, which has never been used until now, can provide a source for artificial intelligence and machine learning independent of place and time and can be used in clinical practice (Babu and Kanaga, 2022, Owusu et al., 2021).

Without using the criteria of the DSM or other diagnostic systems, it is now possible to immediately derive diagnostic conclusions from labelled data with the use of artificial intelligence. Latent Semantic Analysis (LSA) is a natural language processing method that uses statistical methods to find associations between words. LSA is a diverse technique with many applications. LSA was successfully used to identify schizophrenia patients and healthy controls (Elvevag et al., 2007). In addition, speech analysis combined with LSA has been used to detect subtle deviations between the speech of first-degree relatives of schizophrenia patients and healthy individuals (Elvevag et al., 2010). Another study using electroencephalograph (EEG) signals based on event-related potential tried to distinguish between schizophrenia and healthy controls. It has been found that adding features extracted from EEG signals can improve classification accuracy (Zhang, 2019).

This article focuses on the relationship between artificial intelligence and psychiatric diagnosis. But beyond diagnosis, artificial intelligence also plays a significant role in selecting the best treatment plan for psychiatric disorders, anticipating potential episodes, and monitoring the progression of such disorders. In particular, the determination of patient characteristics also provides benefits for the prediction of treatment success in addition to diagnosis. A recent study sought to determine whether a combination of pre-treatment patient characteristics would be more predictive of who would benefit from a placebo or medication. The study found that interactions between pre-treatment patient characteristics were indeed better predictors than a single-variable solution. This finding has important implications for the way we treat patients with medication (Zilcha-Mano et al., 2018).

Precision psychiatry

Precision medicine is an emerging approach for both treatment and prevention. It takes the variability of each individual's genes, environment, and lifestyle into account. This applies not just to healthcare but also to determining the risks for developing certain diseases and who would benefit from specific treatments. The main purpose of precision psychiatry is to provide personalised treatment option for patients with psychiatric disorders. The goal is to maximise therapeutic outcomes based on biological and clinical data. This approach will enable us to determine the optimal treatment for everyone (Fernandes et al., 2017).

AI, machine learning, and deep learning technologies are playing an increasingly critical role in the new era of precision psychiatry by analysing large amounts of data with minimal bias and high accuracy. It would not be possible to process the excessive and complex data generated by precision medicine applications in a meaningful way without AI. Along with personalised treatment and prognosis prediction, precision psychiatry seems to have an important place in diagnostic processes as well. New biomarkers and neuroimaging findings related to psychiatric disorders are constantly being discovered. With these personalised data, it is possible to achieve much more accurate diagnostic results (Nielsen et al., 2020). Digital phenotyping is a relatively new field of research that is gaining popularity, especially within the field of psychiatry. The goal of digital phenotyping is to create a comprehensive picture of an individual by integrating data from digital devices, medical records, and lived experiences. This information can then be used to more effectively monitor, intervene, and diagnose various psychiatric conditions (Davidson, 2022).

Advantages of artificial intelligence in psychiatry

AI represents a new shift in healthcare and has the potential to impact areas of diagnosis, treatment, monitoring, and prevention. The advantages of AI in healthcare include cost effectiveness, the ability to tailor treatments for specific individuals, and the removal of time-related barriers. Another advantage is that it can be applied to those who have mobility problems or who cannot come to the hospital for various reasons. On the other hand, it offers 24/7 evaluation and follow-up capability by exceeding the evaluation performed during the doctor's examination. In addition, it can be used in a hybrid way with all classical methods. Finally, it is very important for psychiatry that artificial intelligence does not tire, does not discriminate, or does not show any prejudice (Blease et al., 2020).

AI can make inferences in data that are larger than humans' capacity to evaluate. It has an important place in determining the risk of certain psychiatric disorders. For example, for women in early pregnancy, electronic health records and machine learning can successfully determine the risk of postpartum depression. Therefore, it will be possible to take necessary precautions, intervene on time, and minimize negative consequences (Zhang et al., 2021). A study was recently conducted to develop and validate machine learning-based models for predicting depression symptoms in individuals who took part in a survey during the outbreak of COVID-19 in China. The findings indicated that such prediction models could be useful for making predictions about mentally at-risk healthcare workers during public health emergencies (Zhou et al., 2022).

Another important advantage of AI over humans is that it can detect stimuli that humans cannot perceive or that are beyond their perceptual capacity. It will be possible for AI to detect possible patterns between stimuli and psychiatric disorders. For example, humans cannot see infrared light; they can only feel some of it as heat (Jagadev and Giri, 2020). However, an AI application that records data with an infrared camera may well detect infrared changes in the facial capillaries related to anxiety or arousal (Ancillon et al., 2022). Similarly, very fast or very mild muscular contractions of the human face can be used as data using high-capacity cameras, or sensitive changes in speech content and physical sound characteristics that humans cannot hear and detect can be detected.

AI can be used to monitor a person's physical and mental health by collecting an excessive amount of data from numerous sources, including wearable technology and electronic health records (Sabry et al., 2022). Apart from that, the social norms of a society can be established using information gathered from other people and society, and it is then possible to assess whether individuals and groups deviate from the norm.

In addition to its benefits, using artificial intelligence in psychiatry may also present some challenges. Artificial intelligence can work faster than human beings and has enough memory to store huge volumes of information. This, to some, is a big threat to the humans who are currently involved in the medical field, both in research and treatment. It can be thought that those working in the field of mental health will lose their jobs (Stringaris, 2019). Contrary to common belief, new fields of study can be developed by combining computer science and psychiatry. Fewer people will be required to perform some repetitive activities, but there will be a need for personnel who will work in a wide variety of new areas related to software and hardware, the transfer of artificial intelligence to psychiatry, and the remote follow-up and treatment of patients. Machine learning is primarily driven by large amounts of data, but the quantity, quality, and location of that data are fundamental to determining results. If machine learning is trained with data that is not representative of the general population or other cultures, or is insufficient, the results can lead us to the wrong conclusions (Phillips et al., 2022). Artificial intelligence applications won't be complete until they incorporate a broad evaluation of the person's social, psychological, and cultural characteristics (Erol and Erol, 2019).

Conclusion

It seems that the practice of psychiatry, like all other branches, is on the eve of change. Artificial intelligence will provide significant benefits for both psychiatrists and patients. With the help of artificial intelligence, psychiatrists can more easily and rapidly collect data on their patients, as well as make treatment decisions. It will allow the psychiatrist to focus more on the issues that are critical to their patients, thus increasing their efficiency in serving others. Artificial intelligence will also enable psychiatrists to explore new ways of helping people with mental health problems. In addition to these, it will help to overcome the inadequacy of psychiatrists in society (Allen, 2020).

This article focuses on the role artificial intelligence contributes to psychiatric diagnosing methods. It can be expected that artificial intelligence, which is obvious to provide important benefits in other fields of psychiatry, will be used in the diagnostic field at the very beginning. Artificial intelligence will be able to evaluate some signs and symptoms more successfully than humans and will be able to evaluate diagnostically digitalizable physiological changes, signs, and symptoms that humans do not evaluate today. Reducing diagnostic errors and increasing diagnostic accuracy are crucial goals for the healthcare system. To achieve these goals, we need to increase diagnostic success rates, especially in psychiatry. By using artificial intelligence, we can reduce unnecessary examinations and laboratory tests, and prevent wrong treatments, and economic losses (Phillips, 2014).

However, artificial intelligence cannot directly diagnose psychiatric disorders, which are products of the human brain, that we do not know precisely how it works today, and whose aetiology we do not know exactly. Current research focuses on the recognition of psychiatric disorders with some datasets that are generally diagnosed and labelled by humans. In other words, it will be possible to improve the current descriptive psychiatric diagnosis systems, use them faster, and strengthen them with different data sets. Furthermore, more accurate reconstitution of diagnostic clusters will be possible, and measurable objective data can be introduced into diagnostic evaluation. With machine learning methods, it will be possible to determine which clinical data is more important. In addition, with the help of cameras, microphones, various sensors, smartphones, and other biological sensing devices, data can be collected and included in diagnostic processes not only in the hospital or consulting room, but also at home, at work, on the road, or while socialising.

Artificial intelligence techniques and artificial intelligence applications in medicine will continue to grow and develop. This development is evident in both basic and clinical sciences. It can be predicted that artificial intelligence techniques, artificial intelligence applications, and their transfer to the field of psychiatry will have an important place in medical education and psychiatric specialisation. Considering that this serious change has already begun, the use of artificial intelligence should be included in medicine and psychiatric education as soon as possible. Perhaps new fields of study and even new professions may be created by integrating psychiatry with fields such as computer science, artificial intelligence, programming, and big data.

A robot that can do a thorough assessment comparable to a human psychiatrist will soon be necessary. For this reason, the clinical evaluation procedure will also include chatbots that can interact successfully with humans. A chatbot is a computer program that simulates human conversation, allowing humans to interact with digital devices as if they were communicating with a real person. Artificial intelligence chatbots use machine learning and natural language processing to enable humans to communicate with computers. Chatbots can be used to communicate with people, answer common questions, and perform specific tasks. AI-based chatbots will be able to be used to automate psychiatric interviews and diagnostic processes in the future. In this way, by minimising the use of psychiatrists, a fast, reliable, and more comfortable service will be provided at a much lower cost (Pham et al., 2022).

Although artificial intelligence cannot entirely replace the DSM diagnostic system anytime soon, it could improve this system by creating objective diagnostic clusters and providing objective detection of certain symptoms. Though other medical fields have long been using laboratory tests, special tests, and radiological tools for diagnosis, psychiatrists can also start to use these tools to speed up and improve the sensitivity and accuracy of diagnosis.

References

AHUJA, A. S. 2019. The impact of artificial intelligence in medicine on the future role of the physician. *PeerJ,* 7, e7702.

ALLEN, S. 2020. Artificial Intelligence and the Future of Psychiatry. *IEEE Pulse,* 11, 2-6.

ANCILLON, L., ELGENDI, M. & MENON, C. 2022. Machine Learning for Anxiety Detection Using Biosignals: A Review. *Diagnostics (Basel),* 12.

AWAYSHEH, A., WILCKE, J., ELVINGER, F., REES, L., FAN, W. & ZIMMERMAN, K. L. 2019. Review of Medical Decision Support and Machine-Learning Methods. *Vet Pathol,* 56, 512-525.

BABU, N. V. & KANAGA, E. G. M. 2022. Sentiment Analysis in Social Media Data for Depression Detection Using Artificial Intelligence: A Review. *SN Comput Sci,* 3, 74.

BAE, Y. J., SHIM, M. & LEE, W. H. 2021. Schizophrenia Detection Using Machine Learning Approach from Social Media Content. *Sensors (Basel),* 21.

BLEASE, C., LOCHER, C., LEON-CARLYLE, M. & DORAISWAMY, M. 2020. Artificial intelligence and the future of psychiatry: Qualitative findings from a global physician survey. *Digit Health,* 6, 2055207620968355.

BOETTCHER, L. N., HSSAYENI, M., ROSENFELD, A., TOLEA, M. I., GALVIN, J. E. & GHORAANI, B. 2020. Dual-Task Gait Assessment and Machine Learning for Early-detection of Cognitive Decline. *Annu Int Conf IEEE Eng Med Biol Soc,* 2020, 3204-3207.

BOSE, S. K., TURKHEIMER, F. E., HOWES, O. D., MEHTA, M. A., CUNLIFFE, R., STOKES, P. R. & GRASBY, P. M. 2008. Classification of schizophrenic patients and healthy controls using [18F] fluorodopa PET imaging. *Schizophr Res,* 106**,** 148-55.

DAVIDSON, B. I. 2022. The crossroads of digital phenotyping. *Gen Hosp Psychiatry,* 74**,** 126-132.

DE BRUIJNE, M. 2016. Machine learning approaches in medical image analysis: From detection to diagnosis. *Med Image Anal,* 33**,** 94-97.

DELIC, V., PERIC, Z., SECUJSKI, M., JAKOVLJEVIC, N., NIKOLIC, J., MISKOVIC, D., SIMIC, N., SUZIC, S. & DELIC, T. 2019. Speech Technology Progress Based on New Machine Learning Paradigm. *Comput Intell Neurosci,* 2019**,** 4368036.

ELVEVAG, B., FOLTZ, P. W., ROSENSTEIN, M. & DELISI, L. E. 2010. An automated method to analyze language use in patients with schizophrenia and their first-degree relatives. *J Neurolinguistics,* 23**,** 270-284.

ELVEVAG, B., FOLTZ, P. W., WEINBERGER, D. R. & GOLDBERG, T. E. 2007. Quantifying incoherence in speech: an automated methodology and novel application to schizophrenia. *Schizophr Res,* 93**,** 304-16.

EROL, K. & EROL, A. 2019. A New Era in Psychiatry: Influence of Technology and Artificial Intelligence. *Noro Psikiyatr Ars,* 56**,** 84-85.

ESTEVA, A., CHOU, K., YEUNG, S., NAIK, N., MADANI, A., MOTTAGHI, A., LIU, Y., TOPOL, E., DEAN, J. & SOCHER, R. 2021. Deep learning-enabled medical computer vision. *NPJ Digit Med,* 4**,** 5.

FAKHOURY, M. 2019. Artificial Intelligence in Psychiatry. *Adv Exp Med Biol,* 1192**,** 119-125.

FERNANDES, B. S., WILLIAMS, L. M., STEINER, J., LEBOYER, M., CARVALHO, A. F. & BERK, M. 2017. The new field of 'precision psychiatry'. *BMC Med,* 15**,** 80.

HAINES, N., BELL, Z., CROWELL, S., HAHN, H., KAMARA, D., MCDONOUGH-CAPLAN, H., SHADER, T. & BEAUCHAINE, T. P. 2019. Using automated computer vision and machine learning to code facial expressions of affect and arousal: Implications for emotion dysregulation research. *Dev Psychopathol,* 31**,** 871-886.

HOSNY, A., PARMAR, C., QUACKENBUSH, J., SCHWARTZ, L. H. & AERTS, H. 2018. Artificial intelligence in radiology. *Nat Rev Cancer,* 18**,** 500-510.

JAFRI, M. J. & CALHOUN, V. D. 2006. Functional classification of schizophrenia using feed forward neural networks. *Conf Proc IEEE Eng Med Biol Soc,* Suppl**,** 6631-4.

JAGADEV, P. & GIRI, L. I. 2020. Human respiration monitoring using infrared thermography and artificial intelligence. *Biomed Phys Eng Express,* 6, 035007.

MOMENI, N., DELL'AGNOLA, F., ARZA, A. & ATIENZA, D. 2019. Real-Time Cognitive Workload Monitoring Based on Machine Learning Using Physiological Signals in Rescue Missions. *Annu Int Conf IEEE Eng Med Biol Soc,* 2019, 3779-3785.

NA, K. S., CHO, S. E. & CHO, S. J. 2021. Machine learning-based discrimination of panic disorder from other anxiety disorders. *J Affect Disord,* 278, 1-4.

NIAZI, M. K. K., PARWANI, A. V. & GURCAN, M. N. 2019. Digital pathology and artificial intelligence. *Lancet Oncol,* 20, e253-e261.

NIELSEN, A. N., BARCH, D. M., PETERSEN, S. E., SCHLAGGAR, B. L. & GREENE, D. J. 2020. Machine Learning with Neuroimaging: Evaluating Its Applications in Psychiatry. *Biol Psychiatry Cogn Neurosci Neuroimaging,* 5, 791-798.

OLVERES, J., GONZALEZ, G., TORRES, F., MORENO-TAGLE, J. C., CARBAJAL-DEGANTE, E., VALENCIA-RODRIGUEZ, A., MENDEZ-SANCHEZ, N. & ESCALANTE-RAMIREZ, B. 2021. What is new in computer vision and artificial intelligence in medical image analysis applications. *Quant Imaging Med Surg,* 11, 3830-3853.

OWUSU, P. N., REININGHAUS, U., KOPPE, G., DANKWA-MULLAN, I. & BARNIGHAUSEN, T. 2021. Artificial intelligence applications in social media for depression screening: A systematic review protocol for content validity processes. *PLoS One,* 16, e0259499.

PHAM, K. T., NABIZADEH, A. & SELEK, S. 2022. Artificial Intelligence and Chatbots in Psychiatry. *Psychiatr Q,* 93, 249-253.

PHILLIPS, J. 2014. Detecting diagnostic error in psychiatry. *Diagnosis (Berl),* 1, 75-78.

PHILLIPS, S. P., SPITHOFF, S. & SIMPSON, A. 2022. Artificial intelligence and predictive algorithms in medicine: Promise and problems. *Can Fam Physician,* 68, 570-572.

POPURI, K., MA, D., WANG, L. & BEG, M. F. 2020. Using machine learning to quantify structural MRI neurodegeneration patterns of Alzheimer's disease into dementia score: Independent validation on 8,834 images from ADNI, AIBL, OASIS, and MIRIAD databases. *Hum Brain Mapp,* 41, 4127-4147.

SABOO, K. V., VARATHARAJAH, Y., BERRY, B. M., KREMEN, V., SPERLING, M. R., DAVIS, K. A., JOBST, B. C., GROSS, R. E., LEGA, B., SHETH, S. A., WORRELL, G. A., IYER, R. K. & KUCEWICZ, M. T. 2019. Unsupervised machine-learning

classification of electrophysiologically active electrodes during human cognitive task performance. *Sci Rep,* 9, 17390.
SABRY, F., ELTARAS, T., LABDA, W., ALZOUBI, K. & MALLUHI, Q. 2022. Machine Learning for Healthcare Wearable Devices: The Big Picture. *J Healthc Eng,* 2022, 4653923.
SAVOVA, G. K., DANCIU, I., ALAMUDUN, F., MILLER, T., LIN, C., BITTERMAN, D. S., TOURASSI, G. & WARNER, J. L. 2019. Use of Natural Language Processing to Extract Clinical Cancer Phenotypes from Electronic Medical Records. *Cancer Res,* 79, 5463-5470.
STRINGARIS, A. 2019. Editorial: Are computers going to take over: implications of machine learning and computational psychiatry for trainees and practising clinicians. *J Child Psychol Psychiatry,* 60, 1251-1253.
WANG, C., PUN, T. & CHANEL, G. 2018. A Comparative Survey of Methods for Remote Heart Rate Detection from Frontal Face Videos. *Front Bioeng Biotechnol,* 6, 33.
YAN, B., XU, X., LIU, M., ZHENG, K., LIU, J., LI, J., WEI, L., ZHANG, B., LU, H. & LI, B. 2020. Quantitative Identification of Major Depression Based on Resting-State Dynamic Functional Connectivity: A Machine Learning Approach. *Front Neurosci,* 14, 191.
YOUNG, A. T., XIONG, M., PFAU, J., KEISER, M. J. & WEI, M. L. 2020. Artificial Intelligence in Dermatology: A Primer. *J Invest Dermatol,* 140, 1504-1512.
ZANG, J., HUANG, Y., KONG, L., LEI, B., KE, P., LI, H., ZHOU, J., XIONG, D., LI, G., CHEN, J., LI, X., XIANG, Z., NING, Y., WU, F. & WU, K. 2021. Effects of Brain Atlases and Machine Learning Methods on the Discrimination of Schizophrenia Patients: A Multimodal MRI Study. *Front Neurosci,* 15, 697168.
ZHANG, H., ZHOU, Z., DING, L., WU, C., QIU, M., HUANG, Y., JIN, F., HSU, L., YANG, Y., SHEN, T., WANG, J., ZHANG, H., SHEN, D. & PENG, D. 2022. Divergent and convergent imaging markers between bipolar and unipolar depression based on Machine Learning. *IEEE J Biomed Health Inform,* PP.
ZHANG, L. 2019. EEG Signals Classification Using Machine Learning for The Identification and Diagnosis of Schizophrenia. *Annu Int Conf IEEE Eng Med Biol Soc,* 2019, 4521-4524.
ZHANG, Y., WANG, S., HERMANN, A., JOLY, R. & PATHAK, J. 2021. Development and validation of a machine learning algorithm for predicting the risk of postpartum depression among pregnant women. *J Affect Disord,* 279, 1-8.

ZHOU, Z., LUO, D., YANG, B. X. & LIU, Z. 2022. Machine Learning-Based Prediction Models for Depression Symptoms Among Chinese Healthcare Workers During the Early COVID-19 Outbreak in 2020: A Cross-Sectional Study. *Front Psychiatry,* 13, 876995.

ZILCHA-MANO, S., ROOSE, S. P., BROWN, P. J. & RUTHERFORD, B. R. 2018. A Machine Learning Approach to Identifying Placebo Responders in Late-Life Depression Trials. *Am J Geriatr Psychiatry,* 26, 669-677.

ZULUETA, J., PISCITELLO, A., RASIC, M., EASTER, R., BABU, P., LANGENECKER, S. A., MCINNIS, M., AJILORE, O., NELSON, P. C., RYAN, K. & LEOW, A. 2018. Predicting Mood Disturbance Severity with Mobile Phone Keystroke Metadata: A BiAffect Digital Phenotyping Study. *J Med Internet Res,* 20, e241.

CHAPTER FOUR

FORMAL THOUGHT DISORDER AND ITS NEUROSCIENTIFIC CORRELATES

ERIK DORNELLES[A] AND DIOGO TELLES-CORREIA[B]
[A] CENTRO HOSPITALAR UNIVERSITÁRIO LISBOA NORTE – SERVIÇO DE PSIQUIATRIA E SAÚDE MENTAL, LISBON, PORTUGAL
[B] FACULDADE DE MEDICINA, CLINICA UNIVERSITARIA DE PSIQUIATRIA E PSICOLOGIA MEDICA, UNIVERSIDADE DE LISBOA, LISBON, PORTUGAL

Abstract

Even though the concept of Formal Thought Disorder (FTD) is an ambiguous and disputed one, it has endured as a core psychopathological construct in the clinical coalface of Psychiatry. FTD can be summarised as a multidimensional construct, reflecting difficulties or idiosyncrasies in thinking, language, and communication in general. It is usually subdivided into positive versus negative, and objective versus subjective. In this chapter, we begin by shedding light on the conceptual limits of FTD and then set out to explore the latest neuroscientific findings regarding its putative biological substrate. Ranging all the way from the synaptic and neurotransmitter level to the anatomical and functional one, whilst also considering their linguistic and neuropsychological implications.

Keywords: Thought disorder, language, neuroscience, psychopathology

Introduction

The concept of Formal thought disorder (FTD) is a long-standing one in the history of Psychiatry, and it has followed the advances of this branch of medicine through a winding and sometimes confusing path. At its core is the concept of thought itself, a complex and evasive phenomenon through which our understanding of ourselves, the world and reality itself is woven. If even the description of ordinary, everyday "normal" thought process can be perplexity-inducing, one can expect that the concept of the disordered thought would be a difficult one to pin down. As Berrios points out, it is hard to separate theories of thought from the concept of thought disorder (Berrios, 2010).

While Esquirol was the first author to hint at the presence of a primary disorder of the faculty in charge of coordinating ideas (Jerónimo, Queirós, Cheniaux, & Telles-Correia, 2018), the modern descriptions of FTD can be traced back more directly to the works of Wilhelm Griesinger, Jules Séglas and Renée Masselon (Berrios, 2010). Later, Emil Kraeplin, Carl Gustav Jung, and especially Eugen Bleuler refined the symptom descriptions and tied them with the concept of schizophrenia (Kircher, Brohl, Meier, & Engelen, 2018). In his seminal work on the "group of Schizophrenias", Eugen Bleuler put particular emphasis on the concept of "loosening of associations", which he considered a primary – closely related to the theorized organic substrate of the disorder – and fundamental symptom – always present over the course of the disorder (Bleuler, 1911).

However, FTD has been repeatedly shown to be present in other diagnosis, even though different disorders might have distinct FTD patterns (Andreasen N. , 1979) (Docherty, DeRosa, & Andreasen, 1996) (Yalincetin, et al., 2016). Nevertheless, the prevalence rates are highest in schizophrenia (50-80%), followed by schizoaffective disorders (60%), and depression (53%) (Cavelti, Kircher, Nagels, Strik, & Homan, 2018); the rates reported in mania are mixed, with some studies reporting higher rates and other lower or similar rates to schizophrenia (Roche, Creed, MacMahon, Brennan, & Clarke, 2015).

FTD is affected by the emotional state and thought content expressed (Docherty, Evans, Sledge, Seibyl, & Krystal, 1994), and exists on a continuum with normal speech; it is present, albeit in a milder form, in about 6% of healthy subjects (Kircher, et al., 2014) (Adreasen, 1986).

Nowadays, FTD is considered a multidimensional and heterogenous group of signs and symptoms, one which reflects not only peculiarities and difficulties in thinking, but also in language and communication in general (Hart & Lewine, 2017). This broadening of the concept of FTD was put forward by Nancy Andreasen, who argued that if we view it from an empirical perspective, most of the particular signs and symptoms of which FTD is comprised could be better described as disorders in communication as a whole, and that the notion of thought would have to be invoked to explain only a few of them (Adreasen, 1986). Indeed, since FTD is usually diagnosed in the dialectic interaction of the doctor-patient dyad, it can be hard to separate the disordered thought processes of the patient from the larger medium of communication. Andreasen also originally proposed the subdivision of FTD into "positive" (pressure of speech, tangentiality, derailment, incoherence, and illogicality) and "negative" (poverty of speech and poverty of content) factors (Andreasen & Grove, 1979), something which has endured in the literature and been shown to be a consistent finding in meta analyses (Yalincetin, et al., 2017).

More recently, Kircher and colleagues have argued that the available FTD rating scales didn't fully capture the whole spectrum of symptoms which are classified under that umbrella term (Kircher, et al., 2014). Specifically, they argued that the most neglected dimension of FTD was the subjective one, meaning the subtle changes in the patient's thought process as reported by the patient himself. In order to fill this gap, Kircher and colleagues developed the Thought and Language Disorder (TALD) scale, a convenient 30-item scale encompassing most if not all FTD symptoms reported form the early 20th century forward and subdivided into 4 factors, namely Objective Positive, Objective Negative, Subjective Positive and Subjective Negative. The first factor, Objective Positive, was said to represent the so-called "disorganisation factor" reported by other factor-analysis studies of FTD (Peralta, Cuesta, & de Leon, 1992) and best represented by the phenomena of *derailment* and *crosstalk*. The Objective Negative factor consisted of *poverty of speech, slowed thinking* and *concretism*, and correlated with TLC's "emptiness factor". The Subjective Positive factor included *pressure/rush of thought* and *thought interference*. Finally, the Subjective Negative factor was best represented by *poverty of thought, inhibited thinking* and *dysfunction of thought initiative and intentionality* phenomena.

This effort to classify FTD signs and symptoms into different subgroups is relevant because the relative impact of the distinct FTD groupings on diagnosis and prognosis might be different. For example, Morgan and colleagues showed that "deviant verbalisations" – a concept which captures stilted or awkward word usage (e.g. "the outform of the map" or "posterior pronunciations") and could be said to be part of the Positive subgroup – might be used to differentiate chronic schizophrenia patients from patients with remitted bipolar disorder (Morgan, et al., 2017), hinting at the idea that different diagnosis might spur different types of FTD. Regarding prognosis, Wilcox and colleagues showed that patients with psychotic depression who experienced FTD are more likely to relapse within a 7-year period (Wilcox, A.L., & Baida-Fragoso, 2000). It has also been shown that Negative FTD at follow-up is related to poor social functioning (Harvey, Docherty, M.R., & Rasmussen, 1990), and that FTD in general is inversely associated with social functioning (Marggraf, Lysaker, Salyers, & Minor, 2020). In ultra-high risk individuals, persistent Positive FTD increases the risk of progression to schizophrenia (DeVylder, et al., 2014), but Negative FTD might better predict the transition to schizophrenia than Positive FTD (Ott, Roberts, Rock, Allen, & Erlenmeyer-Kimling, 2002).

Pathogenesis of FTD

Several different theoretical approaches to FTD exist. Two of the more influential hypotheses explaining the overarching neurocognitive pathogenesis of different FTD symptom are called the "dyssemantic" and "dysexecutive" hypotheses, and, far from being mutually exclusive, might account for different degrees or subtypes of FTD.

The "dyssemantic" hypothesis places emphasis on abnormalities in language-processing related brain regions and functional networks (Goldberg, et al., 1998). Indeed, dysfunctions in the semantic network explain some of the language difficulties in patients exhibiting Positive FTD. The semantic fields – the set of meanings or signifiers which are activated when a particular word is thought or heard – of patients with Positive FTD are wider, and the meanings of words are more loosely connected. This can be tested with the so-called "semantic priming" tests (Manschreck, et al., 1988). In them, participants are first very briefly subjected to a prime word and then are tasked to quickly indicate whether a particular sequence of letters forms a word or a non-word. The prime word can either be related or unrelated with the target word (also called the probe word). In healthy controls, the reaction time is shorter when the prime and target words are semantically related (e.g., "dog" and "cat"). However, if the participant exhibits Positive FTD, the prime word is flashed in a way it can't be consciously read and the words are only indirectly related (e.g., "lemon" and "sweet", mediated by the word "sour"), the patient tends to exhibit "hyperpriming" (Spitzer, et al., 1994) and react faster than healthy controls. This could indicate a quicker and/or wider spread of information in the semantic network in patients with Positive FTD (Moritz, et al., 2001). Interestingly, Bleuler also placed a particular emphasis upon indirect, or mediated, associations which he believed played a major role in the formation of schizophrenic symptomatology (Spitzer, Braun, Maier, Hermle, & Maher, 1993). This is likely associated with the recruitment of the right temporal lobe in the processing of remote semantic information in patients with Positive FTD (Kiefer, Weisbrod, Kern, Maier, & Spitzer, 1998) (Kircher T. , et al., 2002).

Those findings, however, are far from consistent. Some studies report, for example, that depending on the stimulus onset asynchrony (the amount of time between the prime and probe words), patients with schizophrenia might exhibit hypopriming effects or be comparable to healthy controls (Barch, et al., 1996), even though they didn't specifically target the role of FTD. Many studies suggested that the problem might involve higher-order semantics, for instance affecting long distance associations while sparing naming (Barrera, McKenna, & Berrios, 2005), lexical co-occurrences and sequences of discourse (Elvevåg, Foltz, Weinberger, & Goldberg, 2007) (Hella, et al., 2013). Other studies have focused on more complex aspects of meaning interpretation involving figurative language such as idiomatic expressions (Schettino, et al., 2010) and metaphors (Champagne-Lavau & Stip, 2009). This difficulty in comprehension of non-literal language has usually been ascribed to deficits in higher-order semantics or even pragmatics, discourse or poor Theory of Mind.

Some studies have also focused on the syntactic component of language, challenging the classical view that even when the organisation of discourse has completely broken down, the syntax of schizophrenic speech remained unaffected. Thomas and colleagues reported the presence of different syntactic errors, linked to negative symptoms (Thomas, King, Fraser, & Kendell, 1987) and more severe in chronic patients (Thomas, King, Fraser, & Kendell, 1990). More recently, Moro and colleagues attempted to dissociate syntactic and semantic tests and reported a specific impairment in the former but not in the latter, in patients with schizophrenia (Moro, et al., 2015). It has also been proposed that abnormalities in the inferior frontal gyrus and its connections with the temporal lobe might be of particular importance in difficulties of syntactic comprehension (den Ouden, et al., 2019).

The "dysexecutive" hypothesis, in turn, proposes that impaired planning and monitoring might lead to the speech of patients with FTD being poorly formulated or prone to errors, which are then allowed to go unnoticed and uncorrected (Fuentes-Claramonte, et al., 2020). McGrath published one of the most detailed theoretical articulations of the frontal/dysexecutive hypothesis to date (McGrath, 1991), where he speculated that different executive functions might be linked to specific FTD symptoms. He suggested that poverty of speech and content of speech might be related to difficulties in forming a general intention to talk or in establishing a specific focus to guide communication; perseveration, clang associations and rigidity of theme might be related to an inability to change sets, to "re-focus" or "disattend" from an action or cognition; and failures in planning, editing and error-monitoring might underlie many other items such as derailment, loss of goal or pressure of speech. In favour of this hypothesis is the well-established link between the "disorganization syndrome" – of which the main symptom is FTD – and impaired performance on a range of different executive tests (Dibben, Rice, Laws, & McKenna, 2009).

Other recent studies, however, have put forward a more integrative view, suggesting that FTD might be related to a combination of both executive dysfunction and impaired semantic processing. Stirling and colleagues reported that patients with higher FTD severity performed at a lower level on tests sensitive for executive dysfunction and semantic impairments; however, there was little evidence for a relation between FTD and syntactic psycholinguistic function (Stirling, Hellewell, Blakey, & Deakin, 2006). Remberk et al. also showed a correlation between FTD and both executive and semantic disfunctions in a population of early-onset schizophrenic patients (Remberk, Namyslowska, & Rybakowski, 2012). A meta-analysis by Bora and colleagues showed a significative association between both Positive and Negative FTD and executive disfunctions, semantic processing abnormalities, and neurocognitive deficits, but found that syntactic comprehension deficits were more specific to Positive FTD (Bora, Yalincetin, Akdede, & Alptekin, 2019). Also, the pattern of relationship between distinct domains of executive functions and FTD was shown to be different for Positive and Negative FTD: while deficits in planning and working memory were significantly associated with Negative FTD, inhibition was significantly associated with Positive FTD. They speculated that FTD might be of clinical-level reflections of an underlying disfunction in executive and linguistic processes, rather than being an independent construct.

However, these aetiological theories carry important shortcomings. They generally fail to provide a unifying account of the many cognitive abnormalities that have been implicated and tend to ignore the already mentioned multidimensional and heterogenous nature of the concept of FTD (Sumner, Bell, & Rossell, 2018). For instance, Barch and Berenbaum explored the relationship between four different individual aspects of FTD and the performance in three language production tasks, a heterogenous pattern was found: errors in self-monitoring were associated with derailment and illogicality, errors in grammatical-phonological encoding were associated with neologisms and word approximations, and selecting irrelevant information during discourse planning was associated with incompetent references (Barch & Berenbaum, 1996). Another common issue with studies investigating the relationship between specific cognitive processes and FTD is that the independence of those same specific processes from each other and from more general intellectual, educational, and clinical influences remain controversial (Sumner, Bell, & Rossell, 2018).

Structural Brain Changes

Some of the most consistent and well-stablished findings in meta- and mega-analyses of structural MRI studies in patients with schizophrenia are volume reductions of regional grey matter in the frontal operculum and the language-related lateral temporal cortices, namely the left superior temporal gyrus and middle temporal gyrus (Shepherd, 2012) (Fusar-Poli, 2011). These alterations in the language-related Wernicke's and Broca's areas have also been found in first-degree relatives of patients with schizophrenia (Hu, 2013), something that could indicate both neurodevelopmental and genetic causes. Sans-Sansa and colleagues, also reported a relationship between volume reduction in Broca's and Wernicke's areas and *fluent disorganisation* (which could be said to be related to Positive FTD), while *poverty of content of speech* (related to Negative FTD) was correlated to reductions in bilateral medial frontal and orbito-frontal cortical regions (Sans-Sansa, et al., 2013).

Another consistent finding in the literature is the so-called reversed lateralisation of the temporal cortices. While the two brain hemispheres exhibit a high degree of functional (and anatomical) symmetry in areas responsible for sensorimotor control, perception, and higher mental functions, they also show a considerable degree of functional specialisation. In most people, the left hemisphere is more strongly involved in language perception and production, tool use, complex motor actions, and arithmetic. While the right hemisphere specializes in attention, visuo-spatial abilities, and face recognition, among other things(Ocklenburg & Güntürkün, 2012) (Ocklenburg, Güntürkün, Hugdahl, & Hirnstein, 2015). There is a considerable amount of evidence pointing to the fact that patients with schizophrenia often deviate from this typical laterality pattern. For example, two meta-analyses reported that individuals with schizophrenia are more often non-right-handed than controls (Sommer, Ramsey, Kahn, Aleman, & Bouma, 2001) (Dragovic & Hammond, 2005), which suggests that they display an atypical (or reversed) lateralisation. In healthy controls, the volumes of the superior temporal gyrus and middle temporal gyrus are larger in the left than the right hemisphere, however in patients with FTD this distribution is symmetrical or even inverted (Sun J. , Maller, Guo, & Fitzgerald, 2009) (Oertel-Knochel, Knochel, Stablein, & Linden, 2012). These findings are somewhat reminiscent of Timothy Crow's influential theory regarding the relationship between brain laterality and schizophrenia (Crow, 1997). According to him, about 100.000-250.000 years ago a genetic mutation arose which "lateralized" the human brain and gave rise to language; with this new ability, however, also came the risk of developing psychosis in cases where normal language lateralisation failed.

Interestingly, volume reduction of the superior temporal gyrus is also related to auditory hallucinations (Sun J. , Maller, Guo, & Fitzgerald, 2009), and it has been suggested that at least a subset of this phenomena could be related to subtle changes in the form of anticipating and attending to specific thought contents (Ratcliffe, 2017), indicating a possible link between FTD and auditory hallucinations. 2 Negative FTD has also been linked to reductions in bilateral medial frontal and orbitofrontal cortices (Sans-Sansa, et al., 2013). Positive FTD was shown to be inversely related with left amygdala volume, left hippocampus volume, and bilateral hippocampus length (Rajarethinam, et al., 2001). Shenton and colleagues were the first to report a relation between FTD and a reduction in the grey matter volume of the posterior superior temporal region (Shenton, 1992), a finding that was subsequently replicated in other independent studies (Horn, et al., 2010) (Horn, et al., 2009).

Other structurally implicated regions are the left and/or right orbitofrontal cortex (Sans-Sansa, et al., 2013) (Nakamura, et al., 2008), the left amygdala-hippocampus complex (Spalletta, et al., 2010) (Sallet, et al., 2003), the bilateral nucleus accumbens (Spalletta, et al., 2010) (Ballmaier, et al., 2004), the cerebellar vermis (Sandyk, Kay, & Merriam, 1991), and the corpus callosum (Arnedo, et al., 2015).

Another line of research focuses on alterations in interhemispheric connectivity and its relationship with FTD. This can be traced all the way back to Wilhelm Griesinger's speculations that a dysfunction in interhemispheric information processing might be responsible for difficulties in thinking (Griesinger, 1861). Somewhat more recently, Bopp and colleagues reported a negative correlation between Positive FTD and fractional anisotropy – an indirect measure of white-matter integrity – along the right dorsal cingulate bundle (Bopp, et al., 2016). Another study showed an inverted correlation between Positive FTD and the left white-matter fibre bundle of the middle longitudinal fascicle (Asami, et al., 2013). A long association fibre connecting the superior temporal gyrus and temporal pole with the angular gyrus and thought to be related to language and thought processing functions in the left hemisphere.

Functional Brain Changes

Some studies have explored the neural underpinnings of naturally occurring speech in patients with FTD using PET or functional MRI (fMRI), the so-called symptom-catching approach. In this approach, patients are asked to speak freely while simultaneously recording indirect measures of brain activation; in this way, psychopathological phenomena can be potentially assessed, evaluated, and accurately time-locked with specific changes in brain signalling.

Two independent studies have shown a negative correlation between the degree of Positive FTD and activation in the left superior temporal gyrus (McGuire, et al., 1998) (Kircher, et al., 2001). A positive correlation was reported between semantic paraphasias (the "Peculiar words" item in the Thought and Language Index, a positive FTD sign) and blood oxygen level-dependent (BOLD) contrast enhancements in the left anterior cingulate cortex, which is associated with error monitoring and decision-making, and the right middle temporal gyrus, which is connected to the processing of associative fields and the retrieval of semantic information (Kircher T. , 2003). Kircher and colleagues also reported positive correlations between Negative FTD and activation of the right inferior parietal lobe, left posterior cingulate, middle frontal gyrus and cuneus, and a negative correlation between Negative FTD and activity in the left hippocampal and fusiform region (Kircher T. , Liddle, Brammer, Murray, & McGuire, 2003).

A meta-analysis by Wensing and colleagues, using activation likelihood estimation (ALE), reported overall hyperactivation of the left ventral-posterior medial temporal gyrus and left dorsal-posterior medial temporal gyrus clusters, and hypoactivation of the left superior temporal gyrus cluster in FTD patients (Wensing, et al., 2017). They noted that while the superior temporal gyrus was associated with the behavioural domains of speech and auditory processing, the medial temporal gyrus was not only involved in the semantic processing of language-related information, but also in aspects of social cognition and theory of mind through its more dorsally located cluster. They also reported that disruptions in the left inferior frontal gyrus, which is involved in working memory functions and the resolution of conflicting information, might result in disorganised or distorted speech, arguing that this may be the result of a deficit in the integration of basic language and higher order cognitive processing.

Another meta-analysis of fMRI data also highlighted the role of the left (and to a lesser degree the right) inferior frontal gyrus in speech comprehension in patients with thought disorder and argued that schizophrenia was associated with the under-activation of a predominantly left-lateralised "frontotemporal network", as well as increased and possibly compensatory dual hemispheric activation (Rapp & Steinhäuser, 2013).

Horn and colleagues reported a connection between FTD and the disruption in the left-lateralised semantic network, which included the pars orbitalis and pars triangularis of the left inferior frontal gyrus as well as parts of the left superior temporal gyrus and left middle temporal gyrus, continuing into the left lower parietal lobe (Horn, et al., 2012). They highlighted the hypothesis that the left pars orbitalis activates with increasing demands on semantic retrieval in the context of semantic conflict, modulating the temporal semantic areas through top-down control; they further speculated that in patients with FTD this same control function might be disturbed, resulting in difficulties in the semantic constraints of language comprehension and production (citing as examples the loss of goal and semantic paraphasia commonly observed in thought-disordered speech).

Kircher and colleagues reported a reversed functional laterality of activation (right greater than left) in the superior temporal gyrus in patients with FTD during continuous speech (Kircher T. , et al., 2002).

Fuentes-Claramonte et al. described a correlation between presence of FTD and reduced activation of the dorsolateral prefrontal cortex and the inferior lateral frontal cortex bilaterally, as well as in the left temporal cortex (Fuentes-Claramonte, et al., 2020). Further analysis indicated that this correlation reflected an association with the alogia factor (Negative FTD), but not with the fluent disorganisation factor (Positive FTD). Patients with schizophrenia, when compared with healthy controls, also showed a reduced de-activation, in the medial prefrontal cortex, and no de-activation in the amygdala, hippocampus, or posterior temporal cortex.

A resting state perfusion study reported a positive association between perfusion within the superior temporal gyrus and Negative FTD, while Positive FTD was associated with perfusion within the supplementary motor area and inferior frontal gyrus (Stegmayer, et al., 2017). They speculated that this might indicate different underlying pathophysiology: Negative FTD might reflect defective access to semantic memory while Positive FTD likely reflects impaired suppression of irrelevant information during increased speech production.

Chen and colleagues recently used the three brain regions implicated in FTD (previously identified in the already cited meta-analysis by Welsing et al.) as seeds to generate whole-brain resting-state Functional Connectivity (rsFC, which may be defined as a significant temporal correlation between functionally related brain regions in the absence of any stimulus or task) maps, which were then used for predictive modelling in order to investigate their predictive capacities for individual FTD dimensional scores (Chen, et al., 2021). They identified several brain regions with differential rsFC with the seeds: the left fusiform gyrus, left medial temporal gyrus, right medio-superior frontal gyrus, thalamus, inferior parietal lobule, and middle frontal gyrus. These clusters were robustly associated with the severity of Positive FTD only and allowed for individual prediction of Positive FTD severity in an independent dataset. They concluded that the Positive FTD dimension was found to associate with higher-order cognitive function, suggesting a dysexecutive contribution to the pathophysiology of Positive FTD in patients with schizophrenia.

Sumner and colleagues published a qualitative meta-analysis on the available literature of fMRI studies of FTD (Sumner, Bell, & Rossell, 2018), and concluded that amongst the most common functional correlates of FTD were the bilateral superior and middle temporal gyrus, the fusiform gyrus, the inferior frontal gyrus, as well as the cingulate cortex, the caudate nucleus, and the cerebellum.

Neurotransmitter Changes

In order to study the role of alterations in the neurotransmitter systems in the pathogenesis of FTD, some studies have administered psychoactive substances to healthy volunteers. These substances, such as ketamine, LSD, psylocibin or PCP, can bring about symptoms which resemble those experienced in naturally occurring psychoses (Gouzoulis-Mayfrank, et al., 1998), such as perceptual distortions, hallucinations, delusions, and thought disorders (Vollenweider & Kometer, 2010). This line of research can be traced back to Moreau de Tours' experiments with hashish (Moreau, 1845) and is inextricably linked to the progression of our understanding of psychosis and schizophrenia (Paparelli, Di Forti, Morrison, & Murray, 2011).

The administration of ketamine, a NMDA receptor antagonist, can elicit FTD and negative symptoms which resemble a schizophrenic-like psychosis (Abi-Saab, D'Souza, Moghaddam, & Krystal, 1998). It can bring about both Positive and Negative FTD (Adler, et al., 1999). The severity of ketamine-induced FTD has been shown to correlate with ketamine-induced deficits in working memory (Adler, Goldberg, Malhotra, Pickar, & Breier, 1998), but not with deficits in semantic performance, even though ketamine does produce abnormalities in indirect priming similar to those seen in schizophrenia (Adler, Goldberg, Malhotra, Pickar, & Breier, 1998) (Neill, et al., 2011).

A positive correlation between activation in the left superior temporal gyrus and ketamine-produced FTD symptoms during a verbal fluency test has been reported (Nagels, Kirner-Veselinovic, Krach, & Kircher, 2011). Nagels and colleagues also showed, in a later study, an association between the amount of articulation during ketamine administration and neural responses in right-hemispheric inferior and middle temporal gyri (Nagels, et al., 2018), and noted that their results were strikingly similar to those observed in an earlier study with patients with schizophrenia (Kircher T. , et al., 2002). They reported that the right middle temporal gyrus showed a positive correlation with Positive FTD factor of the TLI scale, which resulted in a reversed functional lateralisation during speech in the ketamine branch. Therefore, glutamate dysfunction in the middle and superior temporal gyri has been implicated in the pathophysiology of at least the Positive domain of FTD (Kircher, Brohl, Meier, & Engelen, 2018).

The dopamine system has also been linked to FTD. The co-administration of amphetamine and ketamine has additive effects on FTD in healthy individuals (Krystal, et al., 2005). In a study examining the effects of dopamine on semantic priming, the administration of L-Dopa accelerated responses to incongruent targets and subordinate targets of ambiguous words, similarly to the hyperpriming observed in schizophrenic patients

(Andreou, Veith, Bozikas, Lincoln, & Moritz, 2014). Another study reported a positive correlation between baseline D2/3 receptor availability in the caudate nucleus, thalamus, and dorsolateral prefrontal cortex and the severity of FTD elicited during ketamine administration (Vernaleken, et al., 2013); the authors speculated that high D2/3 receptor availability might grant benefits with regard to cognitive flexibility, but at the same time increase the risk of maladjustment of information processing in the face of environmental, pathological, or pharmacological stresses.

Finally, the serotoninergic system may also be implicated. 5-HT2A agonists such as LSD, mescaline or dimethyltryptamine (DMT) have also been used as pharmacological models of psychosis (Paparelli, Di Forti, Morrison, & Murray, 2011) (De Gregorio, Comai, Posa, & Gobbi, 2016). Gouzoulis-Mayfrank and colleagues reported the advent of Positive FTD in healthy subjects after administration of ketamine or DMT, with higher scores of Positive FTD with DMT (Gouzoulis-Mayfrank, et al., 2005).

The use of substances in order to induce model psychosis also carry important limitations, however. They model acute psychotic episodes (Adler, et al., 1999), whereas most clinical FTD studies use patients with chronic or residual psychotic symptoms, which could be caused by different neurobiological or cognitive dysfunctions. They also don't account for the complex interactions between the different neurotransmitter systems in the brain.

Conclusion

As we have seen, the concept of FTD has evolved through time and followed the progression of Psychiatry and the neurosciences in general. Historically, it has been conceptually tied to the diagnosis of schizophrenia, something which still lingers surreptitiously in current research on FTD, which as we have seen is predominantly done with samples of patients with schizophrenia. Additionally, it is inextricably tied to the different theories of thought, language, and communication and of how these concepts might influence each other. Just like other signs or symptoms, the "psychiatric objects", the concept of disordered thought cannot be properly grasped apart from the nature of consciousness or subjectivity (Parnas, Sass, & Zahavi, 2013), and cannot be neatly separated from other constructs such as affectivity, attention, intelligence, etc.

With this in mind, FTD is best described as a multidimensional and heterogenous concept, rather than a uniform sign or symptom, and one which appears on a continuum with normal speech. It also carries important diagnostic and prognostic information.

Many areas of the brain have been implicated in the pathogenesis of FTD, some more consistently than others. The superior temporal, middle temporal, and inferior frontal gyri in particular have repeatedly revealed both structural and functional alterations in patients with FTD. A reversed lateralisation has also been observed at both structural and functional levels. The different neurotransmitter systems have also been connected with FTD, with the glutamate system being the one more thoroughly explored. However, the direction of causality between changes in the brain and FTD, and the influence of potential mediators remain largely unknown.

While disfunctions in both semantic and executive cognitive faculties have been independently explored as potential explanations for the pathogenesis of FTD, a more integrative account has surfaced in more recent research. Instead of pitting them against each other, it speculates that FTD might actually be the behavioural or subjective reflections of a combination of different proportions of underlying disfunctions in the executive and/or linguistic processes. For instance, Positive FTD might be more related to deficits in the inhibition of different cognitive processes, while Negative FTD might be connected to a deficient access to semantic information or difficulties in setting an intention. One must keep in mind, however, that thinking about FTD through the lenses of individual cognitive processes or faculties might distort or obscure certain aspects of how thinking functions in the larger context of intersubjective communication.

In any case, future research should make an effort to at least differentiate between the Positive and Negative domains of FTD, and ideally between individual items. It is also important to be mindful of further developments in the philosophy of Mind, Thought, and Language, in order to elaborate increasingly subtle ways of conceptualising thought disorder.

Structural changes	**Volume reductions of the left superior temporal gyrus, left middle temporal gyrus, inferior frontal gyrus, orbito-frontal cortex** **Reversed lateralisation of the temporal cortices** **Volume reduction of white-matter responsible for interhemispheric connectivity**

Functional changes	**Underactivation of the left superior temporal gyrus and left inferior frontal gyrus,** **Hyperactivation of the medial temporal gyrus** **Reversed functional lateralisation**
Neurotransmitter changes	**Dysfunction of the Ketamine, Dopamine and Serotonin systems**

Table 1: Main brain changes implicated in FTD

References

Abi-Saab, W., D'Souza, D., Moghaddam, B., & Krystal, J. (1998). The NMDA antagonist model for schizophrenia: promise and pitfalls. *Pharmacopsychiatry* , 31: 104-109.

Adler, C. M., Goldberg, T. E., Malhotra, A. K., Pickar, D., & Breier, A. (1998). Effects of ketamine on thought disorder, working memory, and semantic memory in healthy volunteers. *Biological psychiatry*, 43(11): 811–816.

Adler, C. M., Malhotra, A. K., Elman, I., Goldberg, T., Egan, M., Pickar, D., & Breier, A. (1999). Comparison of ketamine-induced thought disorder in healthy volunteers and thought disorder in schizophrenia. *The American journal of psychiatry*, 156(10): 1646–1649.

Adreasen, N. (1986). Scale for the Assessment of Thought, Language, and Communication (TLC). *Schizophrenia Bulletin*, 12:473–82.

Andreasen, N. (1979). Thought, language, and communication disorders: II. Diagnostic significance. *Arch Gen Psychiatry*, 36:1325–1330.

Andreasen, N., & Grove, W. (1979). Thought, language, and communication in schizophrenia: diagnosis and prognosis. *Schizophr Bull*, 12: 348–59.

Andreou, C., Veith, K., Bozikas, V. P., Lincoln, T. M., & Moritz, S. (2014). Effects of dopaminergic modulation on automatic semantic priming: a double-blind study. *Journal of psychiatry & neuroscience*, 39(2): 110–117.

Arnedo, J., Mamah, D., Baranger, D., Harms, M., Barch, D., Svrakic, D., . . . Zwir, I. (2015). Decomposition of brain diffusion imaging data uncovers latent schizophrenias with distinct patterns of white matter anisotropy. *Neuroimage*, 120: 43-54.

Asami, T., Saito, Y., Whitford, T. J., Makris, N., Niznikiewicz, M., McCarley, R. W., . . . Kubicki, M. (2013). Abnormalities of middle longitudinal fascicle and disorganization in patients with schizophrenia. *Schizophrenia research*, 143(2-3), 253–259.

Ballmaier, M., Toga, A., Siddarth, P., Blanton, R., Levitt, J., Lee, M., & Caplan, R. (2004). Thought disorder and nucleus accumbens in childhood: a structural MRI study. *Psychiatry Res*, 130: 43-55.

Barch, D., & Berenbaum, H. (1996). Language production and thought disorder in schizophrenia. *J Abnorm Psychol*, 105: 81-88.

Barch, D., Cohen, J., Servan-Schreiber, D., Steingard, S., Steinhauer, S., & Van Kammen, D. (1996). emantic priming in schizophrenia: An examination of spreading activation using word pronunciation and multiple SOAs. *J. Abnorm. Psychol.* , 592-601.

Barrera, A., McKenna, P., & Berrios, G. (2005). Formal thought disorder in schizophrenia: an executive or a semantic deficit? *Psychological Medicine*, 121-132.

Berrios, G. (2010). *The History of Mental Symptoms: Descriptive Psychopathology since the Nineteenth Century.* Cambridge University Press.

Bleuler, E. (1911). *Dementia praecox oder Gruppe der Schizophrenien. Handbuch der Psychiatrie.* Leipzig: Deuticke.

Bopp, M., Zöllner, R., Jansen, A., Dietsche, B., Krug, A., & Kircher, T. (2016). White matter integrity and symptom dimensions of schizophrenia: A diffusion tensor imaging study. *Schizophrenia Research.*

Bora, E., Yalincetin, B., Akdede, B., & Alptekin, K. (2019). Neurocognitive and linguistic correlates of positive and negative formal thought disorder: A meta-analysis. *Schizophrenia Research*, 209: 2-11.

Cavelti, M., Kircher, T., Nagels, A., Strik, W., & Homan, P. (2018). Is formal thought disorder in schizophrenia related to structural and functional aberrations in the language network? A systematic review of neuroimagin findings. *Schizophrenia Research*, 199, 2–16.

Champagne-Lavau, M., & Stip, E. (2009). Pragmatic and executive dysfunction in schizophrenia. *J. Neurolinguistics*, 23, 285–296.

Chen, J., Wensing, T., Hoffstaedter, F., Cieslik, E. C., Müller, V. I., Patil, K. R., . . . Nickl-Jockschat, T. (2021). Neurobiological substrates of the positive formal thought disorder in schizophrenia revealed by seed connectome-based predictive modeling. *Neuroimage Clin.*

Crow, T. (1997). Is schizophrenia the price that Homo sapiens pays for language? *Schizophr Res*, 28(2-3):127-41.

De Gregorio, D., Comai, S., Posa, L., & Gobbi, G. (2016). d-Lysergic Acid Diethylamide (LSD) as a Model of Psychosis: Mechanism of Action and Pharmacology. *International journal of molecular sciences*, 17(11): 1953.

den Ouden, D., Malyutina, S., Basilakos, A., Bonilha, L., Gleichgerrcht, E., Yourganov, G., . . . Fridriksson, J. (2019). Cortical and structural-connectivity damage correlated with impaired syntactic processing in aphasia. *Human brain mapping,*, 40(7): 2153–2173.

DeVylder, J. E., Muchomba, F. M., Gill, K. E., Ben-David, S., Walder, D. J., Malaspina, D., & Corcoran, C. M. (2014). Symptom trajectories and psychosis onset in a clinical high-risk cohort: the relevance of subthreshold thought disorder. *Schizophrenia research*, 159(2-3), 278–283.

Dibben, C. R., Rice, C., Laws, K., & McKenna, P. J. (2009). Is executive impairment associated with schizophrenic syndromes? A meta-analysis. *Psychological medicine*, 381–392.

Docherty, N., DeRosa, M., & Andreasen, N. (1996). Communication disturbances in schizophrenia and mania. *Arch Gen Psychiatry*, 53:358–364.

Docherty, N., Evans, I., Sledge, W., Seibyl, J., & Krystal, J. (1994). Affective reactivity of language in schizophrenia. *The Journal of nervous and mental disease*, 182(2), 98–102.

Dragovic, M., & Hammond, G. (2005). Handedness in schizophrenia: A quantitative review of evidence. *Acta Psychiatrica Scandinavica*, 111(6), 410–419.

Elvevåg, B., Foltz, P. W., Weinberger, D. R., & Goldberg, T. E. (2007). Quantifying incoherence in speech: an automated methodology and novel application to schizophrenia. *Schizophrenia research*, 93(1-3), 304–316.

Fuentes-Claramonte, P., López-Araquistain, L., Sarró, S., Sans-Sansa, B., Ortiz-Gil, J., Maristany, T., . . . Pomarol-Clotet, E. (2020). Brain functional correlates of formal thought disorder in schizophrenia: examining the frontal/dysexecutive hypothesis. *Psychological Medicine*, 1-8.

Fusar-Poli, P. R. (2011). Neuroanatomical Maps of Psychosis Onset: Voxel-wise Meta-Analysis of Antipsychotic-Naive VBM Studies. *Schizophrenia Bulletin*, 1297–1307.

Goldberg, T. E., Aloia, M. S., Gourovitch, M. L., Missar, D., Pickar, D., & Weinberger, D. R. (1998). Cognitive substrates of thought disorder, I: the semantic system. *The American journal of psychiatry*, 155(12), 1671–1676.

Gouzoulis-Mayfrank, E., Habermeyer, E., Hermle, L., Steinmeyer, A., Kunert, H., & Sass, H. (1998). Hallucinogenic drug induced states resemble acute endogenous psychoses: results of an empirical study. *European psychiatry : the journal of the Association of European Psychiatrists*, 13(8): 399–406.

Gouzoulis-Mayfrank, E., Heekeren, K., Neukirch, A., Stoll, M., Stock, C., Obradovic, M., & Kovar, K. A. (2005). Psychological effects of (S)-ketamine and N,N-dimethyltryptamine (DMT): a double-blind, cross-over study in healthy volunteers. *Pharmacopsychiatry*, 38(6): 301–311.

Griesinger, W. (1861). *Die Pathologie und Therapie der psychischen Krankheiten, für Aerzte und Studirende.* Stuttgart: Krabbe.

Hart, M., & Lewine, R. (2017). Rethinking Thought Disorder. *Schizophr Bull* , 43(3): 514–522.

Harvey, P., Docherty, N., M.R., S., & Rasmussen, M. (1990). Cognitive deficits and thought disorder: II. An eight month. *Schizophr Bull*, 16: 147–56.

Hella, P., Niemi, J., Hintikka, J., Otsa, L., Tirkkonen, J., & Koponen, H. (2013). Disordered semantic activation in disorganized discourse in schizophrenia: a new pragma-linguistic tool for structure and meaning reconstruction. *International Journal of Language and Communication Disorders*, 320-328.

Horn, H., Federspiel, A., Wirth, M., Müller, T., Wiest, R., Walther, S., & Strik, W. (2010). Gray matter volume differences specific to formal thought disorder in schizophrenia. *Psychiatry Research: Neuroimaging*, 183-186, 182(2).

Horn, H., Federspiel, A., Wirth, M., Müller, T., Wiest, R., Wang, J., & Strik, W. (2009). Structural and metabolic changes in language areas linked to formal thought disorder. *British Journal of Psychiatry*, 194(2), 130-138.

Horn, H., Jann, K., Federspiel, A., Walther, S., Wiest, R., Müller, T., & Strik, W. (2012). Semantic Network Disconnection in Formal Thought Disorder. *Neuropsychobiology*, 66:14-23.

Hu, M. L. (2013). Decreased left middle temporal gyrus volume in antipsychotic drug-naive, first-episode schizophrenia patients and their healthy unaffected siblings. *Schizophrenia research*, 144(1-3), 37–42.

Jerónimo, J., Queirós, T., Cheniaux, E., & Telles-Correia, D. (2018). Formal Thought Disorders–Historical Roots. *Front Psychiatry.*, 9: 572.

Kiefer, M., Weisbrod, M., Kern, I., Maier, S., & Spitzer, M. (1998). Right hemisphere activation during indirect semantic priming: evidence from event-related potentials. *Brain and language*, 64(3), 377–408.

Kircher, T. (2003). *Neuronale Korrelate von Sprach- und Denkprozessen bei Gesunden und Patienten mit Schizophrenie.* Darmstadt: Steinkopff.

Kircher, T. T., Bulimore, E. T., Brammer, M. J., Williams, S. C., Broome, M. R., Murray, R. M., & McGuire, P. K. (2001). Differential activation of temporal cortex during sentence completion in schizophrenic patients with and without formal thought disorder. *Schizophrenia Research*, 50(1-2):27-40. doi.

Kircher, T., Brohl, H., Meier, F., & Engelen, J. (2018). Formal thought disorders: from phenomenology to neurobiology. *Lancet Psychiatry*, 5: 515–26.

Kircher, T., Krug, A., S. M., Ghazi, S., Schales, C., Frauenheim, M., . . . & Nagels, A. (2014). . A rating scale for the assessment of objective and subjective formal Thought and Language Disorder (TALD). *Schizophrenia research*, 160(1-3), 216–221.

Kircher, T., Liddle, P. F., Brammer, M. J., Williams, S. C., Murray, R. M., & McGuire, P. K. (2002). Reversed lateralization of temporal activation during speech production in thought disordered patients with schizophrenia. *Psychological medicine*, 32(3), 439–449.

Kircher, T., Liddle, P., Brammer, M., Murray, R., & McGuire, P. (2003). Neuronale Korrelate "negativer" formaler Denkstörungen. *Nervenarzt*, 74:748-54.

Krystal, J. H., Perry, E. B., Gueorguieva, R., Belger, A., Madonick, S. H., Abi-Dargham, A., . . . D'Souza, D. C. (2005). Comparative and interactive human psychopharmacologic effects of ketamine and amphetamine: implications for glutamatergic and dopaminergic model psychoses and cognitive function. *Archives of general psychiatry*, 62(9): 985–994.

Manschreck, T. C., Maher, B. A., Milavetz, J. J., Ames, D., Weisstein, C. C., & Schneyer, M. L. (1988). Semantic priming in thought disordered schizophrenic patients. *Schizophrenia research*, 1(1), 61–66.

Marggraf, M. P., Lysaker, P. H., Salyers, M. P., & Minor, K. S. (2020). The link between formal thought disorder and social functioning in schizophrenia: A meta-analysis. *Eur Psychiatry.*, 63(1) e34.

McGrath, J. (1991). Ordering thoughts on thought disorder. *British Journal of Psychiatry*, 158, 307–316.

McGuire, P., Quested, D., Spence, S., Murray, R., Frith, C., & Liddle, P. (1998). Pathophsysiology of "positive" thought disorder in schizophrenia. *Br J Psychiatry*, 173: 231–35.

Moreau, J. (1845). *Du hachisch et de l'aliénation mentale : études psychologiques.* Paris: De Fortin, Masson et Cie.

Morgan, C. J., Coleman, M. J., Ulgen, A., Boling, L., Cole, J. O., Johnson, F. V., . . . Levy, D. L. (2017). Thought Disorder in Schizophrenia and Bipolar Disorder Probands, Their Relatives, and Nonpsychiatric Controls. *Schizophr Bull*, 43: 523–35.

Moritz, S., Mersmann, K., Kloss, M., Jacobsen, D., Wilke, U., Andresen, B., . . . Pawlik, K. (2001). 'Hyper-priming' in thought-disordered schizophrenic patients. *Psychological Medicine*, 31(2), 221–229.

Moro, A., Bambini, V., Bosia, M., Anselmetti, S., Riccaboni, R., Cappa, S. F., . . . Cavallaro, R. (2015). Detecting syntactic and semantic anomalies in schizophrenia. *Neuropsychologia*, 79: 147-157.

Nagels, A., Cabanis, M., Oppel, A., Kirner-Veselinovic, A., Schales, C., & Kircher, T. (2018). S-Ketamine-Induced NMDA Receptor Blockade during Natural Speech Production and Its Implications for Formal Thought Disorder in Schizophrenia: A Pharmaco-fMRI Study. *Neuropsychopharmacology : official publication of the American College of Neuropsychopharmacology*, 43(6): 1324–1333.

Nagels, A., Kirner-Veselinovic, A., Krach, S., & Kircher, T. (2011). Neural correlates of S-ketamine induced psychosis during overt continuous verbal fluency. *NeuroImage*, 54(2): 1307–1314.

Nakamura, M., Nestor, P., Levitt, J., Cohen, A., Kawashima, T., & Shenton, M. (2008). Orbitofrontal volume deficit in schizophrenia and thought disorder. *Brain*, 131: 180-195.

Neill, E., Rossell, S., McDonald, S., Joshua, N., Jansen, N., & Morgan, C. (2011). Using ketamine to model semantic deficits in schizophrenia. *Journal of clinical psychopharmacology*, 31(6): 690–697.

Ocklenburg, S., & Güntürkün, O. (2012). Hemispheric asymmetries: the comparative view. *Front. Psychol.*

Ocklenburg, S., Güntürkün, O., Hugdahl, K., & Hirnstein, M. (2015). Laterality and mental disorders in the postgenomic age – A closer look at schizophrenia and language lateralization. *Neuroscience & Biobehavioral Reviews*.

Oertel-Knochel, V., Knochel, C., Stablein, M., & Linden, D. (2012). Abnormal functional and structural asymmetry as biomarker for schizophrenia. *Curr Top Med Chem*, 12(21):2434-51.

Ott, S., Roberts, S., Rock, D., Allen, J., & Erlenmeyer-Kimling, L. (2002). Positive and negative thought disorder and psychopathology in childhood among subjects with adulthood schizophrenia. *Schizophrenia research*, 58(2-3), 231–239.

Paparelli, A., Di Forti, M., Morrison, P. D., & Murray, R. M. (2011). Drug-Induced Psychosis: How to Avoid Star Gazing in Schizophrenia Research by Looking at More Obvious Sources of Light. *Front Behav Neurosci*, 5: 1.

Peralta, V., Cuesta, M., & de Leon, J. (1992). Formal thought disorder in schizophrenia: A factor analytic study. *Comprehensive Psychiatry*, 105-110.

Rajarethinam, R., DeQuardo, J., Miedler, J., Arndt, S., Kirbat, R., Brunberg, J., & Tandon, R. (2001). Hippocampus and amygdala in schizophrenia:

assessment of the relationship of neuroanatomy to psychopathology. *Psychiatry Res*, 108(2):79-87.

Rapp, A., & Steinhäuser, A. (2013). Functional MRI of sentence-level language comprehension in schizophrenia: A coordinate-based analysis. *Schizophrenia Research*, 150: 107-113.

Ratcliffe, M. (2017). *Real Hallucinations: psychiatric illness, intentionality, and the interpersonal world.* Cambridge, MA: MIT Press.

Remberk, B., Namyslowska, I., & Rybakowski, F. (2012). Clinical and cognitive correlates of formal thought disorder in early onset schizophrenia . *Neuro Endocrinol Lett*, 33(3): 347-55.

Roche, E., Creed, L., MacMahon, D., Brennan, D., & Clarke, M. (2015). The Epidemiology and Associated Phenomenology of Formal Thought Disorder: A Systematic Review. *Schizophrenia Bulletin*, 951–962.

Sallet, P., Elkis, H., Alves, T., Oliveira, J., Sassi, E., Campi de Castro, C., . . . Gattaz, W. (2003). Reduced cortical folding in schizophrenia: an MRI morphometric. *Am J Psychiatry*, 160: 1606-1613.

Sandyk, R., Kay, S., & Merriam, A. (1991). Atrophy of the Cerebellar Vermis: Relevance to the Symptoms of Schizophrenia. *International Journal of Neuroscience*, 57: 205-212.

Sans-Sansa, B., McKenna, P. J., Canales-Rodríguez, E. J., Ortiz-Gil, J., López-Araquistain, L., Sarró, S., . . . Pomarol-Clotet, E. (2013). Association of formal thought disorder in schizophrenia with structural brain abnormalities in language-related cortical regions. *Schizophrenia Research*, 308-313, 146(1-3).

Schettino, A., Lauro, L. R., Crippa, F., Anselmetti, S., Cavallaro, R., & Papagno, C. (2010). The comprehension of idiomatic expressions in schizophrenic patients. *Neuropsychologia*, 48, 1032–1040.

Shenton, M. E. (1992). Abnormalities of the left temporal lobe and thought disorder in schizophrenia. A quantitative magnetic resonance imaging study. *The New England journal of medicine*, 327(9), 604–612.

Shepherd, A. L. (2012). Systematic meta-review and quality assessment of the structural brain alterations in schizophrenia. *Neuroscience & Biobehavioral Reviews*, Volume 36, Issue 4.

Sommer, I., Ramsey, N., Kahn, R., Aleman, A., & Bouma, A. (2001). Handedness, language lateralisation and anatomical asymmetry in schizophrenia: meta-analysis. *Br J Psychiatry*, 178:344-51.

Spalletta, G., Spoletini, I., Cherubini, A., Rubino, I., Siracusano, A., Piras, F., & Caltagirone. (2010). Cortico-subcortical underpinnings of narrative processing impairment in. *Psychiatry Res*, 182: 77-80.

Spitzer, M., Braun, U., Maier, S., Hermle, L., & Maher, B. (1993). Indirect semantic priming in schizophrenic patients . *Schizophrenia Research*, 11: 71-80.

Spitzer, M., Weisker, I., Winter, M., Maier, S., Hermle, L., & Maher, B. A. (1994). Semantic and phonological priming in schizophrenia. *Journal of abnormal psychology*, 103(3), 485–494.

Stegmayer, K., Stettler, M., Strik, W., Federspiel, A., Wiest, R., Bohlhalter, S., & Walther, S. (2017). Resting state perfusion in the language network is linked to formal thought disorder and poor functional outcome in schizophrenia. *Acta psychiatrica Scandinavica*, 136(5): 506–516.

Stirling, J., Hellewell, J., Blakey, A., & Deakin, W. (2006). Thought disorder in schizophrenia is associated with both executive dysfunction and circumscribed impairments in semantic function. *Psychological Medicine*, 36(4): 475-484.

Sumner, P., Bell, I., & Rossell, S. (2018). Sumner, Philip J.; Bell, Imogen H.; Rossell, Susan L. (2018). A Systematic Review of Task-Based Functional Neuroimaging Studies Investigating Language, Semantic and Executive Processes in Thought Disorder. . *Neuroscience & Biobehavioral Reviews*.

Sun, J., Maller, J., Guo, L., & Fitzgerald, P. (2009). Superior temporal gyrus volume change in schizophrenia: a review on region of interest volumetric studies. *Brain Res Rev*, 61: 14–32.

Sun, J., Maller, J., Guo, L., & Fitzgerald, P. (2009). Superior temporal gyrus volume change in schizophrenia: a review on region of interest volumetric studies. *Brain Res Rev.*, 61(1):14-32.

Thomas, P., King, K., Fraser, W., & Kendell, R. (1987). Positive and negative symptoms of schizophrenia and linguistic performance. *Acta Psychiatr. Scand.*, 76(2): 144-151.

Thomas, P., King, K., Fraser, W., & Kendell, R. (1990). Linguistic performance in schizophrenia: a comparison of acute and chronic patients. *Br. J. Psychiatry*, 156: 204-210.

Vernaleken, I., Klomp, M., Moeller, O., Raptis, M., Nagels, A., Rösch, F., . . . Gründer, G. (2013). Vulnerability to psychotogenic effects of ketamine is associated with elevated D2/3-receptor availability. *The international journal of neuropsychopharmacology*, 16(4): 745–754.

Vollenweider, F., & Kometer, M. (2010). The neurobiology of psychedelic drugs: implications for the treatment of mood disorders. *Nat Rev Neurosci*, 11: 642–651.

Wensing, T., Cieslik, E. C., Müller, V. I., Hoffstaedter, F., Eickhoff, S. B., & Nickl-Jockschat, T. (2017). Neural correlates of formal thought disorder: An activation likelihood estimation meta-analysis. *Human brain mapping*, 38(10), 4946–4965.

Wilcox, J., A.L., R., & Baida-Fragoso, N. (2000). The prognostic value of thought disorder in psychotic depression. *Ann Clin Psychiatry*, 12(1):1-4.

Yalincetin, B., Bora, E., Binbay, T., Ulas, H., Akdede, B., & & Alptekin, K. (2017). Formal thought disorder in schizophrenia and bipolar disorder: A systematic review and meta-analysis. *Schizophrenia research*, 185, 2–8.

Yalincetin, B., Bora, E., Binbay, T., Ulas, H., Akdede, B., & Alptekin, K. (2016). Formal thought disorder in schizophrenia and bipolar disorder: a systematic review and meta-analysis. *Schizophr Res*.

CHAPTER FIVE

AGE-RELATED DYNAMICS IN THE NEUROPSYCHOLOGICAL PROFILE IN DEPRESSION

VANYA MATANOVA &
ZLATOMIRA KOSTOVA
INSTITUTE FOR MENTAL HEALTH AND DEVELOPMENT

Abstract

Many different factors influence the neuropsychological profile in depression, and the relationships between them are very complex. There is much empirical data on the neuropsychological functioning in depression. However, a comprehensive framework for understanding the disorder remains unclear. The interaction between different factors determines the age-related dynamics of the neuropsychological profile. Factors with impact on depression have been studied many times, but age-related changes in the neuropsychological profile remain poorly understood. To understand this dynamic, it is important to determine whether neuropsychological deficits are conditional or trait factors in individuals vulnerable to depression.

The main issues refer to whether the neuropsychological deficits in depression are specific and whether they are related to the severity of depressive symptoms. In this regard, it is necessary to clarify the neural substrates of the neuropsychological deficits in depression.

Keywords: depression, neuropsychological profile, mental development

Introduction

It is known that cognitive impairment is one of the main characteristics of depression, which can be both primary and secondary to the symptoms of low mood and hypoactivity. An important part of the diagnosis and intervention in depression is the clarification of the cognitive profile.

There is evidence that depression is associated with deficits in several cognitive areas: attention, memory, and executive functions (Tyrrell, M., & Elliot, R., 2015). There is also data of possible differential sensitivity in difficult tasks, depending on the function of the prefrontal cortex. The exact profile of the deficit can be influenced by a number of clinical and demographic factors, including the severity of depression, the age of patients, and the effects of medications. Evidence from neuroimaging shows that abnormal functioning of the frontal lobes, and especially the medial prefrontal cortex, may be at the root of cognitive impairment and low mood in depression.

Neuropsychological profile of depression in childhood and adolescence

Maladaptive cognitive and attributional models are the main characteristics of depressive disorders in childhood. Depressed children report significantly more hopelessness and dysfunctional attributional styles. A greater part of children with depression shows maladaptive cognitive models, suggesting that depressive disorders in childhood may be heterogeneous with respect to cognitive models.

A meta-analysis of the neuropsychological functioning of children and adolescents diagnosed with depression found expressed impairments of executive functions in the field of verbal fluency, inhibitory ability, sustained attention, verbal memory, and planning (Wagner S, Müller C, Helmreich I, Huss M, Tadić A., 2015).

Depression in childhood is commonly associated with learning problems and academic failures. In the presence of depressive symptoms, such as low self-esteem, depressed mood or feelings of inefficiency, a direct link with executive dysfunction and impaired attention is seen, which have a negative impact on academic performance (Ciuhan GC, Iliescu D., 2021).

Depression in adolescents is a heterogeneous condition with different symptoms associated with abnormalities in the functioning of different brain circuits. (Oliver, A., Pile, V., Elm, D., & Lau, J. Y., 2019). It negatively affects cognitive and social functioning as well as academic achievement. A study of Brooks, B. L., Iverson, G. L., Sherman, E. M., & Roberge, M. C. (2010) found that children and adolescents aged 9-17 years with depression had neurocognitive impediments, which were demonstrated as reduced speed of information processing, impaired verbal memory, and executive dysfunctions. Probably due to this heterogeneity in the symptoms of depression in adolescents, there are controversial studies related to adolescents' bias regarding intentional attention to (or from) negative stimuli, compared to those that do not have a negative affective cathexis. This presupposes functioning through a maladaptive style of information processing and in this sense, it maintains and impacts depressive affectivity (Oliver, A., Pile, V., Elm, D., & Lau, J. Y., 2019).

Adolescent major depressive disorder reports abnormalities in the activation of the ventromedial prefrontal region, anterior cingulate cortex, and amygdala, which correspond to the presumed role of medial areas in the pathophysiology of depression (Kerestes R, Davey CG, Stephanou K, Whittle S, Harrison BJ., 2013). A number of studies confirm the presence of abnormalities of the fronto-parietal network during the processes of executive control and attention control in depressed adolescents. Functional magnetic resonance imaging was used to compare brain activity between 20 medically untreated adolescents with a first episode of depression aged 13-18 years, and 21 healthy controls conformant to gender, age, and IQ. The participants completed an attention task with and without a cash reward to assess the impact of the reward on attention maintenance networks. It was found that the reward regulated frontostriatal and hippocampal/temporal activation in control subjects, but deactivated these regions in depression, with opposite compensatory effects in the cerebellum. The medically untreated adolescents showed abnormalities in the regulation of the fronto-striato-cerebellar brain regions involved in attention and reward during motivated attention, however not during unmotivated attention. This presumes a dysfunctional interaction between motivation and cognition, as motivation in depressed adolescents seems less capable of regulating attention networks as compared to healthy controls (Chantiluke K., Halari R., Simic M., Pariante C.M., Papadopoulos A., Giampietro V., Rubia K., 2012).

With depressed adolescents and healthy controls aged 13-17 years, the activity of the anterior cingulate cortex during a Stop Signal Task was examined using functional magnetic resonance. Significantly higher activation of the area was found in depressed adolescents compared to controls. These results established for the first time the abnormal functioning of that area in depressed adolescents and had important implications for understanding the underlying neural correlates and potential treatment of depression in adolescents (Yang T.T., Simmons A.N., Matthews S.C., Tapert S.F., Frank G.K., Bischoff-Grethe A., Lansing A.E., Wu J., Brown G.G., Paulus M.P., 2009).

Compared to healthy controls, adolescents with depression are more incapable of reducing the negative affect during cognitive judgement i.e., they rarely use adaptive strategies to regulate emotions like reassessing the meaning of a negative stimulus or event. This process corresponds to blunt modulation of amygdala activity. While in healthy controls the activation of the amygdala is modulated by age, in individuals with depression such relation is not observed. In the depressed group, increased activation of the ventromedial prefrontal cortex and decreased activation of the dorsal cortex in the midline were also found. In general, these findings suggest that the brain systems that support cognitive judgement are functionally altered in adolescent depression - reduced regulation of amygdala responses to aversive images. Depression in adolescents appears to be characterised by disorders in both the ventral prefrontal-subcortical "generative" and dorsal "regulatory" systems, which contribute to adaptive emotional processing (Stephanou K, Davey CG, Kerestes R, Whittle S, Harrison BJ., 2017).

Depression at the age of 4-24 years (average age 18.3 years) shows hyperactivation in the left prefrontal cortex, right anterior insula, bilateral thalamus, left parahippocampal gyrus, and left upper temporal cortex, as well as hypoactivity within the right caudate. There is hypersensitivity to emotional stimuli from overactivation of the anterior cingulate cortex and thalamus, which lead to a cascade of other symptoms - ineffective regulation of emotions despite increased activation of the dorsolateral prefrontal cortex and ventrolateral prefrontal cortex during affective processing, which may change during development or clinical course. As well as maladaptive rumination and weak executive control due to difficulties in switching from network activity in default mode to positive network activity during cognitively difficult tasks, and anhedonia due to hypoactivation of the posterior insula during processing of rewards (Miller CH, Hamilton JP, Sacchet MD, Gotlib IH., 2015).

A study aimed at examining neuropsychological deficits in adolescents (12-18 years) suffering from depressive disorders shows that the deficit in the speed of processing - cognitive and motor - may depend on the subtype of depression or the severity of the affective disorder, as a substantial delay in cognitive and motor functions was only found in the group of major depressive episode (Klimkeit, E. I., Tonge, B., Bradshaw, J. L., Melvin, G. A., & Gould, K., 2011).

When comparing depressive adolescents with healthy controls using functional magnetic resonance imaging (fMRI), it was found that adolescents with suicidal experience showed increased brain activity in attention control patterns when exposed to angry faces, and less capacity to regulate attention when processing emotionally strong stimuli (Pan LA, Hassel S, Segreti AM, Nau SA, Brent DA, Phillips ML., 2013).

Functional magnetic resonance imaging (fMRI) studies showed that adolescents at 12-15 years of age, with a history of peer rejection, were thought to be sensitive to future new rejection experiences. The results of this study showed higher activity in the dorsal anterior cingulate cortex during social exclusion, and higher activity in the anterior prefrontal cortex, even when they were accidentally excluded from a social interaction in which they were generally included (Will GJ, van Lier PA, Crone EA, Güroğlu B., 2016).

Neuropsychological profile in depressed adults

A greater part of studies reported a generalised profile of impairment in depressed adults. In most cases, impaired cognition can have diagnostic value, especially in elderly patients. Cognitive deficits are often severe in elderly patients; they affect daily functioning and complicate the differential diagnosis of depression/dementia. It is crucial to determine how neuropsychological deficits in depression may be related to clinical factors and whether there are specific neuropsychological deficits in depression.

The crucial question is whether depression in the elderly is a separate disorder, aetiologically and symptomatically. Existent theories support the existence of this distinction, with cognitive deficits in elderly patients being considered a key feature. The neuropsychological profile of elderly patients with depression is comparable to that observed in organic dementias, in particular Alzheimer's disease. In fact, the term "pseudodementia" has traditionally been used to characterise the cognitive profile of geriatric depression. There is a relation between the symptoms and the subsequent cognitive decline in those who already show mild impairment. The neuropsychological profile of depressive elderly is significantly different from that of younger patients. Attempts to test whether there is an interaction between depression and age in determining cognitive deficits are unconvincing. For example, Tarbuck, A. F., & Paykel, E. S. (1995) compare depressed and recovered patients under and over 60 years of age. Patients at an average age under 40 years show significant impairment of executive functions. Middle-aged patients about 50 years old show impairments concerning memory and executive functions. Patients over the age of 70 show delayed cognitive functioning, as well. The interaction between depression, age and cognitive impairment does not justify the establishment of a specific neuropsychological profile in geriatric depression, given the impact of normal ageing on cognitive performance.

Depression is not a single disorder; this gives a reason to distinguish different subtypes based on the clinical profile. Patients with bipolar disorder have been found to show multiple neuropsychological deficits in both the manic and depressive phases of their disease, however some subtle differences between the two phases of bipolar disorder exist. Murphy et al (2001) confirm that mania is associated with a generalised profile of impairment similar to that seen in depression. In patients with mania, the ability to inhibit behavioural responses to previous significant stimuli is impaired, a disorder also observed in patients with anterior lobe injuries.

The difference between unipolar and bipolar depression is generally accepted but attempts to delineate subtypes in the spectrum of unipolar depression are controversial. The question arises as to whether unipolar and bipolar depression can be neuropsychologically distinguished. The debate focuses on whether the more severe form of unipolar depression can be clinically distinguished from the milder form. Attempts to determine the neuropsychological validity of this distinction are relatively unconvincing, revealing quantitative rather than qualitative differences. For example, Nelson et al (2017) affirm that there are poorer features of attention in psychotic depressed patients than in non-psychotic patients, comparable to that seen in schizophrenia. Similarly, Simpson et al (1998) found that psychotic depressed patients showed more pronounced impairment of executive function and processing speed than non-psychotic ones. Basso et al (1999, 2001, 2013) describe a similar pattern in younger patients.

To assess whether clinical severity of depression is an important predictor of neuropsychological impairment, it is necessary to measure the correlations between the cognitive deficits and the severity of depression. More severe depression in the morning is associated with more significant cognitive impairment than milder depression in the evening. It should not be overlooked that the relationship between clinical severity of depression and neuropsychological deficit may be influenced by the rating scales used.

Another factor that affects the neuropsychological performance of depression is hospitalisation. It is still not clear whether hospitalisation is such an important indicator of severity in cases of neuropsychological impairment, and whether hospitalisation factors may exacerbate the cognitive deficit.

The extent to which antidepressants affect cognitive function is not clearly established. Although the cognitive effects of drugs have not been reliably distinguished, it appears that a greater part of the traditional tricyclic antidepressants may impair aspects of cognition, especially processing speed. Less pronounced effects have been reported with selective serotonin reuptake inhibitors (SSRIs) or monoamine oxidase inhibitors (MAOIs). The differential effects of different antidepressants on cognitive abilities present important data relevant to the treatment of depression.

The main question is whether neuropsychological deficits in depression are factors of the condition observed only during a current depressive episode, or factors of traits present in individuals vulnerable to depression. Most studies show that there is an expressed improvement in cognitive performance during symptomatic recovery, but residual disturbances are also reported in comparison to healthy controls. Kuny & Stassen (1995) describe the dynamics of cognitive impairment in recovering patients and conclude that cognitive and clinical recovery are largely independent. According to them, cognitive impairment can be an independent symptom in depression. Neuropsychological deficits in depression are likely to be factors in both condition and traits. Discussion of how cognitive deficits are affected by different clinical parameters is based on the rather general neuropsychological profile that is usually observed. However, it is important to consider whether any specificity can be established in the generalised pattern of impairment; an issue that becomes particularly relevant when considering the neural basis of cognitive deficits.

Patients with depressive disorder may be differently sensitive to negative information and the processing thereof. Bias to negative information can exacerbate depressed mood. Deviations in information processing have been particularly studied in the context of memory, and it has been established that patients with depression show a tendency to remember negatively coloured material. Watkins et al (2002) found that patients with depression showed a greater bias to negative than positive words, contrary to the pattern manifested by the healthy controls. The approach to studying emotional bias has the advantage of linking mood and cognition, which correlates to the cognitive-behavioral theories of depression on which treatment strategies are commonly based.

Some of the clinical symptoms of depression may have a direct causal effect on working capacity. It is common for patients to report difficulty in attention focusing. Lack of motivation is one of the clinical symptoms of depression and can play a causal role in a range of neuropsychological disorders. Cognitive deficits in depression can also be due to motivational factors. In a study of elderly patients with depression, Beats et al (1996) described a "catastrophic response to perceived failure" where, after patients made an initial mistake, subsequent performance deteriorated. According to Elliott et al (1998, 2002), the patients probably fail to use negative feedback as a motivational stimulus to improve their subsequent performance. Healthy controls, neurological and neurosurgical patients with similar general deficits were much less likely to make a mistake after a previous failure. This difference may be a result of the expectations of failure and feelings of worthlessness that are part of the clinical profile of depression. Channon (1996, 1998) also reported ineffective use of feedback to improve coping in patients with dysphoria. Specific motivational deficits form an important way to associate clinical symptoms with neuropsychological deficits. However, these factors may only explain some aspects of the cognitive profile in depression.

The neuropsychological profile of primary depression also addresses the question of whether depression deficits may be domain-specific. Evidence of selective deficit in one area or another may have neurobiological and neuropsychological implications for the theories of depression. Numerous neuropsychological studies of patients with depression have clearly established that some aspects of memory and learning (visual and verbal, short-term and long-term) are impaired, as well as of executive functions. Impairment is usually seen in a wide range of cognitive areas. The key question is not whether deficits exist in some areas, but whether deficits are more pronounced in a particular domain. There is empirical data that neuropsychological deficits in depression are not more pronounced in any aspect of function but are "consistent with global diffuse brain injury." Degl'Innocenti et al (1998) report differential deficits in tests for executive functions, and Channon and Green (1998) suggest that that these cases of impairment may be a failure when using appropriate strategies. Interestingly, deficits in executive functions have been demonstrated in untreated patients, indicating that they are unlikely to be due to medications. Patients with depression have a difficulty performing a wide range of tasks, as deficits of executive functions are particularly pronounced. The concept of "executive function" is used interchangeably with "frontal lobe function" and therefore specific deficits in these areas would suggest prefrontal pathology in depression.

Neural correlates of neuropsychological deficits in depression

There has been much discussion over the years about whether depression can be associated with structural changes in the brain. Empirical evidence suggests that there may be structural abnormalities in elderly patients that are associated with the degree of cognitive impairment (Robbins et al, 1998), although the evidence is less convincing in younger patients. Structural abnormalities may be related to the duration of depression rather than age. Sheline et al (2002) found that the duration of the disease, not age, predicted a loss of volume in the hippocampus. Hickie et al (2005) found a correlation between subcortical hyperintensity of white matter and psychomotor retardation. White matter is also associated with various indicators of learning and memory, as well as aspects of language and executive functions. Meanwhile, Shah et al (2002) demonstrated a link between verbal memory and grey matter density in the left hippocampus, a structure that is commonly associated with memory function. These various findings suggest a link between neuropsychological deficits and structural abnormalities in some patients with depression.

Bench et al (1993) used factor analysis to link regional cerebral blood flow to clinical features. One of the factors has a high load on cognitive efficiency and is positively associated with the blood flow in the medial prefrontal cortex. In the follow-up of this study Dolan et al (2021) analysed the main components of neuropsychological data. The main components appear with high loads on memory and attention. Goodwin (1997) described a correlation between cognitive impairment and hypofrontality.

Therefore, the most reliable finding in literature refers to prefrontal abnormalities, especially in the medial areas, anterior cingulate to the medial orbitofrontal cortex. This is obviously a plausible description of the neuropsychological evidence of severe executive dysfunction in depression. However, prefrontal dysfunction can also contribute to memory deficits, especially in more difficult memory tasks. The prefrontal cortex is involved in aspects of working memory and memory-related control processes. However, patients with depression also show deficits in simple recognition tasks, commonly associated with the function of the temporal lobes, which are important substrates of recognition memory. The medial prefrontal cortex is involved in the function of attention, mostly with the difficulty in attention focusing. It is known as a region that is associated with emotional reactions in both healthy controls and depressed patients. Fundamental pathology in the regions of the medial prefrontal cortex may be the basis of both clinical features and cognitive deficits in depression. It is possible that this pathology includes both functional and structural abnormalities. A study of Drevets et al (2000, 2008) reported both types of abnormality in the ventromedial area. The medial prefrontal cortex is an area with extensive interconnections and available neurotransmitters, especially serotonin. It is therefore possible that dysfunction in this region may be fundamental to depression, a disorder characterised by a complex interaction of affective and cognitive impairments. However, it remains to be clarified whether the medial prefrontal abnormality is a predisposing factor to depression or manifests itself with the onset of the disorder. This is one of the many issues that remain to be addressed in the search for a consistent framework for understanding depression.

Conclusion

In the last decades, functional neuroimaging by the means of positron emission tomography (PET), single photon emission computed tomography (SPECT), and functional magnetic resonance imaging (fMRI) has been used to identify functional abnormalities associated with depression. Studies using this approach have identified several regions that are uncommon in patients with depression. Probably the most widely discussed finding is hypofrontality, involving abnormal blood flow in the prefrontal cortex. The medial regions of the anterior cortex are particularly involved. Another functional abnormality is a reduced striatum blood flow. These striatum findings, combined with prefrontal abnormalities, provide support for the popular theory that depression may involve dysfunction of the anterior-subcortical chains. This description would be consistent with the neuropsychological evidence of particularly expressed difficulties in tests for executive function. The cognitive effort hypothesis would also predict prefrontal abnormality, as the increasing difficulty of the task is related to prefrontal activity. Findings of prefrontal and striatum abnormalities in studies of depression at rest were consistent with the neuropsychological profile.

Clarifying how cognitive deficits are associated with low mood and hypoactivity has important implications for the treatment of depression. At a theoretical level, understanding cognitive deficits and their interaction with affective symptoms and neuronal substrates is essential for an overall understanding of depression.

References

Basso, M. R., & Bornstein, R. A. (1999). Relative memory deficits in recurrent versus first-episode major depression on a word-list learning task. *Neuropsychology*, *13*(4), 557.

Basso, M. R., Bornstein, R. A., Carona, F., & Morton, R. (2001). Depression accounts for executive function deficits in obsessive-compulsive disorder. *Cognitive and Behavioral Neurology*, *14*(4), 241-245.

Basso, M., Combs, D., Purdie, R., Candilis, P., & Bornstein, R. (2013). Neuropsychological correlates of symptom dimensions in inpatients with major depressive disorder. *Psychiatry research*, *207*(1-2), 61-67.

Beats, B. C., Sahakian, B. J., & Levy, R. (1996). Cognitive performance in tests sensitive to frontal lobe dysfunction in the elderly depressed. *Psychological medicine*, *26*(3), 591-603.

Bench, C. J., Frith, C. D., Grasby, P. M., Friston, K. J., Paulesu, E., Frackowiak, R. S., & Dolan, R. J. (1993). Investigations of the functional anatomy of attention using the Stroop test. *Neuropsychologia*, *31*(9), 907–922. https://doi.org/10.1016/0028-3932(93)90147-r

Brooks, B. L., Iverson, G. L., Sherman, E. M., & Roberge, M. C. (2010). Identifying cognitive problems in children and adolescents with depression using computerized neuropsychological testing. *Applied neuropsychology*, *17*(1), 37–43

Channon, S., & Green, P. S. S. (1998). Executive dysfunction in depression: The use of performance strategies. In *Proceedings of the British Psychological Society* (Vol. 6, No. 2, pp. 104-104).

Chantiluke, K., Halari, R., Simic, M., Pariante, C. M., Papadopoulos, A., Giampietro, V., & Rubia, K. (2012). Fronto-striato-cerebellar dysregulation in adolescents with depression during motivated attention. *Biological psychiatry*, *71*(1), 59-67.

Ciuhan, G. C., & Iliescu, D. (2021). Depression and learning problems in children: Executive function impairments and inattention as mediators. *Acta psychologica*, *220*, 103420.

Degl'Innocenti, A., Agren, H., & Bäckman, L. (1998). Executive deficits in major depression. *Acta psychiatrica Scandinavica*, *97*(3), 182–188. https://doi.org/10.1111/j.1600-0447.1998.tb09985.x

Dolan, N., Simmonds-Buckley, M., Kellett, S., Siddell, E., & Delgadillo, J. (2021). Effectiveness of stress control large group psychoeducation for anxiety and depression: Systematic review and meta-analysis. *British Journal of Clinical Psychology*, *60*(3), 375-399.

Drevets, W. C. (2000). Functional anatomical abnormalities in limbic and prefrontal cortical structures in major depression. *Progress in brain research*, *126*, 413-431.

Drevets, W. C., Price, J. L., & Furey, M. L. (2008). Brain structural and functional abnormalities in mood disorders: implications for neurocircuitry models of depression. *Brain structure and function*, *213*(1), 93-118.

Elliott, R. (1998). The neuropsychological profile in unipolar depression. *Trends in Cognitive Sciences*, *2*(11), 447-454.

Elliott, R., Rubinsztein, J. S., Sahakian, B. J., & Dolan, R. J. (2002). The neural basis of mood-congruent processing biases in depression. *Archives of general psychiatry*, *59*(7), 597-604.

Goodwin, G. M. (1997). Neuropsychological and neuroimaging evidence for the involvement of the frontal lobes in depression. *Journal of Psychopharmacology*, *11*(2), 115-122.

Hickie, I., Naismith, S., Ward, P. B., Turner, K., Scott, E., Mitchell, P., ... & Parker, G. (2005). Reduced hippocampal volumes and memory loss in patients with early-and late-onset depression. *The British journal of psychiatry*, *186*(3), 197-202.

Kerestes, R., Davey, C. G., Stephanou, K., Whittle, S., & Harrison, B. J. (2014). Functional brain imaging studies of youth depression: a systematic review. *NeuroImage: Clinical*, *4*, 209-231.

Klimkeit, E. I., Tonge, B., Bradshaw, J. L., Melvin, G. A., & Gould, K. (2011). Neuropsychological deficits in adolescent unipolar depression. *Archives of clinical neuropsychology*, *26*(7), 662-676

Kuny, S., & Stassen, H. H. (1995). Cognitive performance in patients recovering from depression. *Psychopathology*, *28*(4), 190–207. https://doi.org/10.1159/000284922

Miller, C. H., Hamilton, J. P., Sacchet, M. D., & Gotlib, I. H. (2015). Meta-analysis of functional neuroimaging of major depressive disorder in youth. *JAMA psychiatry*, *72*(10), 1045-1053.

Murphy, F. C., Rubinsztein, J. S., Michael, A., Rogers, R. D., Robbins, T. W., Paykel, E. S., & Sahakian, B. J. (2001). Decision-making cognition in mania and depression. *Psychological medicine*, *31*(4), 679-693.

Nelson, J., Klumparendt, A., Doebler, P., & Ehring, T. (2017). Childhood maltreatment and characteristics of adult depression: meta-analysis. *The British Journal of Psychiatry*, *210*(2), 96-104.

Oliver, A., Pile, V., Elm, D., & Lau, J. Y. (2019). The cognitive neuropsychology of depression in adolescents. *Current Behavioral Neuroscience Reports*, *6*(4), 227-235.)

Pan, L. A., Hassel, S., Segreti, A. M., Nau, S. A., Brent, D. A., & Phillips, M. L. (2013). Differential patterns of activity and functional connectivity in emotion processing neural circuitry to angry and happy faces in adolescents with and without suicide attempt. *Psychological medicine*, *43*(10), 2129-2142.

Robbins, T. W., James, M., Owen, A. M., Sahakian, B. J., Lawrence, A. D., McInnes, L., & Rabbitt, P. M. (1998). A study of performance on tests from the CANTAB battery sensitive to frontal lobe dysfunction in a large sample of normal volunteers: implications for theories of executive functioning and cognitive aging. Cambridge Neuropsychological Test Automated Battery. *Journal of the International Neuropsychological Society : JINS*, *4*(5), 474–490. https://doi.org/10.1017/s1355617798455073

Shah, P. J., Glabus, M. F., Goodwin, G. M., & Ebmeier, K. P. (2002). Chronic, treatment-resistant depression and right fronto-striatal atrophy. *The British Journal of Psychiatry*, *180*(5), 434-440.

Sheline, Y. I., Mittler, B. L., & Mintun, M. A. (2002). The hippocampus and depression. *European psychiatry : the journal of the Association of European Psychiatrists*, *17 Suppl 3*, 300–305. https://doi.org/10.1016/s0924-9338(02)00655-7

Simpson, S., Baldwin, R. C., Jackson, A., & Burns, A. S. (1998). Is subcortical disease associated with a poor response to antidepressants? Neurological, neuropsychological and neuroradiological findings in late-life depression. *Psychological Medicine*, *28*(5), 1015-1026.

Stephanou, K., Davey, C. G., Kerestes, R., Whittle, S., & Harrison, B. J. (2017). Hard to look on the bright side: neural correlates of impaired emotion regulation in depressed youth. *Social cognitive and affective neuroscience*, *12*(7), 1138-1148.

Tarbuck, A. F., & Paykel, E. S. (1995) Effects of major depression on the cognitive function of younger and older subjects. *Psychological Medicine*, *25*(2), 285-295.

Tyrrell, M., & Elliot, R. (2015). The Depression Learning Path. *What you need to know about how depression works and how to beat it.*

Wagner, S., Müller, C., Helmreich, I., Huss, M., & Tadić, A. (2015). A meta-analysis of cognitive functions in children and adolescents with major depressive disorder. *European child & adolescent psychiatry*, *24*(1), 5-19.

Watkins, P. C. (2002). Implicit memory bias in depression. *Cognition & Emotion*, *16*(3), 381-402.

Will, G. J., van Lier, P. A., Crone, E. A., & Güroğlu, B. (2016). Chronic childhood peer rejection is associated with heightened neural responses to social exclusion during adolescence. *Journal of abnormal child psychology*, *44*(1), 43-55.

Yang, T. T., Simmons, A. N., Matthews, S. C., Tapert, S. F., Frank, G. K., Bischoff-Grethe, A., ... & Paulus, M. P. (2009). Depressed adolescents demonstrate greater subgenual anterior cingulate activity. *Neuroreport*, *20*(4), 440.

CHAPTER SIX

CIRCADIAN RHYTHM IN PSYCHIATRIC DISORDERS

NADEJDA MADJIROVA
MEDICAL UNIVERSITY PLOVDIV

The human being is the most complex computer, and all our cells and functions have a special place in this complex machine. But who made the program and who controls it? I doubt if anyone can give us the exact answer.

Abstract

The regulation of a given process will be determined by an integration of multiple internal and external timing influences. The human circadian system is highly complex and regulates numerous processes, many of which maintain characteristic phase differences from each other and from the earth's day-night cycle. It involves a large number of autonomous oscillators entrained by a master clock and a range of different zeitgebers (Germain & Kupfer, 2008).

The circadian timing system controls all the internal physiological and behaviour rhythms, synchronises them to the external environment, and ensures temporal isolation in incompatible physiological or behavioural processes. Many scientists tried to arrange the puzzle of the circadian rhythm of the various psychiatric disorders and seek the roots of their disturbances. One of the main hypotheses was that the circadian (daily) timing system is one of the most important for the mental disturbances. Karatsoreos (2014) in his review described its function in various psychiatric disorders such as depression, anxiety, and schizophrenia (SCH). Almost all biological processes in organisms related to life, lasting longer than 24 h, display circadian rhythms. The most obvious of these is the regulation of the rest-activity cycle. The common and highly disruptive co-morbid problem in many psychiatric conditions, including depression, schizophrenia (SCH), and obsessive-compulsive disorder, is a disturbed sleep-wake-cycle. Disruption in physiological and psychological symptoms is typical for depressive disorders (Karatsoreos, 2014; Turek, 1986, Mendlewicz, 2009). The link between circadian function and depression occurs at many levels (Wirz-Justice, 2009). An interesting example of this multi-level interaction is evident in the development and use of agomelatine, a melatonin agonist that also has serotonergic activity.

Keywords: chronobiology, circadian rhythms, psychiatry

Introduction

In this chapter the types of circadian rhythms in our population and in some selected psychiatric disorders will be discussed.

> *For this reason, our questionnaire evaluated the circadian rhythm of mood/vigour in 1503 healthy controls (647 males and 856 females) aged between 3 and 85 years. We did a distribution according to sex, age, profession, and social position.*

Following the generally accepted basic types of rhythms, described by Hampp (1961) and other authors (Madjirova 2006 and references therein), we decided upon the following types: arrhythmic, morning, evening, as described in the first chapter. During our study we found "**fluctuating**" type rhythm. In a small percentage (9%) Hampp detected fluctuation in the impulses and emotions, which were affected by different hours of the day and night and depended on various external/internal factors. He determined they were "individuals with reactive change in condition of drives and emotions". Middelhoff (1967) described a similar group in depressed patients. In our study, the group of fluctuating type are people who registered fluctuations in their mood/vigour without serious life events or physical/somatic problems. All the participants were asked in detail about their daily fluctuation of mood/vigour. Without the presence of any external/internal factors, the participants recorded and evaluated the fluctuations, indicating that their rhythm cannot be regarded as one of the generally accepted types (arrhythmic, morning, evening).

The percentage distribution of the types of the circadian rhythms of mood/vigour of the whole group, shows that almost half of them are arrhythmic type (51.36% for mood; 51.90 for vigour), followed by fluctuating (17.45%; 10.78%), evening (14.50%; 13.37%), and morning (16.65%; 23.95%). We did not find differences by sex.

In order to clarify some of the differences between the two questionnaires, 156 of the studied people were investigated by both methods simultaneously. The participants in Hampp's study showed a significantly higher percentage of rhythmic type, whereas the arrhythmic type dominated in our group.

Upon questioning the studied people, it was found that some of them with mild morning/evening type according to Hampp, fell into the group of arrhythmic type in our questionnaire. This also could explain the greater frequency of the evening type in his questionnaire.

Also of interest is the percentage of coincidence between the rhythm of impulses and emotions; we established that for both sexes it occurs in 75.73% of the healthy controls. In both there is a tendency for this percentage to increase with the advance of the age (56.9% up to 20 years, 71.63% up to 30 years, 80.0% up to 60 years, and 89.40% after 60 years).

We did not try to evaluate emotional rhythm in people younger than 14 years, because it is not stable.

Arrhythmic type is more frequently observed in mature age (between 30-50 years), the morning type is more frequent in advanced age (after 50 years), while the evening type was common for the younger group (before 30 years). These results are almost the same for mood and vigour.

In the distribution of the type of circadian rhythms according to their profession, the data regarding the rhythm of impulses was of greater interest. The relative part of arrhythmic type is the greatest (79.07%) and it is significantly higher in comparison with the other groups (students, white-collar workers, blue-collar workers, and pensioners). Among the pensioners, the morning type (40.78%) is the most common in comparison with all other groups ($0.05 > p < 0.001$), whereas the evening type is more typical for students (18.55%) and is significantly higher ($p<0.001$) in comparison with white-collar workers ($t=4.45$), manual workers ($t=5.96$), agricultural workers ($t=5.96$), and pensioners ($t=6.00$).

The fluctuation type has a greater relative share among the students, and it speaks of an inadequate stability of rhythm at this age. No differences according to sex were found. Hampp (1961) established a higher percentage of arrhythmic type among people doing manual labour and higher percentage of evening type among intellectuals. The evening type, as in most publications, is most frequent among graduates and there is a statistical difference against those with primary education ($t=4.58$; $p<0.001$) and secondary education ($t=2.33$; $p<0.05$). There is a statistical reliability also between individuals with secondary and primary education – more frequent among individuals with secondary education ($t=2.33$; $p<0.05$).

In order to establish the differences between the rural and urban populations, a comparison of the inhabitants of towns and villages was made. Here it must be noted that the group living in the rural areas included those who up to the time of investigation, have lived and worked in the village, while the group of urban dwellers was made up of individuals who have, for many years, lived and worked in towns. The groups of pupils and students were excluded because for the first period there is a tendency for an irregular way of life, which results in desynchronisation of the rhythm (Hildebrandt, Stratmann, 1979).

Knowledge of the circadian rhythms in healthy controls is necessary for the clarification of some pathological mechanisms in affective disorders (AD). During the last six decades many papers support the hypothesis about circadian rhythm dysfunction in psychiatric disorders (Madjirova 2006 and references therein).

Circadian rhythms in psychiatric patients

Kirov (1967), Stoyanov (1971) and Meninnger-Lerhenthal (1960) reported that at the end of the 19th century and at the beginning of the 20th century, more attention was being paid to periodic schizophrenia by Kirn (1878), Pilz (1901), Ustein (1909), and Kraepelin (1909). In his monograph, Menninger-Lerhenthal announced that at the end of 19th century some psychiatrists observed daily fluctuations of mood in psychiatric patients: Kraftt-Ebing (1888), Kraepelin (1898), Fleck & Kraepelin (1922) mentioned that patients with depression feel better in the evening, whereas patients with neuroses feel better in the morning. Menninger-Lerhenthal supported the same idea, whereas Kretchmer (1940) stressed on the fact that the difference between healthy individuals and psychiatric patients with neuroses and depression, was only in their degree. For the first time Beck (1962), by the use of his own scale, found that SCH patients had an inversion of their circadian rhythm. Hale (1964), through the use of a self-rating scale in 70 depressive patients, established that 24% were evening type and 29% were of morning type rhythm (cited in 189). Middelhoff (1967), by modification of Hampp's questionnaire, studied 81 patients and established that 35% were evening type and 49% were morning type. J. Martin (2001) spoke about the inversion of the rhythm during the depressive phase (250). According to Waldmann (1970), the rhythm of patients is changed only during their depressive state. Weitbrecht (1973) noticed that the improvement of the depression came in the afternoon or in the evening. Knorring, et al. (1977) studying 199 patients, found that 45% were evening and 16% were morning type. Tashev (1979) and Milenkov (1982) by their questionnaire, remarked that evening type rhythm was typical among AD.

> The circadian rhythm of mood was determined in 667 patients (155 with AD, 401 with neurotic disorders (ND), and 112 with SCH) by our inquiry. The comparison with healthy controls (HC), examined in the same inquiry, shows that 51.40% were arrhythmic, type which is significantly higher than in the patients - 29.09% ($t=4.49$ and $p<0.001$). 44.89% of the patients were fluctuating type and the values were significantly higher ($t=3.76$; $p<0.001$) in comparison with HC (17.45%).

As the evaluation by the method of inquiry is not very objective for patients, we used a scale, and the fluctuation of emotions was registered each hour of the day with various degrees (light degree – 1; moderate– 2; heavy – 3; very heavy - 4). Using this questionnaire, 919 psychiatric patients were evaluated: 329 with AD, 156 – SCH, and 434 – ND. The correlation between 1072 healthy controls, aged between 17 and 85 years, and patients shows that arrhythmic type is significantly higher for healthy controls ($t=6.86$; $p<0.001$), whereas evening type is significantly higher for patients ($t=4.73$; $p<0.001$).

- Arrhythmic type is the dominant in healthy controls (approximately half of them).
- Morning type is higher in neuroses and schizophrenia.
- Evening type is typical for depression.
- Fluctuating type is higher in neuroses.

Kivelä et al. (2018) stress the importance of evening type. Eveningness is related to AD and especially depression. Among depressed individuals, evening types tend to exhibit worse symptom severity and report increased psychological distress, higher suicidality, and more impairment in their daily lives (including work). Eveningness has previously been associated with depressive symptoms in university students. The evening chronotype has also recently been associated with compulsive internet use. Evening type adolescents have been found to report higher mood seasonality. Eveningness has been associated with trait anxiety in females-adolescents morning and intermediate types. Morning type individuals tend to exhibit healthier and more regular eating habits and have higher control over eating, compared to evening type personality disorders.

Typical for the patients in the three groups is that the percentage of arrhythmic type is significantly decreased, and the parts of evening type in AD, and morning and fluctuating types in ND, are increased (fig.2-1).

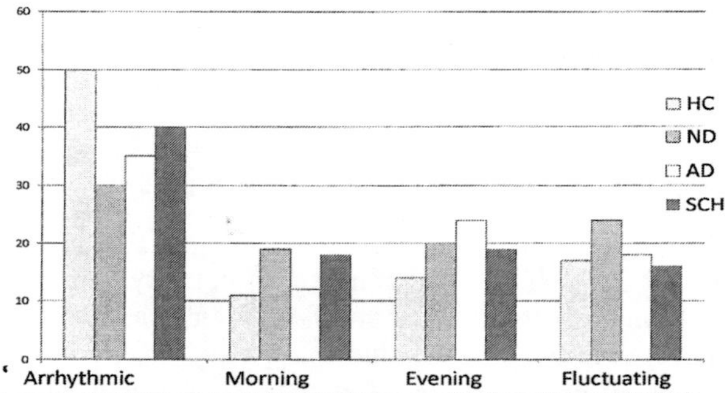

T & p between	t & p	t & p	t & p	t & p
Healthy & HD	t=8.22 p<0.001	t = 2.39; p< 0.02	t = 2.10; p < 0.05;	t = 2.03; p < 0.05
Healthy & AD	t=4.29; p<0.001	t = 0.13; p >0.05	t = 4.89; p < 0.001	t = 0.48; p > 0.05
Healthy & Sch	t=2.64; p<0.01	t = 1.94; p> 0.05	t = 1.50; p > 0.05	t = 0.27; p > 0.05
ND & AD	t=1.52; p>0.05	t = 2.00; p < 0.05	t = 1.97; p < 0.05	t = 1.88; p > 0.05
ND & Sch	t=1.69; p>0.05	t = 0.2; p > 0.05	t = 0.02; p > o.05	t = 2.2; p< 0.05
Sch & AD	t=0.58; p>0.05	t = 1.73; p >0.05	t = 1.62; p > 0.05	t = 0.76; p > 0.05

Fig. 2-1 Percentage distributions of the various types of circadian rhythms in patients with ND, AD and SCH

We must mention that arrhythmic type for HC means a good mood and good working capacity throughout the whole day. Typical for arrhythmic type in psychiatric patients, is that they are depressive and their mood and working capacity is poor during the whole day.

*In the group of ND according to ICD-10 were included: F4 (F40 – phobic anxiety disorders; F41 – other anxiety disorders; F42 – obsessive compulsive disorders; F44 – reaction of heavy stress and disturbances in adaptation; F44 – dissociative disturbances; F 45 – somatoform disorders; F48 – neurasthenia. According to DSM- 5 the codes are: 300.23 - Social anxiety disorder (Social Phobia); 300.01 (F41.0) – Panic Disorder; 300.22

(F40.00) – Agoraphobia; 300.02 (F41.1) – Generalised Anxiety Disorder; 300.3 (F42) – Obsessive Compulsive Disorder; 309.81 (F43.10) – Posttraumatic Stress Disorder; 300.14 (F44.81) – Dissociative Identity Disorder.

We must pay a special attention to the fluctuating type. We also found that some people registered fluctuation of their circadian rhythm without any serious psychological/environmental reasons. Among healthy controls (HC), 17.45% were of fluctuating type for emotional rhythm and 11.85% for the rhythm of vigour.

The examination of 410 patients with ND showed that arrhythmic types are 36.12% for vigour and 29.03% for mood; fluctuating type are 34.88% and 43.9%, respectively. The fluctuating type is significantly higher in comparison to the group of HC.

We tried to attempt the retrospective assessment of these types of rhythms prior to the neurosis affection, showing that fluctuating type of impulses (22.68%) and emotions (34.39%) is higher in comparison with the healthy controls. This fact indicates that there is instability of the impulses and emotions in this contingent (see fig.2-2).

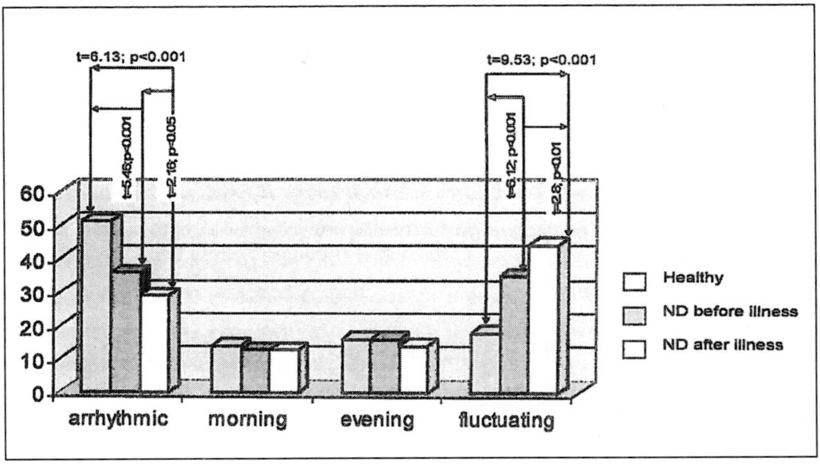

Fig. 2-2. Percentage distributions of the circadian rhythms in neurotic patients before and during their illness

Because the method of questionnaire is not objective, a control group of 103 patients with ND was formed, and the circadian rhythm of their impulses/emotions were examined every hour from 7.00am to 10.00pm. Data were processed using variation analyses. The percentage distribution of arrhythmic and fluctuating type rhythms was almost the same. These data show that healthy people with fluctuating type rhythm have a predisposition to neurotic disorders.

A reasonable question may be posed, whether or not the fluctuating type of rhythm in healthy people could be one of the risk factors predisposing to neurotic disorders development. We can use these data for prophylaxis and prevention of neuroses.

Characteristics of the various types of circadian rhythms

As we determined "a fluctuating" type rhythm, we must prove it through the use of some psychological methods (the intensity of their temperament) and the values of some vegetative parameters as temperature, pulse rate, and blood pressure.

The intensity of the temperament components:
Our investigation of 379 HC and 149 psychiatric patients (ND, AD, SCH) shows that the four types of circadian rhythm have different intensities of the temperament components (Madjirova, Vlahova-Nikolova, 1987; Madjirova, Balabanova, 1981). For these reasons we used Tashev's temperament-behaviour questionnaire. This test reveals the structure of the temperament, represented by the four basic groups of temperament features – sanguine, choleric, phlegmatic, and melancholic, the relation between them and the intensity of the separate temperament components. This questionnaire also includes a fifth group of contents, which outline the prenatal depressive-personality tendencies. The various types of circadian rhythm showed different intensity of the temperament components in HC and in psychiatric patients.

The expression of the temperament components in HC and psychiatric patients:

379 HC are characterised by:

Arrhythmic type – phlegmatic and sanguine components.

Morning type – phlegmatic and choleric components.

Evening type – phlegmatic components.

Fluctuating type - choleric, phlegmatic and sanguine components.

149 psychiatric patients are characterised by:

Arrhythmic type - Phlegmatic, followed by depressive tendencies and choleric components.

Morning type - Phlegmatic and depressive components.

Evening type – It is like morning type but the values are significantly higher.

Fluctuating type - Phlegmatic and depressive tendencies.

This permits the assertion of these four types of circadian rhythms. It is obvious that the depressive tendencies in psychiatric patients presented in all four types of circadian rhythm and phlegmatic features.

1. Vegetative parameters (temperature, pulse, blood pressure)

In HC temperature varies as a part of the circadian cycle:

Minimum body temperature= most sleepy (usually this is sometime in the very early morning). Typically, this is a couple hours after peak production of the hormone melatonin. Maximum body temperature= Most awake (usually afternoon)

According to this study, morning people have an earlier temperature peak (corresponding to the time of day when one is most awake), while evening people have a later peak. Many authors reported that the circadian rhythm of HC with morning/evening type rhythm have different daily fluctuation of temperature/pulse rhythm (Hildebrandt & I. Stratmann, 1979). These daily fluctuations of the rhythm correlate with their activity and mood during the day. Body temperature in evening type is increased very gradually from the time of waking throughout the day until the peak reached later in the evening. This explains the fact that they are very slow during the day and activate in the evening. Foret et al. (1985) followed the body temperature in "morning", "evening", and "neither", type people with normal sleep. They recorded sleep and rectal temperature under three conditions: baseline nights, sleep deprivation, and sleep on the recovery night after one night and one day of sleep deprivation. They established that temperature increased earlier in "morning" and "neither type" people, and decreased in "evening" type after sleep deprivation. They did not find any differences in temperature during their normal sleep, nor in the period of recovery of their sleep, after sleep deprivation. The circadian phase of the subjects was estimated in the laboratory using dim-light melatonin onset in saliva and the body temperature minimum (Goulet et al., 2007). The authors established that the morning type have earlier sleep schedules than the evening type. Morning and evening types differ in their endogenous circadian phase, but whether this is the cause or the consequence of the difference in light exposure remains controversial. The conclusion is that morning types are exposed to more light in the morning than night type.

Lack et al. (2009) studied 20 young, healthy students (8 -morning type, and 12 – evening type). The typical sleep onset, arising times, circadian phase markers for temperature and melatonin, and objective sleepiness were all 2-3 hours later for evening type than in the morning type. Although morning types had earlier temperature rhythm, they slept at a relatively later temperature rhythm phase than evening types.

Most studies were about the temperature rhythm of morning/evening type rhythm in HC but data about psychiatric patients are insufficient.

> *The temperature, pulse, mood, and activity were measured by our special questionnaire at each hour (from 7:00 am to 11:00 pm) in 68 HC, 288 with RDD, 144 with ND with depressive syndrome and 196 with SCH. All participants were examined in the period of 1984-1989. The four groups were divided according to their circadian rhythm, determined by our questionnaire. We measured the BP in 143 patients with AD. We will comment on the circadian rhythm of temperature. Synchronisation is typical for HC, but it is not so in psychiatric patients. We find that most expressed are the changes of the medial daily temperature for the various circadian rhythm of the four groups.*

- ***Affective disorders:*** The temperature/pulse MESORs of morning type were higher (36.52+/-0.08; 83.94+/-0.089), followed by arrhythmic, evening, and fluctuating type rhythms.
- ***Neurotic disorders:*** Pulse rate in arrhythmic type was significantly faster ($t=6.51$; $p<0.001$), whereas it was significantly slower in morning type ($t=8.95$; $p<0.001$).

BP - the average values of SBP and DBP were the highest for fluctuating type, and the lowest for evening type ($t=4.00$; $p<0.001$).

We established that the various types of circadian rhythms (arrhythmic, morning, evening, and fluctuating types) have different daily rhythms of temperature and pulse in the two groups examined patients.

- ***Schizophrenia:*** *Temperature*: Arrhythmic type had the lowest medial temperature (36.44) and it was highly significant ($p<0.001$) in comparison with the others ($t=5.47$ for evening; $t=3.88$ for fluctuating, and $t=3.47$ for morning type). *Pulse*: Fluctuating type was with significantly higher mediate pulse ($p<0.001$) in comparison with the others ($t=5.77$ for evening, $t=6.83$ for morning, and $t=7.17$ for arrhythmic type).

The pulse rate did not accelerate with the increase of the temperature whereas for HC, there was a correlation between these two parameters.

Temperature and pulse chronograms in AD and ND: We established that their daily fluctuations were different for the two groups and for the various types of circadian rhythms.

Temperature rhythm of evening type in ND was significantly higher at 9:00 am., 1:01 am, 07:00 pm, 8:00 pm, and 11:00 pm, and at 4:00 pm for fluctuating type ($p<0.05$). Morning and arrhythmic types were with almost the same circadian rhythm of these parameters for the two groups.

Pulse rate was significantly frequent in AD for morning type, whereas for ND it was arrhythmic type during most hours of the day ($p<0.001$). The chronograms of evening and fluctuating type varied for the two groups without any significance during the different hours.

The chronograms of the various types of circadian rhythms were different for the two diseases.

The different types of circadian rhythms were with different temperature/ pulse MESORs.

Healthy controls: The temperature/pulse chronograms were different for the various types of circadian rhythms. The MESOR of the fluctuating type was the highest, whereas for the morning type it was the lowest. Synchronisation between the two vegetative parameters was typical for HC for the various types of circadian rhythm. We paid a special attention to their temperature chronogram: it was different for the various types of circadian rhythms and quite different in comparison with the patients with AD, ND and SCH.

These data support our thesis for determination of the fluctuating type rhythm.

2. Correlation between age and the temperature and pulse chronogram

The temperature and pulse MESORs were different in the young and adult people. The changes of the temporal organisation with the age caused changes in the human circadian rhythms (Davis, 1981). The rhythm amplitude decreased and temperature MESOR decreased with age (Cahn et al., 1968). Witting et al. (1994) discussed the effect of old age on the free running period of circadian rhythms in rats. Carrier et al. (1996) found amplitude reduction of the circadian temperature and sleep rhythm in the elderly. Biryukevich (1972) reported on changes of heart-rate frequency of rhythms in newborn children until 18 years of age. Zanghi et al. (2016) measured day-night activity patterns, core body temperature, and actigraphy-generated behavioural sleep, in aged canines with their cognitive dysfunction. Weiner & Waterhouse (2006) observed the effect of core temperature, physical activity and ageing.

Our study included 544 people (66 – HC, 278 - AD, 200 - ND). Temperature and pulse of all participants were registered. Typical for these groups was that in all ages, the middle temperature and pulse were lower in HC.

- ***Healthy controls***– the temperature was higher in almost all hours of the day in younger people (under the age of 40) in comparison with the older adults (over the age of 40), whereas the pulse was more frequent between 40 and 50 years. Synchronisation was obvious at almost all hours of the day.

    - ***Neurotic disorders*** – temperature and pulse MESORs were higher for younger patients in comparison with adults older than 40 years in almost all hours of the day. The average daily temperature of adult patients between 40 and 51 (36.45+/-0.05) and over 50 years (36.397+/-0.02) was significantly lower in comparison with the middle (36.59+/-0.05) and the youngest group (36.61+/-0.01) with high significance ($p<0.001$). We found the same result in pulse MESORs: $t=2.14$ between the group of adults and the middle-aged $t=3.68$ ($0.05<P<0.001$).

Synchronisation between the two parameters was in almost all hours of the day.

- ***Affective disorders*** – temperature and pulse MESORs were higher for the younger patients, but their MESORs increased after 60 years, and it is more obvious for pulse.

These results speak to the difference between temperature and pulse chronogram between the two disorders (ND, AD) and the healthy controls.

3. Seasons of the year and the temperature and pulse chronogram

The temperature of the environment influences our rhythms. The studies of the seasonal rhythmic processes in humans began at the end of the 19th century. According to Aschoff (1981) the pioneer of this examination was R. Mailling-Hansen (1886), who established the fluctuation of the height of children during the different seasons. Hildebrandt in 1962 described over 30 seasonal rhythms in humans.

Many researchers proved the influence of the environmental temperature on the body temperature (Krauchi, et al., 1997; Krauchi & Wirz-Justice, 1987;, Nikolov & Solakova, 1984). Some scientists established different values of temperature, blood pressure, pulse, and heart rate during the different months of the year (Madjirova 2006 and references therein). Menshikov et al. (1980), in 240 healthy people, registered seasonal fluctuation of the excretion of epinephrine, nor-epinephrine, and dopamine. Swade & Coppen (1980) thought that the medication of depression must consider the seasons and according to some authors, the soporific effect is quicker in spring than in summer (Madjirova 2006 and references therein).

In order to prove this connection, the participants were determined according to the seasons of the year.

We examined 471 people in the period 1985-1988: we measured their temperature, pulse, and blood pressure, compared to 145 patients with AD, every hour from 7:00 am. to 10:00 pm.

- ***75 healthy people*** (23 in winter, 14 in spring, 28 in summer, and 10 in autumn). The average daily temperature was the highest in spring (36.484+/-0.0034) and it was significant in comparison with winter (36.372+/-0.00070) and summer (t=3.5; t=3.3; $p<0.001$). The pulse MESOR in autumn (78.82+/-0.306) was highly significant ($p<0.001$) according to the other seasons of the year (t=9.78 for winter; t=5.10

for spring, and t=3.62 for summer). Their peaks were at different hours – temperature peak in winter was at 3:00 pm, and the minimum value was at 8:00 am, the peak for summer was at 9:00 pm, whereas the values were higher in the afternoon in spring and autumn. The pulse peaks were at 8:00 pm for winter, 3:00 pm for spring, 3:00 pm and 6:00 pm for summer, and 10:00 am for autumn.

- ***142 patients with SCH*:** 44 in spring; 16 in autumn; 41 in summer and 41 in winter. Synchronisation between temperature and pulse chronograms was absent during the four seasons. The temperature values were lower in spring, and their peak was in the afternoon. Winter and summer values were higher in the afternoon, but the peak in autumn was in the morning and the chronogram was unstable. The pulse chronograms were almost the same during the four seasons, but the frequencies were higher in autumn and lower in spring. The temperature and pulse MESORs were the highest in autumn (36.61+/-0.00028; 95.34+/-0.23) and highly significant for temperature ($p<0.001$; t=8.9) and pulse ($p<0.05$; t=19.3) in comparison with spring (36.39+/-0.00038; 82.592+/-0.11).

- ***254 patients with AD*:** 60 in winter; 79 in spring; 76 in summer; 39 in autumn. The daily temperature rhythm was almost the same during the various seasons. The values were higher in spring and lower in autumn without any significance. Pulse was with peaks at 9:00 am, 2:00 pm and 8:00 pm, the winter peak was at 9:00 am, and the minimum was at 6:00 pm, whereas in spring and summer there was not a peak. The average daily values of temperature were higher in spring and lower in autumn.

- ***246 patients with ND*:** 87 in winter; 57 in spring, 36 in summer, 66 in autumn. The average daily temperature and pulse rate were with significantly higher values ($p<0.001$) in autumn (36.61+/-0.0035; 85.37+/-0.15) in comparison with spring and summer (36.43+/-0.0022; 36.467+/-0.0022; 81.518+/-0.10; 80.91+/-0.06).

Desynchronisation between temperature/pulse was obvious during all seasons of the year.

Seasonal distribution of the peak-hours and minimum in ND:

Spring: Temperature peak-hour/minimum was 3:00 pm/7:00 am
Pulse peak-hour/minimum was 8:00 pm/ 9:00 pm

Summer: Temperature peak-hour/minimum was 4:00 pm/7:00 am; 10:00 am
Pulse peak-hour/minimum was 9:00 am; 8:00 pm/10:00 pm

Autumn: Temperature peak-hour/minimum was 8:00 am/7:00 am
Pulse peak-hour/minimum was 7:00 am/7:00 pm

Winter: Temperature peak-hour/minimum was 5:00 pm & 7:00pm/ 7:00am & 6:00pm
Pulse peak-hour/minimum was 2:00 pm/7:00 am

Conclusion

- *Healthy controls and patients with AD, ND and SCH have different chronograms of temperature and pulse during the 4 seasons.*
- *The values of temperature and pulse in HC are lower in all hours and seasons in comparison with the patients with AD, ND &SCH.*
- *We did not find synchronisation between temperature and pulse during the various seasons in patients with AD, ND and SCH.*

4. Circadian rhythm and sleep disturbances in depression

Patients with serious psychiatric problems commonly complain of troubled sleep. Disturbed sleep is considered as a nonspecific prodromal symptom of nearly all mental illness. Ward (1960) reported that 80.4% of all psychiatric inpatients have some type of sleep disturbance (cited in Williams & Karacan, 1985). Many scientists have written about the role and the significance of sleep in the regulation of the circadian rhythms (Madjirova 2006 and references therein) and discussed the adaptive possibilities of man after a change in the sleep/wakefulness rhythm. Monk (1997) made the connection between the suppressed mood and frequent disturbances in sleep in healthy individuals during spring and autumn (cited in Monk, et al., 1997). Sleep disturbances present the most in patients with psychiatric problems and so they are treated with sleep-promoting psychopharmacological agents (benzodiazepines or newer hypnotics).

Primary chronobiological postulate is that the integrity of the circadian sleep-wake cycle, as the most obvious output of the biological clock, promotes healthy functioning in all psychiatric disorders. Tsujimoto et al. (2014) noted that clinical signatures that correlate with rhythm disturbances include decreased need for sleep, disturbances in content of thought and formal thought disorder, increase in rate and amount of speech, and increased motor activity and energy. These results are suggestive of a possible commonality or shared pathophysiology between sleep disruption and disturbed circadian rhythm.

Sleep disturbances are classic signs and symptoms of depression. Tashev (1979) and Buysse (1998) reported that about 3/4 of ED complained of sleep disturbances: 40% suffered from insomnia, and 15% had somnolence. Murray & Harvey (2010) established the link between circadian sleep and emotional regulation in BAD.

> *Our study in 1995 showed that only 418 from the examined 1255 healthy controls and 226 of the psychiatric patients by our inquiry, answered the question connected with their rhythm after a disturbed night's sleep (237). Most of them (91.55%) declared a change in their circadian rhythm on the next day. The number of arrhythmic type decreased and the number of fluctuating type increased to 27.43%. About 28.5% marked changes in the degree, and only 6.68% did not find any changes in their circadian rhythm.*

The disturbed sleep-wake cycle in schizophrenics correlated with poor cognitive function, whereas in borderline personality disorder it correlated with atypical depressive symptoms and daytime sleepiness. Most of the scientists paid a special attention to the connection between sleep disturbances and depression. About 80% of SCH patients have sleep disturbances (Wulff et al., 2018), but very little is known about the contribution of circadian coordination to this prevalent disruption. Undoubtedly there are physiological mechanisms underlying the sleep-wake cycle. According to Wever (cited in Wirz-Justice & Campbell, 1982) the human circadian system has been moulded by two endogenous self-sustained coupled oscillators: a strong one controlling body temperature, REM sleep propensity, and cortisol secretion. Srivansan et al. (2009) found that disturbance in sleep architecture occurred in major depressive disorders and in BAD. Reduction of slow wave sleep decreased latency of rapid eye movement sleep and abnormalities in the timing of REM/non-REM sleep cycles have all been documented in patients with major depressive disorders. It is thus evident that an understanding of the basic mechanisms of sleep regulation is essential for an analysis of some pathophysiological mechanisms of depressive disorders. Many publications stress on the connection between the depression/schizophrenia and sleep disturbances and consider the correlation between sleep and some hormonal disturbances (Madjirova 2006 and references therein) Germain & Kupfer (2008) reviewed many articles in order to understand the role of the circadian rhythm and sleep disturbances in the pathogenesis and treatment of depression. They concluded that sleep and waking were the most obvious circadian rhythms in mammals and that circadian and sleep disturbances were very important in the pathophysiology of mood disorders. Depressed patients often show altered circadian rhythms, sleep disturbances, and diurnal variation. Some of the most successful chronotherapeutic methods for non-seasonal and seasonal depression are bright light exposure, melatonin therapy; dark therapy; sleep deprivation and social rhythm therapies, somatic therapy (Madjirova 2006 and references therein). Antidepressant drugs have marked effects on circadian processes and sleep. Strian et al. (1979), Surgue (1981) and Brown & Seggie (1988) discussed the effect and various mechanisms of action of antidepressants on the circadian rhythm in ED. Wu et al. (2004) considered the effect of co-medication of SSRIs and mood stabilizers. The application of fluvoxamine on rats provoked a specific chronobiological effect on pineal serotonin and melatonin (Demish et al., 1996). Rush et al. (1989) reported that reduced REM latency predicted the response to TCA in depressed outpatients. Saleem (1984) searched the relationship between dexamethasone suppression test and its relationship to anxiety states.

In 1995 we measured cortisol plasma levels in 122 depressed patients at 8:00 am and 11:00 pm on the first day and at 8:00 am, 4:00 pm, and 11:00 pm the second day after oral administration of dexamethasone. Some of the patients were studied before/after medication so the total number of plasma cortisol level examination came to 173 (92 were with AD, the others were with SCH and ND with depressive syndrome). All of them had to describe the state of their sleep by the help of our questionnaire. The temperature and pulse were taken hourly from 7:00 am to 11:00 pm for two consecutive days where the total measurements came to 34. The blood pressure was measured on 27 of them. Data were compared with a control group of 65 healthy controls without somatic and mental disorders, tested at the same time. Plasma levels of cortisol were examined by the method of Ziegler et al. as modified by Ankov et al. (1970). The cortisol values were determined by a Perkin-Elmer (Australia) spectrofluorometer. Data of vegetative parameters were computed by the method of cosinor rhythmometry by F. Halberg (1969; 1980) and Nelson et al. (1979).

In processing data, it was established that plasma cortisol levels before/after oral administration of dexamethasone the first day at 11:00 pm were significantly higher in patients with disturbed sleep at 8:00 am on the first day ($t=2.02$; $p<0.05$) and at 11:00 pm on the second day ($t=2.35$; $p<0.02$). The distribution by sex was almost the same. Males/females with disturbed sleep had higher plasma cortisol levels in comparison with males/females with good sleep. The significance for males appeared at 11:00 pm on the first day, whereas in females it appeared at 8:00 am, 4:00, pm and 11:00 pm on the second day. Comparison by sex showed that plasma levels at 8:00 am and 11:00 pm on the first day in patients with disturbed sleep and at 8:00 am and 4:00 pm on the second day in patients with good sleep were significantly higher for males. Differences by sex were noted by Tashev & Bakalova (1984) and in our previous study (Madjirova et al., 1992). We found that the percentage distribution of suppressors/non-suppressors was almost the same in patients with good/disturbed sleep. The number of suppressors was significantly higher in females with good sleep ($t=2.09$; $p<0.05$). In the suppressor group were individuals with plasma cortisol levels no higher than 5.0 nmol/I. According to Saleem (1984) age and sex did not correlate with abnormal DST. Christensen et al. (1988) found that spontaneous and suppressed cortisol levels significantly correlated with age, type of severity of depression, and with stress/distress events. Comparison of patients younger than 40 and those over 40 with good sleep showed that plasma cortisol levels were significantly higher in older patients at 8:00 am ($t=2.83$; $p<0.02$) on the second day. The distribution by age and sex (19-40 and over 40 years of age) showed that patients with disturbed sleep in all groups had higher cortisol levels in plasma. These differences were more expressed in younger patients (37 have disturbed sleep and 18 have good sleep). Comparison of patients with good/disturbed sleep showed a statistical significance at 8:00 am ($t=2.01$, $p<0.05$) on the first day and at 8:00 am ($t=2.84$; $p<0.01$), 4:00 pm ($t=2.1$; $p<0.05$) and 11:00 pm the second day. These differences were more expressed in females at 8:00 am and 4:00 pm ($t=2.49$; $p<0.02$, $t=2.20$; $p<0.05$) on the first day and at 8:00 am and 11:00 pm ($t=6.94$; $p<0.001$; $t=4.2$; $p<0.02$). Still, one must not overlook the fact that the male group with good sleep consisted of only 2 patients. Concerning patients aged over 40, there was a statistical significance only in females at 4:00 pm ($t=2.5$; $p<0.02$) on the second day. Values of plasma cortisol levels in younger patients with disturbed sleep were almost the same as those of older patients with disturbed sleep. The plasma levels in older group were significantly higher at 08:00 am ($t=2.83$; $p<0.02$) on the second day. Suppressors among younger patients with disturbed/good sleep were 48.65% and 61.11%, and for the older group with disturbed/good sleep were 53.95% and 50.0%.

The abnormality of DST is highly specific for ED (Carroll et al., 1976; Carroll, 1980).

As our group was heterogenous, we formed another group in which were included only the patients with AD (Major depressive disorder, recurrent episode and BAD, current depressive episode). It numbered 134 (40 males, 94 females), 50 (20 males, 30 females) of them were with good night sleep, the remaining 84 (20 males, 64 females) had disturbed sleep. Once again patients with disturbed sleep had higher cortisol levels, which were more expressed on the second day after administration of dexamethasone, and the values are significantly higher for males.

Many authors (Madjirova 2006 and references therein) supported the idea for the interrelationship between cortisol plasma levels and temperature. Aschoff (1978) reported that synchronisation of the cortisol rhythm came after the 24-hour temperature rhythm. Moiseeva (1978) followed for three consecutive days, the temperature rhythm in healthy controls and her conclusion was that people with better adaptation have more stable rhythms. Dirlich et al. (1982) described a case with 48-hour rhythm of mood, temperature, and cortisol. They established that in their geophysical days the core temperature, the circadian sleep-wake rhythm, and the values of free cortisol rhythm in urine were highly synchronised. Some authors (Madjirova 2006 and references therein) found a tendency of the circadian rhythm in depressive patients to run faster, or they spoke of "Free running rhythm". Tsujimoto et al. (2014) ignored their hypothesis and proposed the main reason for rhythm disturbances in AD was connected with the instability of their temperature rhythm.

> *Our results of population mean COSINOR analysis by Halberg for temperature, pulse, and blood pressure in patients with good/disturbed sleep are given on table 2-1. We established that temperature MESORs were higher in patients with good sleep, followed by the group with disturbed sleep. The values of controls (36.387+/-0.79) were significantly lower in comparison with the patients with good sleep (t=2.36; p<0.02). There was no significant difference between the groups with good/disturbed sleep.*

Parameters	Group	No	Mesor	Ampl/	Phase	Peak-hour	Signif.
Temperature	Good sleep	30	36.419+/-0.08	0.53	-239.57	15.58	No
	Disturbed sleep	62	36.408+/-0/08	1.48	-233.21	**15.33** (13.57-17.38	**Yes**
	Healthy	65	36.387+/-0.79	1.28	-244.62	**16.18** (15.07-18.03)	**Yes**
Pulse	Good Sleep	30	82.85+/-2.60	1.02	-155.07	10.20	No
	Disturbed sleep	62	81.06+/-2.2	1.41	-217.93	**14.32** (11.38-17.50)	**Yes**
	Healthy	59	74.83+/-2.69	2.10	-213.83	**14.15** (11.22-17.39)	**Yes**
RR systolic	Good Sleep	7	118.39+/-14.11	1.24	-169.59	11.18	No
	Disturbed sleep	20	120.58+/-7.58	1.58	-287.69	19.17	No
	Healthy	42	126.54+/-6.80	7.13	-12.35	0.49	No
RR Diastolic	Good Sleep	7	82.39+/-6.89	2.60	-96.63	6.27	No
	Disturbed sleep	20	82.09+/-4.2	1.27	-23.51	1.33	No
	Healthy	42	82.67+/-3.27	1.86	-58.95	**3.58** (0.14-9.24)	**Yes**

Table 2-1 Results of population mean COSINOR analysis (F. Halberg) for temperature, pulse and blood pressure in 92 depressed patients with good and disturbed sleep followed two consecutive days

From this study we concluded that patients with disturbed sleep are characterised with:

- *The higher cortisol plasma values;*
- *The lower temperature MESORs;*
- *The percentage distribution of the suppressors/non-suppressors is almost the same in patients with good/disturbed sleep;*
- *Distribution by sex/age shows that the values are higher in the patients with disturbed sleep, and it is more expressed for the older patients (over 40 years).*

Detailed commentary will be given in part III, where it the interrelationship between the stability of the circadian rhythm and the temperature/pulse MENSORs of patients with good/disturbed sleep is observed.

5. The circadian rhythm of temperature, pulse and blood pressure in some psychiatric disorders

5.1. Circadian rhythm of temperature, pulse and blood pressure in healthy persons and psychiatric patients

We must not neglect the fact that the temperature and pulse values are different at the beginning of the disease, during medication with various medication, and after their recovery. The various psychopharmacological drugs could modulate the circadian rhythm too. Desynchronisation is the most spread hypothesis. Halberg was one of the first scientists to document the importance of chronobiology in psychiatry. In 1953 he stressed on the desynchronisation in SCH, and later in depression (Halberg, 1968, Halberg and Cornelisen, 1994). The body temperature cycle of depressed patients may run on an earlier schedule than the same cycle does in healthy people. Many authors (Madjirova 2006 and references therein) support the idea for desynchronisation in AD and SCH. The abnormal circadian rhythm lays in the pathogenesis of mood disorders concerns diurnal variation (Leibenluft, 1996).

We support the idea for desynchronisation of the circadian rhythm of temperature, pulse, blood pressure, mood and vigour.

For this purpose, we followed the daily rhythmic process of temperature and pulse rate for one minute, hour by hour from 7:00 am to 11:00 pm with 2- or 3-night measurements in 515 psychiatric patients and 65 healthy controls. Some of the patients were examined before/after treatment with various psychopharmacological drugs (neuroleptics, antidepressants, tranquilizers), so the total number of cases was 860 (188 with SCH, 365 with AD, depression in recurrent depression and BAD, and 234 with ND). Data were analysed by Halberg's cosinor method. Comparison between the chronograms of temperature and pulse determined by this method showed that MESORs of SCH were significantly higher than those of healthy controls and AD before medication ($t=2.07$; $t=1.96$; $p<0.05$). The temperature in SCH and AD decreased after medication, but not significantly. Peaks of temperature and pulse were noted at different hours in SCH and AD before/after medication. Desynchronisation of SCH, AD *and ND was more obvious on Fig. 2-3. Wirz-Justice (2008) in healthy controls established that mood follows a circadian rhythm with lowest values around the time the core body temperature is at its minimum.*

The received data speak for different mechanisms in the pathogenesis of these psychiatric disorders. We should not neglect the fact that the groups of patients with SCH, AD, and ND were heterogenous, and their subgroups showed some specific signs.

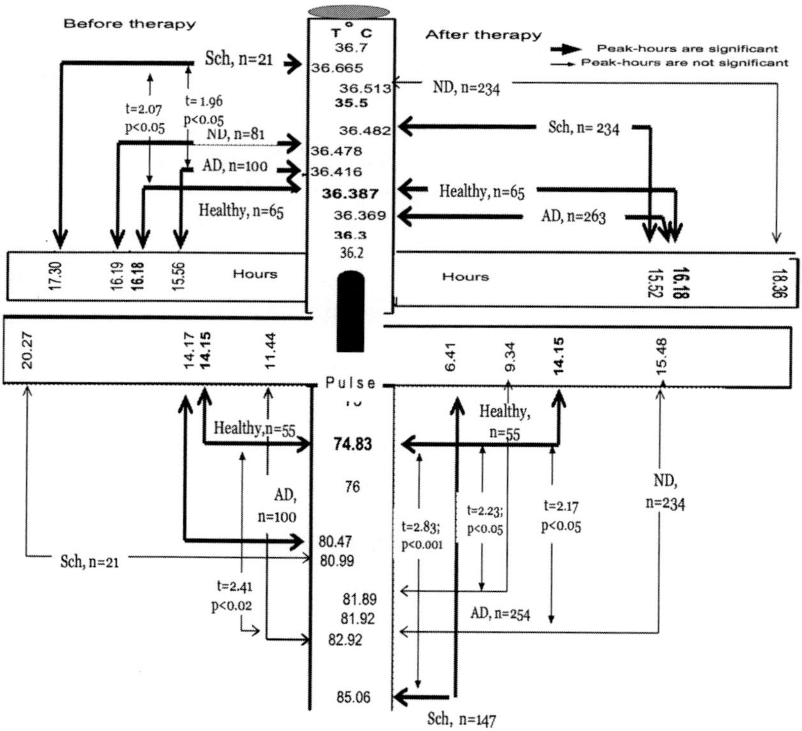

Fig. 2-3. Temperature and pulse MESORs and peak-hours in healthy controls and patients with SCH, AD, and ND before and after therapy.

These data speak for an internal desynchronisation between the rhythms in SCH and AD, and synchronisation in healthy controls. The peaks of patients with ND were synchronised. After therapy they were conditionally synchronised because of the absent peak-hours.

Desynchronisation between the vegetative parameters of SCH and AD were obvious on the population graphic (Fig. 2-4)

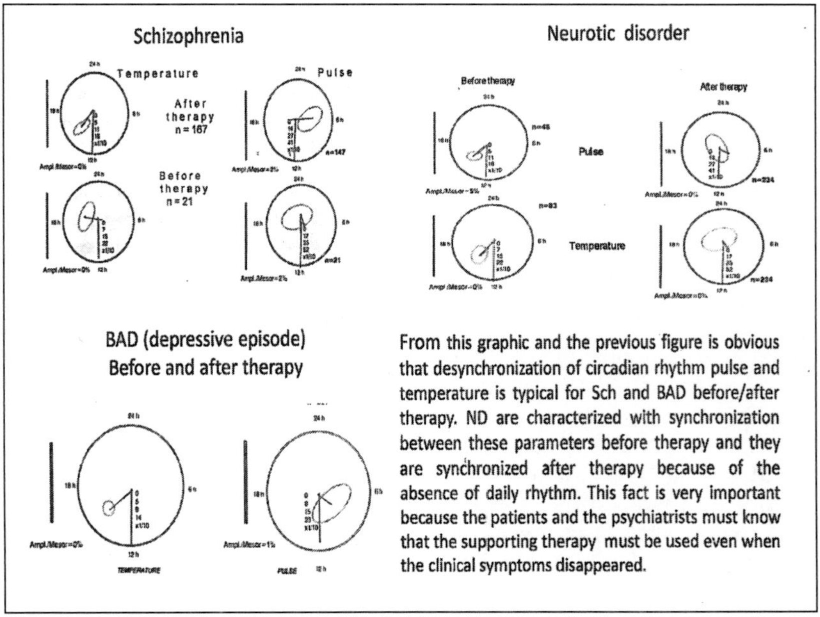

Fig. 2.4. Population graphics in temperature and pulse in patients with SCH, AD and ND

5.2. Schizophrenic disorders

E. Menninger-Lerhenthal (1960) noticed that the temperature during schizophrenic episode was with one degree higher in comparison with the remission period in a female with SCH. Many authors support the hypothesis for desynchronosis in SCH (Madjirova 2006 and references therein) and comment on the necessity of the choice of an appropriate scheme of treatment, an appropriate drug and its diurnal distribution depending on once-daily administration, depending on the drug absorption by the body at the different hours of the day. Thermoregulation in SCH patients is important too (Chong & Castle, 2004). Zarizinskii (1984) advised psychiatrists to have in mind the biological rhythms of the patients during treatment of paranoid SCH.

SCH and disturbed sleep-wake circle is another theory supported by many psychiatrists (Wulff et al., 2012; 2018; Yates, 2016). According to them, the abnormal circadian rhythm in SCH has been associated with sleep disturbances. 30-80% of SCH patients showed such a derangement. They suggested that exogenous melatonin affected both the sleep and the psychic structures. Yates explained the role of sleep and circadian rhythms in regulation of dopamine in psychoses. He supposed that the disturbances in REM-phase were found in SCH and BAD. Sleep played an important role in psychoses predominantly mediated by dopaminergic pathways. Structures of sleep disturbances increased dopamine releasing and sensitivity. His experiments on humans/animals proposed the important role of interplay between sleep and dopamine for psychotic disturbances. The increased dopamine levels disrupted the sleep and the circadian rhythms. Dopamine disruption and psychoses were intricately linked. This suggested that treatment of circadian rhythm is very important for their improvement. Nearly 80% of SCH patients have insomnia, but this connection was neglected.

Wulff et al. (2012), examined the relationship between sleep-wake activity, recorded actigraphically over 6 weeks, along with ambient light exposure and simultaneous circadian clock timing by collecting weekly 48 h profiles of urinary metabolite of melatonin in 20 SCH out-patients and 21 healthy controls matched for age, gender, and employment status. All SCH patients showed significant sleep/circadian disruption. Half of them had severe circadian misalignment raging from phase-advance/delay to non-24 h periods in sleep-wake and melatonin cycles. The other half showed patterns from excessive sleep to highly irregular and fragmented sleep epochs but with normally timed melatonin production. Severe circadian sleep/wake disruptions existed despite stability in mood, mental state, and newer antipsychotics. SCH patients complained of poor sleep and are commonly observed to shift their rest-activity cycle. Even with the introduction of the new antipsychotic drugs, sleep-wake abnormalities are one of the main complaints. Their results show that the circadian timing of the sleep-wake profile and endocrine rhythms were either severely delayed or free running with respect to time of day in SCH patients. Their studies proved that abnormal rest-activity or EEG sleep profiles were associated with increased of psychotic symptoms, decreased cognitive performance, and poor psychosocial outcomes.

Wirz-Justice and al. (1997) remarked that patients with chronic SCH, treated with Haloperidol, had a near-arrhythmic circadian rest-activity cycle, whereas rhythms of 6-sulphatoxy-melatonin and core body temperature were of normal amplitude and phase-advanced. Sleep EEG protocol established a phase-delayed sleep-wake propensity cycle, low sleep continuity (ultradian "boots"), and very little slow-wave sleep and slow-way activity (075-4.5 Hz). Switching the treatment to the atypical neuroleptic clozapine improved both the circadian organisation of the rest-activity cycle and patient's clinical state. High-dose haloperidol treatment may have lowered the circadian alertness threshold, whereas clozapin augmented circadian amplitude (perhaps through its high affinity to dopamine D4 and serotonin 5HT7 receptor in the suprachiasmatic nuclei). Measurements of the circadian rest-activity cycle may be a useful non-invasive method to follow functional consequences of neuroleptic treatment. Bromundt et al. (2011) reported for circadian rest-activity cycles in 3 patients with SCH measured with an actimeter over 48 hours. The range was from highly synchronised to low-amplitude poorly entrained rhythms that they had seen.

> *We established (Madjirova 2006 and references therein) that temperature and pulse in SCH (before/after treatment) were significantly higher than those of the controls (Fig. 2-3). After medication, there were no significant decreases in temperature and increases in pulse. Sex differences were not found. Peaks in temperature and pulse were noted at different times before/after therapy (Fig. 2-4). MESORs and peak-hours for temperature, pulse and blood pressure before/after therapy and controls are given at table 2-2. Thus, it was found an overall internal desynchronisation of physiologic rhythms of SCH, with no correlation of temperature with pulse peaks. This may have implications for the timing of daily treatment (i.e., the importance of circadian rhythm in drug absorption, etc.). Desynchronisation was more demonstrative on the population graphic of population mean cosinor analysis for temperature and pulse on fig. 2-3 and fig. 2-4. However, other factors (such as age, season, sleep disturbances, the stability of circadian rhythm, and the influence of drugs) must first be considered in further studies.*

Maybe the various SCH subgroups could show some specific chronobiological features but such a distribution had not been done as the number of the examined cases before medication is insufficient (21 cases). I suppose that temperature chronograms of SCH and Schizoaffective psychoses will be different too.

At the end of the 19th century, psychiatrists noticed an inversion of the circadian rhythm of vigour in patients with catatonic stupor – these patients became agitated for a short period of time at midnight. The medical staff recognised this inversion of catatonic patients and fed them in the night

(Nadjarov, 1988). We did not prove such inversion in our patients, but we must have in mind the absence of neuroleptics for their treatment at that time. The examination of 6 patients with catatonic stupor, studied for 20 days, showed that their temperature and pulse MESOR was higher, but not significantly compared with the other group SCH patients (see table 2-2). Their peak hours were in the afternoon and not different from the healthy group.

Dg:	Groups	N	Days	MESOR	Peak-hour	Sig-niff.
Temperature						
Healthy		65	65	36.387+/-0.08	**16.18** (15.07-18.03)	**YES**
Sch	Before therapy	21	21	36.665+/-0.116	**17.35** (14.44-17.18)	**YES**
	After therapy	167	167	36.482+/-0.06	**15.52** (14.44-17.18)	**YES**
Stupor	Total group	6	20	36.787+/-0.19	**15.31** (10.17-20.15)	**YES**
Stupors	Febrile catatonia	1	5	37.372+/-0.35	14.48	No
	Catatonic stupor	6	20	36.787+/-0.19	**15.31** (10.17-20.15)	**YES**
	Depressive stupor	1	2	36.133+/-0.26	**13.58**	**YES**
	Psychogenic	1	7	36.684+/-0.23	**17.38**	**YES**
	Organic	1	4	37.785+/-1.32	15.51	No
Pulse rate						
Healthy		55	55	74.83+/-2.69	**14.15** (11.22-17.39)	**YES**
Sch	Before therapy	21	21	80.06+/-1.73	20.27	No
	After therapy	167	167	85.06+/-2.41	**6.41** (3.45-12.47)	**YES**
Stupor	Total group	5	17	91.29+/-5.89	**13.16** (8.16-18.10)	**YES**
Blood Pressure-systolic						
Healthy		42	42	126.0+/-6.80	0.49	No
Sch		14	14	109.0+/-6.83		No
Catatonia		2	2	130+/-9.7	**13.53** (8.16-8.15)	**YES**
Blood Pressure- diastolic						
Healthy		42	42	82.67+/-3.27	**3.58** (0.14-9.24)	**YES**
Sch		14	14	73.43+/-4.71		NO
Stupor	Catatonic stupor	5	17	91.29+/-5.89	**13.16**	**YES**
	Depressive stupor	1	2	82.31	7.40	No

Table 2- 2 Temperature, pulse, and blood pressure MESORs in SCH and catatonic stupor

This study does not support the idea for the inversion of the circadian rhythm in catatonic patients, as reported by Nadjarov (1988). We must not neglect the fact that from one side, the number of this group is not sufficient, and on the other side, and there are the exogenous factors (the medications). Halberg and C. Cornelisen (1994) studied rectal temperature and blood eosinophils in three emotionally disturbed patients before and during 12-hourly electroshocks. One of their patients was in catatonic stupor.

The temperature peaks in our patients with catatonic, depressive, and psychogenic stupor (3.31 pm, 1.58 pm, and 5.38 pm) were not different from the peak-hour of control group (4.18 pm). Common between febrile and organic stupor, was that their temperature was the highest (37.372+/-0.35; 37.785+/-1.32) in comparison with the others and showed no daily fluctuation – they had no expressed peak-hour during the day. The temperature MESOR was lower for depressive stupor.

Psychogenic stupor: We followed twice for 7 days, a young 18-year-old female with psychogenic stupor. Her temperature MESOR (36.684+/-0.132) was also higher in comparison with the other groups and the peak-hour (5.38 pm) was not quite different from the control group. She was followed for about 25 years and in this time, she had several crises. Her clinical picture was characterised with asthenia, decreased working capacity, depressive mood, and disturbed sleep, but she never had psychotic symptoms. She finished university (literature) in Sofia, worked as a librarian, wrote poetry, and published several books. She was married and had one child, but she later divorced.

Exogenous psychoses: We had the chance to follow for 5 days, an 18-year-old girl with exogenous psychosis. Her temperature and pulse were registered hourly for 5 days. Her temperature (37.343+/-0.0638) and pulse (109.64+/-3.02) MESORs were higher in comparison of the other groups. The two parameters did not show daily fluctuation.

Febrile catatonia: The temperature MESOR in a female, 61 years old, with febrile catatonia was not so high (37.372) that we can explain with her age. She had two schizophrenic episodes with catatonic stupor (febrile catatonia). Her first episode was 40 years ago and after that she had a very good remission. Her second episode was again with a febrile catatonia but possibly due to her older age, she did not recover and died.

I would like to pay a special attention to the patient with febrile catatonia. We can see from table 2-2 and fig.2-4 that typical for all psychiatric patients with psychoses, with the exception of exogenous psychoses, febrile catatonia, and organic stupor, is that their temperature was not higher than the temperature in patients with infectious disease. People after serious infectious disease develop immunity until the end of their lives. The high body temperature reflects activation of the immune system. Maybe the same is with the patients that survive after febrile catatonia. In the past, SCH patients were treated with malaria quartana. The increased temperature activated their immune system and their recovery after this therapy. The psychiatrists noticed that some SCH patients improved after serious febrile infection (virus infection with high temperature). These data support the thesis for the disturbed immune system in SCH patients.

The seasonality of SCH was noticed by many scientists (Hare, 1983; Jablenski, 1986; Suvisaari et al., 2001), that most of SCH patients were born in winter/spring. This fact could explain this hypothesis. Seasonal variation of SCH for Europe and USA shows expressed peak in winter and early in spring and the significance is higher (5-11%) in comparison with the total population. Suvisaari et al. (2001) also established that the birth rate among SCH patients in winter and spring months is 5%-8% higher than the birth rate of the general population. Finnish patients with SCH born from 1950 to 1969 (N=15,389) were identified from three nationwide health care registers. Unaffected siblings of these patients born in the same period (N=37,819) were identified from the Finnish National population database. The seasonal variations of birth among patients and siblings were examined by a log-linear model. Explanatory variables were sex, year of birth categorised into four 5-years groups, and seasonal variation, which was analysed by fitting to the monthly birth data. Their conclusion was that seasonal variation of birth among SCH patients may consist of two factors: parental procreation habits, causing a slight excess of births of both patients and unaffected siblings during the winter-spring months; irregular environmental factors that considerably increased the magnitude of the seasonal variation of births among patients but not affect their siblings.

Such seasonality is not found in the other psychic disorders, but it could be spread among other diseases such as diabetes mellitus, malformations of the cardiovascular system, luxatio coxae congenital, and morbus Dawn (Jablensky, 1986). The next lower peak is in autumn. One of the hypotheses is connected with some hormonal cycles in the mother that yet are not established. Jablensky did not exclude internal and prenatal damage of the embryo such as a viral infection. Brain atrophy of some newborn children that develop later SCH resembles the one in children with viral encephalopathy. One of the ideas for SCH is that it is a new disease that appeared in Europe between 17-18th century and its appearance coincides with the measles virus infection (smallpox, chickenpox). One of the last hypotheses is for slow influence virus, and others stress on the association of the human prion gene with SCH (Tsai et al., 2001; D. Stoyanov ,2005).

Pathophysiology of catatonic stupor: Disturbances in sleep and Central Nervous System provoked catatonic states. The cortex brain motor centrums are suppressed during catatonic stupor. Pavlov's opinion for stupor was that at the beginning he analysed the symptoms of the different catatonic states. He realised that patients with stupor fail to react to questions under normal everyday circumstances. On the other hand, he found that if the circumstances were changed, if the same patients were questioned in a soft voice in extremely quiet surroundings, then their reaction was favourable. Pavlov found an analogy here with those phenomena which were seen frequently at the beginning of the experimentally induced sleep, in animals. He noticed that during s. c. "paradoxical" phase the animal loses its reaction to a strong stimulus, while still reacting normally to a weak one. This correlates with the action of the catatonic schizophrenia in a state of stupor, Pavlov interpreted another catatonic symptom, negativism, on the same bases. Many other SCH symptoms similarly bear a striking resemblance to familiar phenomena in normal hypnotised subjects. Among these are stereotypy, echolalia, echopraxia, and catalepsy. Pavlov found a correlation between catatonic stupor and paradoxical phase and negativism and ultra-paradoxical phase.

Saunder (1970) made a commentary about the difference between organic and psychogenic stupor. One of his patients had past history of both cerebrovascular disease and depression, and the other was a 44-year-old female who suffered from left hemiplegia two months before her hospitalisation in a psychiatric department. After slow intravenous application of 5% sodium amilibarbitone their uncommunicativeness was overcome. Their therapy was ECT.

Future perspectives

To be studied were the chronograms of some vegetative/biochemical parameters (temperature, pulse and blood pressure, plasma levels of cortisol, dopamine and melatonin) in various SCH subgroups: paranoid SCH, disorganised SCH (also known as hebephrenic SCH); catatonic SCH, undifferentiated schizophrenia, residual schizophrenia. These data can give us information for their chronograms in understanding their pathogenesis and the best medication for their improvement.

The examination of the circadian rhythm in schizoaffective psychosis will help the psychiatrists to understand its place between SCH and BAD.

5.3.Affective disorders (AD)

From the middle of the 20th century many publications about the circadian rhythm in patients with AD appeared (Madjirova 2006 and references therein). Salvatore et al. (2008) reported about the circadian rhythm abnormalities in ill and recovered bipolar I disorder patients. Linkowski et al. (1985) studied the 24-hour profile of adrenocorticotropin and cortisol in major depression, and ACTH, cortisol, and growth hormone 24-hour profile in major depressive illness. Wood et al. (2009) commented on the different circadian phase between BD and controls. Pflug & Martin (1980) made analysis of circadian temperature rhythm in ED. Pflug et al. (1976) had a long-term study of depression and manic-depressive states and daily temperature. Souêtre et al. (1989) evaluated the circadian rhythms in depression and during recovery: the main chronobiological abnormality is the blunted amplitude. Actigraphic assessments of circadian activity and sleep patterns in BAD were performed by Jones et al. (2003).

The examinations of the circadian rhythms of these patients are very important for the pathogenesis. Di Gaspero in 1927, (cited by Mendlewicz, et al., 1983), E. Menninger-Lerhenthal (1960), B. Pflug et al. (1976), D. Kripke et al. (1979) established that patients with ED had a higher temperature during depression and it then normalised after recovery. Faravelli et al. (1985) did not find any temperature and pulse differences before/after medication. The above-mentioned authors and Beersma et al. (1983) did not establish desynchronisation in patients, while AD. Halberg in 1968 suggested that some, but not all, circadian rhythms in such patients were not synchronised with 24-hour day-night cycle. According to his hypothesis, the interaction between the unsynchronised "free-running" rhythms and the normally synchronised (entrained) rhythms causes switches back and forth between mania and depression. Many authors reported that the abnormal circadian rhythm lies in the pathogenesis of mood disorders concerned with diurnal variation (Madjirova 2006 and references therein). According to Bicakova-Rocher et al. (1996) patients with AD were characterised with a temperature rhythm shorter than 24 hours; this fact explained their desynchronisation. Many scientists supported this idea.

Kuhs et al. (1989) studied 25 patients with ED (according to ICD-9) and 12 healthy controls. The participants had to estimate prospectively a 30-s interval on two successive days at 7.30 am, 11.30 am, 3.30 pm, and 7.30

pm. Even in daily courses with "typical" diurnal variation an increasingly favourable self-assessment of well-being was not accompanied by a corresponding diurnal fluctuation of time estimation. These data cast doubt on the significance of "typical" diurnal variations in depression symptomatology.

Germain & Kupfer (2008), Boyce & Barriball (2010) endorsed the hypothesis for circadian rhythm disruption in depression and stress the role of the circadian and sleep rhythm in their pathogenesis and their treatment. According to them, sleep and waking are the most obvious circadian rhythms of mammals. Depressed patients often showed altered circadian rhythms, sleep disturbances, and diurnal mood variations.

Manic-depressive disorders are linked to disturbances of internal synchronisation of bodily functions in the circadian frequency range (Giedke and Pflug, 1994). Novakova et al. (2015) reported that patients with BAD differ in manic and depressive episodes. Diurnal variation during the depressive phase and healthy periods were investigated in 84 hospitalised depressive patients. They concluded that depression induced rhythmicity: those belonging to the arrhythmic group when healthy, showed a significant increase in rhythmicity when depressed, predominantly the classical form of diurnal variation (morning with improvement towards evening). Age and sex were important factors for diurnal variation. In the course of hospitalisation, the type of diurnal rhythm remained individually constant.

Joug-HoMoon al. (2016) established advanced circadian phase in mania and delayed circadian phase in mixed mania and depression returned to normal after treatment of BAD.

Gonzalez et al. (2014) studied by actigraph, 42 patients with BAD and found interrelationship between affective state & rhythmic activity in BAD. Rhythm disruption was a marker of BAD. The integral conception was that rather than there being a stable change in the absolute timing of the circadian clock, there was an inherent instability in the circadian system and therefore an increased sensitivity toward temporal disorganisation of physiological rhythms. Disturbances in the levels of sleep and inherent locomotor activity were noticed in manic and depressive phase of BAD. They showed less stable circadian activity patterns, a greater inherent activity, and a greater variability by the use of actigraph. The greater severity of affective symptoms and a decrease in the circadian rhythmic activity was typical. Mania showed greater rhythm disturbances than depression. Manic symptoms correlated with a lower degree of rhythmicity and less robust rhythms of locomotors activity, as indicated by lower 24-hour autocorrelation and circadian quotient variables, respectively. This finding shows a relationship between mood state, symptom severity, and rhythm disturbances of locomotors activity in BAD. Carr et al. (2018) wrote of desynchronisation of diurnal rhythms in BAD and borderline personality disorder.

Kivelä et al. (2018) stress on the importance of evening type. Eveningness was related to endogenous depression; these included worse symptoms severity, poorer prognoses, and higher seasonal mood variation among evening types. Among depressed individuals, evening types tended to exhibit worse symptom severity and report increased psychological distress, higher suicidality, and greater impairment in their daily lives (including work). Eveningness has previously been associated with depressive symptoms in university students.

Tsujimoto et al. (2010) did not find a statistically significant differences between medicated/unmedicated patients or either, 24-hour autocorrelation, and circadian quotient scores (cited in Thommen & George, 1972). The particular medications used to treat the illness may exert some of their therapeutic action via their influence on endogenous molecular clocks. For example, both lithium and valproic acid have been shown to influence the rhythmic expression of circadian genes and rhythmic properties of molecular clock. Unmedicated patients, in comparison with medicated patients, showed higher YMRS (Young Mania Rating Scale) score and no differences in locomotor rhythms were observed between the groups. These findings suggest that maybe other factors are related to the manic state. The interrelationship between various markers of rhythms also could be noted. In the 24-hour autocorrelation and circadian quotient scores there was a relationship between the degree of circadian rhythmic processes and the robustness of circadian rhythms. While a correlation between circadian quotient and YMRS score was found, there was established no correlation between the severity of manic symptoms and either amplitude or MESOR in disturbances of rhythm. These data support the conception for the interrelationship between biological rhythm and BAD. The central circadian pacemaker influenced the locomotors activity, while it was affected by many other variables and was not considered a robust marker of the central circadian clock. Future studies would benefit from the use of more refined chronobiological protocols to characterise and quantify rhythm disturbances and functioning of the central circadian clock in bipolar patients. Even with the limitations noted above, actigraphy present a unique method to objectively and longitudinally access chronobiological variables in bipolar patients. Their study supports the concept that there is a significant mood instability associated with affective states in BAD. They found a relationship between mania and rhythm disturbances. They demonstrated the ability to measure rhythm disturbances, utilising actigraphy in patients with BAD. Ambulatory monitoring of activity patterns in conjunction with other chronobiological biomarkers may be valuable assessments that could be potentially serve as physiological biomarkers of the illness and could lead to potential refinement of endophenotypes in bipolar disorder.

Tsujimoto et al. (2014) followed the deep body temperature every two hours for two consecutive days in 65 psychiatric patients, 38 of them were with major depressive episodes. Their results showed that the amplitude of body temperature in depressive patients was significantly less than that of the control group. They found a positive correlation between the MESOR and the severity of the depressive symptoms. The body temperature both in depressive/manic state tended to fluctuate much as not only to fit to sinusoid curves, but also to reduce the periodicity of the circadian rhythm. They concluded that the rhythm disturbances in AD were not the phase shift but the instability of the temperature circadian rhythm.

> *We established that temperature and pulse chronograms are different for the various types of circadian rhythm. We decided to understand the chronogram in patients when the two consecutive days were with the same/different type circadian rhythm. In 1985 from 7:00 am to 7:00 pm, we recorded hourly the temperature and pulse in 39 depressive patients. They were divided into two groups: A –27 patients who were with arrhythmic type rhythm of mood on both days, and B – 12 patients who had different rhythm of mood across the two days. The temperature chronogram in group A was almost the same during the two days, but pulse peak on the first day was at 8:00 pm, and the 2nd day was 4 hours earlier. The chronograms of temperature and pulse in group B were quite different during the following two days. Temperature peak was one hour earlier on the 2nd day. Pulse peaks were at 12:00 am and 6:00 pm the first day and at 10:00 am and 9:00 pm on the second day. Desynchronisation between temperature and pulse was obvious for the two groups.*

New findings on desynchronisation in clock gene expression may illustrate chronobiological vulnerability for depression and affect dysregulation. The clock genes in the SCN gradually adapt to a phase shift of the light-dark cycle (as found in shift work, transmeridian flight), whereas clock genes in the muscle, liver, and lung resynchronise at their own rates. This results in a "double desynchronisation," "internal desynchronisation" between different clocks in the body and brain, and “external desynchronisation” between the timing of body rhythms with respect to the light-dark cycle.

Haug and Fahndrich (1994) did not find any correlation between the severity of depression and any various measures of diurnal mood variation in a group of 70 patients. Their observations did not support theories of chronobiological rhythm disturbances in depression. Haug (1989) reported that diurnal variation of mood predicts sleep deprivation-outcome from one side and commented on the frequency of this variation in various psychiatric patients. Hamon and Boyer (2005) discussed new perspectives in the pathophysiology and give some tendencies in the treatment of depressions.

Kronfeld-Schor & Einat (2012) supported the connection between rhythm and depression. One of the limitations of related research is the lack of good animal models.

Wirz-Justice (2000) established differences between MESORs, peaks, and acrophase of depressive patients with first episode and chronic-depressives. Patients in their first episode showed a decrease in amplitude compared to the controls and there was a reduction in chronic patients with chronic depression. According to her, the amplitude differences are due to the subject's different activity levels because these differences were reduced according to the severity of the illness. The increased circadian amplitude in rest-activity rhythm of healthy subjects could be explained by the increased entrainment to external Zeitgebeger, most likely by the maintenance of robust social and biological Zeitgebers that are essential for life.

Souêtre et al. (1989) established that the comparison between 16 patients with AD, 15 recovered after 3 weeks treatment with antidepressants and 16 HC, shows that the depressed patients showed clear circadian rhythm abnormalities, consisting mainly of amplitude reduction. Normal circadian profiles were restored after recovery when the amplitude, in particular, was increased. Features of the circadian rhythms observed in remission may be associated with antidepressant drug effects, whereas those observed in depression resemble the circadian rhythms observed in normal subjects living under conditions of temporal isolation and those of blind subjects. Our findings suggest that depression may be related both to a weakening of the coupling processes between internal pacemakers and to an abnormal sensitivity to environmental information.

Schulz ***(2007) arguments for and against chronobiological changes in mood*** *(Shuaib & Haq, 1977).*

Arguments for l changes in mood:

- Many functions that are altered during depression are regulated by biological clocks, for example, sleep or feeding.
- The severity of depressive symptoms changes with a daily regular pattern; a few patients with AD suffer from regular cycles of relapse.
- The existence of sad, and the beneficial role of light in sad and in nonseasonal depression.
- The observation that a number of blinded subjects have free running periods and feel depressed when the rhythms are out of phase in relation to the astronomical time, e.g., when hormones that should be secreted during night-time, are secreted during the day.
- The efficacy of sleep deprivation and the possible benefits of advance in sleep phase.
- The changes of the circadian rhythm of many variables during depression.
- The modified sensitivity to the melatonin suppressing effect of light in bipolar patients and in their descendants.
- Most antidepressants and mood stabilisers influence endogenous rhythms in free-running conditions in animals. Sleep deprivation and light therapy also modify biological clock physiology. Lithium might act on biological clocks through its effect on glycogen syntheses 3 (GSK3).
- Circadian genes might be associated with bipolar disorder.
- Polymorphism of the clock gene might correlate with some aspects of sleep in patients with BAD.

Mutation of clock gene in mice renders these animals hyperactive, with little need to sleep and a high threshold for anxiety, i.e., they somewhat resemble a manic patient.

Arguments against chronobiological changes in mood:

- A single administration of a compound such as corticotrophin releasing hormone to animals acutely induces behaviours homogenous to human anxiety and depression.

- Most animal models of depression do not primarily involve biological clocks (however, the chronic mild stress model does not include perturbation in the rhythms of Zeitgebergs exposure).
- Most humans who have glossy perturbed rhythms, for example during jet lag, do not develop clinical depression.
- Melatonin secretion pattern does not show important changes during depression.
- Most subjects with low melatonin levels (cardiac patients on β-blocking drugs, tetraplegics) are not depressed.

In another table the author summarised the findings of the chronotype as a risk factor for psychiatric disorders. According to him eveningness is related to AD and especially depression; these include symptoms severity, poor prognosis, and higher seasonal mood variation among evening types.

Mitsutake et al. in 2000 commented on a clinically healthy 34-year-old male who filled out the PA/NA (positive affect/negative affect) scale (PANAS) five times a day for 86 days. Automatically at 30-minute intervals (19.05-29.06.2000) heat rate (HR) and SBP/DBP were measured by an ambulatory monitor, while different endpoints of heart rate variability (HRV) were determined at 5-minute intervals from beat-to-beat ECG monitoring for 42 days. Saliva samples were collected at the times of mood ratings for one month for later determination of melatonin and cortisol concentrations were recorded at intervals of 24 hours. A positive association was noteworthy between the circadian amplitude of NA and the MESOR of both SBP and DBP, suggesting that BP is raised in the presence of large swings in NA. Needing further validation was a weak association between the MESOR of NA and the circadian SBP amplitude ($r = -0.272$; $P = 0.108$), suggesting a lowering of the circadian SBP amplitude in the presence of a strong NA.

Cornelisen et al. (2015) studied 196 students, who completed a mood rating scale 7 times a day for a week with 3 hours intervals. The mood was registered by PANAS. The circadian/circaseptan acrophases differ between PA/NA as evidenced by the non-overlap of the respective 95% confidence intervals for the acrophase. The 84-hour (half-week) and 12-hour (half-day) component were also detected with statistical significance (except for the 12-hour component in NA), suggesting that the circadian/circaseptan waveforms departed from sinusoidality. The weekly and half-weekly amplitudes were larger than the circadian amplitude for NA, whereas in the case of PA, the circadian variation was most prominent. The patterns in relative data (expressed as a percentage of student's average value), clearly illustrate the differences in relative circaseptan vs. circadian prominence and in the acrophase of each component between PA/NA. In MDD, a circadian rhythm in blood eosinophils may gauge a free-running adrenal cycle and was associated with overt infradian changes in mood as extreme as alternating bipolar states.

Chronobiological characteristic of AD according to Joung-HoMoon et al. (2016), Wirz-Justice (2008) and Son et al. (2016) is:

- *BD in acute mood episodes showed circadian dysregulation due to phase shifts which returned to normal treatment;*
- *Acute manias were ~ 7 h circadian phase advanced;*
- *Mixed manias were > 6 h delayed;*
- *Depressions were 4-5 h delayed compared to the controls;*
- *Circadian dysregulation due circadian rhythm phase shifts might be a pathophysiological mechanism of BD.*

They included 31 mood episodes of 26 BD patients, and 18 controls. All participants wore wrist actigraphs during the studies and cortisol levels in saliva were measured for two consecutive days. One BD patient was observed in both manic/depressive episodes during different hospitalisations. In sum, 31 mood episodes requiring hospitalisation of 26 BD patients were analysed. Their conclusion was that the patients did not show significant differences in any parameters for physical activity in comparison with healthy controls, neither in recovery nor during acute mood exacerbations. *Patients with depression showed about 4-5 hour delayed biochemical circadian acrophases at the start of hospitalisation, and then recovered through advances to the normal ranges of the control group. Significant differences of cortisol and gene expression circadian rhythms were seen in acute depressive states when compared with those of recovered states.*

Azorin & *Kaladjian* (2009) reported that changes in circadian rhythms were an integral part of the clinical features of ED, and particularly of seasonal depressions. The most classical changes were amplitude modifications, fluctuations, and periodicity of the hormonal secretion rhythms. The leading models include free course, phase advance (or instability), and hypnic models, or those on disturbances of the internal clock. The main psychopathological model is those of endokinesis and psychosocial desynchronisation. The therapeutic applications of the pathophysiological models use manipulation of the wake-sleep cycle, phototherapy, and melatonin and its derivatives. Those of the pathophysiological models used time-space management and development of resynchronisation capacities. The question determining whether these adverse changes were a cause or effect of depressive behaviour is unresolved.

Moraes et al. (2013) found lower amplitude in the circadian rhythm activity and light exposure, but a higher amplitude in the rhythm of peripheral temperature in depressed patients. The comparison between the values of temperature and activity of the control group and the depressed patients was that the depressed patients had lowest temperature values during the day.

We have in mind that some psychiatrists found specific clinical and genetic features in patients with ID and patients with PD. According to ICD-8 and ICD-9 they were with different codes (296.0 & 296.2 for ID and 296.13 and 296.2 for PD). In the new DSM-IV, DSM-V, and ICD-10 there is no code for ID.

Tashev in 1979 during the examination of 1173 patients with manic-depressive psychoses, who were followed until their death, determined 6 clinical subtypes: intermittent depression -ID (55.16%); recurrent depressive disorder - RDD (17.31%); one phase depression (3.07%); bipolar type (16.71%), periodic mania (6.56%); one phase mania (1.19%). Approximately 92% of the evaluated patients were ID, RDD and BAD. He established specific clinical signs and inheritance for each group. Several years later T. Tashev proved the same results with another contingent.

Having in mind Tashev's results and the ICD-8 and ICD-9, we decided to study the circadian rhythm of patients with RDD, ID and BAD (depressive phase). By Halberg's cosinor method we determined their peak-hours, MESORs, phases and amplitudes of temperature, pulse and BP in 267 patients with AD, and 110 of them were with RDD, 122 with ID and 35 with BAD (depressive phase). 90 of them were examined before/after therapy (50 with RDD, 25 with ID and 15 with BAD). As we found specific changes in temperature MESORS and peak-hour, the other two parameters (pulse and blood pressure) will not be a subject of discussion. The pulse rate was almost the same in all groups and they did not show an expressed peak-hour during the day. The various subgroups of AD showed some specific chronobiological features of temperature. The temperature MESOR of RDD (36.57 C) before medication was significantly higher in comparison with the MESOR of ID (36.254 C). After medication the temperature MESOR of PD decreased (36.427 C), whereas the MESOR of ID was increased (36.378 C). The patients with BAD (depressive episode) showed no dynamic of MESORs before (36.378 C) and after medication (36.346 C) and were not different from the MESORs of healthy controls (36.387 C). The peak-hours of the patients with RDD and ID before/after therapy were in the afternoon: 5.27 pm/4.03 pm, 4.30pm/4.24pm. Their peaks were not different from the peaks of healthy controls (4.18 pm). Patients with BAD (depressive episode) did not have an express peak-hour before therapy (Figure 2-5).

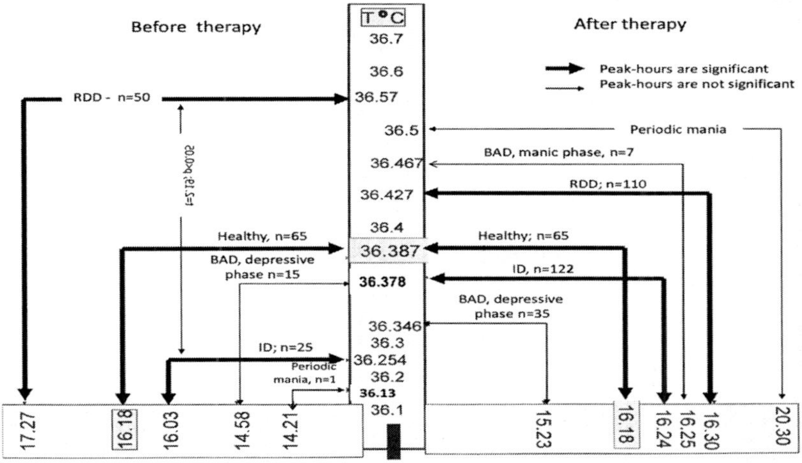

Fig.2-5. Temperature MESORs and peak-hours in RDD (recurrent depressive disorder), ID (involution depression), BAD (depressive phase) and BAD (manic phase).

These data give us the answer why some authors (Pflug et al., 1976; 1985) report that the temperature MESOR was higher in comparison with the healthy group. Others say that it was almost the same as the MESOR of the healthy controls, and a third group (Tricckas et al., 1983; 1984; Faravelli et al., 1985) established that it was lower. The different results could be explained with the fact that the groups were quite heterogeneous, and the sample size too small.

In my clinical practice only one patient (62 years male) with periodic mania was observed. He was followed for two consecutive days before and 2 days after medication. His temperature, pulse, and blood pressure MESORs before therapy were 36.313 C; 75.83 and 160.44/98.64, and after therapy 36.41 C; 78.17; 163.70/100.46. All parameters, with the exception of DBP (peak-hour is in 01.59pm, before therapy), showed no daily fluctuation.

We evaluated the same parameters in 7 patients with BAD (manic phase) and their values were: 36.467C; 86.61; 128.03/89.79. Desynchronosis in this group is obvious: temperature and DBP show no daily rhythm, whereas pulse peak is at 3:09 pm and SBP is at 11.28 am. We did not have the ability to study the patients with BAD (manic phase) before medication.

For periodic mania we could not make any serious conclusion as the number of the observed patients was only one.

The use of psychotropic drugs

Di Gaspero in 1927 (cited in Mendlewicz, et al., 1983) followed the temperature of 3 patients with ED. In that period psychiatrists did not use any psychopharmacological drugs. He established that their temperature during depression was higher, and it decreased after clinical recovery. All of them were in involution age. His data are the opposite of ours. This fact could be explained that their temperature was not measured each hour and from our studies was established that the temperature fluctuated during the day. He did not give any information about the circadian rhythm of mood, their temperament, nor their sleep.

In our previous studies we established that the daily temperature in AD and ND depends on the type of the circadian rhythm (morning, evening, arrhythmic, fluctuating), seasons of the year, sleep problems, temperament, stability of rhythm of mood, and the therapy (Madjirova, 1988; 1995; 1997; 2006; 2013). These factors were not mentioned, but it is certain that they did not use any psychopharmacological drugs.

Davis (1981) thought that the circadian rhythm was transformed with age and supposed that it was connected with the change of the rhythm amplitude in older age, and it could even disappear (Madjirova, 1987; 2006). According to Daan and Ashoff (1974) and Pittendrigh (1981), in old animals a phase advance of the circadian rhythm can be observed. R. Wever (1979) commented that this phenomenon was a predisposition for AD in old people. Most of the scientists and geneticists are sure that phase advance depends on individual genetic predisposition of the persons and their circadian pacemaker (Madjirova 2006 and references therein). Mendlewiich et al. (1979) reported an abnormal 24-hour pattern of melatonin secretion in depression and studied chronobiological neuroendocrine, sleep and EEG parameters. Later in 2009 he announced a disruption of the circadian timing on molecular mechanisms in depression.

The findings of Czeisler et al. (1999) are very important for understanding the pathophysiology of disturbed sleep in older people. According to Weiner & Waterhouse (2006) the circadian rhythm of core temperature depended upon several interacting rhythms of both endogenous/exogenous origins. The observed circadian rhythm of body temperature varied with the age; in comparison with the adults, it was poorly developed in neonates and deteriorated in the older subjects. Comparing masked and purified data enabled the reasons for these differences – whether due to the body clock, the effectors pathways or organs, or irregularities due to the individual's lifestyle – to begin to be understood. Such investigations stress the immaturity of the circadian rhythm in the human neonate and its deterioration in the elderly compared with younger subjects, but they also indicate the robustness of the body clock itself into advanced age, at least in mice.

In order to exclude the influence of the age, *a comparison between the values of RDD in involution age and ID was done. All patients with RDD before 45 years were excluded.* We established that temperature MESOR of RDD in involution age before therapy (36.485C) was higher in comparison with ID (36.254), and after medication it decreased to the values of healthy group. Whereas in ID it increased but again was lower in comparison with healthy and RDD (Fig. 2-5). Their peak-hours were in the afternoon and were not different from the healthy controls. Desynchronosis between temperature and pulse was typical for the whole group of AD before/after therapy (see fig. 2-3; fig. 2-4). Daily fluctuations of pulse disappeared in all groups of patients with AD. Temperature peaks were in the afternoon and were higher or lower in comparison with the healthy controls. Sex distribution was almost the same.

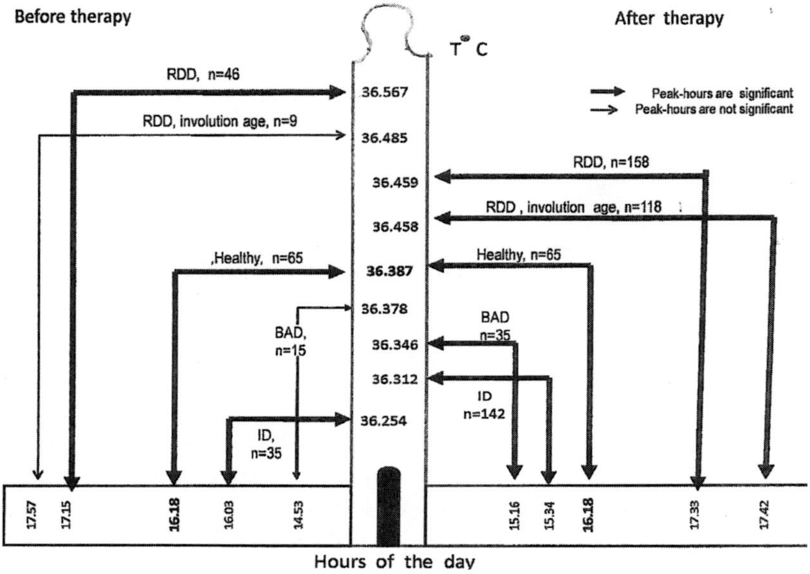

Fig.2-6. Temperature MESORs and the peak-hours before and after therapy in RDD, RDD in involution age, ID and BAD (depressive episode).

Desynchronisation of RDD (in involution age), ID, RDD, and BAD (depressive phase) was more obvious in their population graphic (see fig. 2-7). Typical for all of them was that pulse showed no daily rhythmicity, whereas temperature was with expressed peak-hour in the afternoon for all groups, but at different hours.

These results showed that ID was characterised with some specific chronobiological features and it is necessary to think about its place in the future classifications. The different chronobiological models of ID, RDD, and BAD (depressive phase) could speak also for some specific features in their pathogenesis.

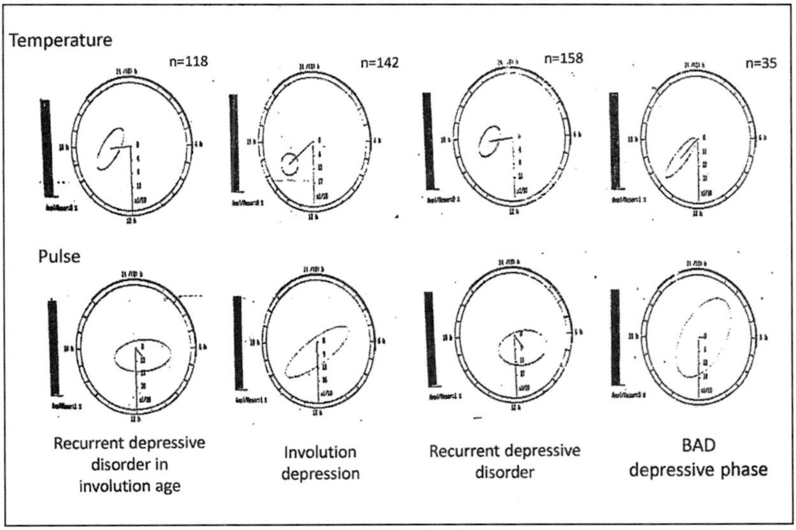

Fig.2-7. Population graphics determined by Halberg's COSINOR method in depressive patients after therapy with RDD in involution age, involution depression, RDD and Bipolar Affective Disorder (depressive phase).

Recommendations for future studies:

- *To examine the chronobiological rhythm of the various subgroups in AD on a greater number of patients who must be examined before, after medication and during their remission period.*
- *The determination of the various subgroups to be proved by the circadian rhythms of other parameters – cortisol plasma levels, melatonin and s.o..*
- *To determine the place of ID in the future classifications.*
- *The examination of the circadian rhythm of BAD-type I, BAD-type II, and cyclothymia provides additional information about their pathogenesis.*

Conclusion

The results suggest that disturbances in biological rhythms present in all ***subgroups of AD, before and after medication.*** *Modern studies can give us information about their pathogenesis and their chronobiological model* *could orient us for the best drug and its use at the most suitable time of the day.*

5.4.Neurotic disorders (ND)

> *My review on the circadian rhythms in psychiatric disorders established that most publications were connected with rhythmicity in AD, followed by SCH. Even chronobiological studies of ND are rare. Psychiatrists at the end of the 19th century and at the middle of the 20th century noticed that patients with ND feel better in the morning (Madjirova 2006 and references therein). Shumilina et al. (1956) used hypothermia in experimental neurosis in dogs. Rose et al. (1982) studied the experimental neuroses and Poppei et al. (1982) advise the supporting therapy to continue 3-6 months after clinical improvement, because the synchronisation of the internal circadian rhythms comes later.*

Gorwood (2012) in his review stressed on the importance of the circadian rhythm in anxiety disorders. Their abnormal rhythms could explain some symptoms and some risk factors that provoke AD. According to him, abnormal cortisol circadian rhythm was proposed as a mediating factor between early stress and later anxiety disorder. It is interesting that anxious patients have more abnormal social rhythms than HC. It is surprising that the circadian variability in anxiety disorders was less obvious than in mood disorders.

Murray et al. (2002) suggested that neuroticism was characterised with a weakened circadian rhythm. They found that HC with high neuroticism was characterised with attenuated circadian amplitudes in unmasked body temperature. Also hypothesized, Positive Affect exhibited a circadian rhythm that was only significant in the Lower group (diurnal rhythm in positive affect). They established a stronger synchronisation between the biological and psychological rhythms that were observed in the group with low neuroticism. The results of their examination on 48 patients with anxiety disorders and 41 controls, showed that patients reported a significantly lower frequency of rhythmicity of daily life activities in comparison with the HC. Considering abnormal circadian rhythms as important factors in anxiety disorders does not only require that sleep disorders are both associated with the risk factors for anxiety but also that these patients have abnormal social rhythm.

Beĭer (2007)'s results showed that the specific activity of anxiolytic and antidepressant drugs and the function of brain structures controlled rhythmical processes.

In the group of ND were included 187 patients: 79 of them were studied before medication and 234 during the treatment with various antidepressant drugs or tranquilizers, others during two or more hospitalisation, so the total number of examined patients was 317 patients. All the patients, from 7:00 am to 11:00 pm with 1-3 night-measurements, had their temperature and pulse, and half of the group had blood pressure, recorded hourly.

Before therapy the temperature MESOR for the whole group patients with ND was significantly higher in comparison with AD (t=2.07; p<0.05) and HC (t=1.96; p<0.05), pulse MESOR was higher in comparison with healthy (t=2.41; p<0.02) and the two vegetative parameters were synchronised (see fig. 2-3; fig. 2-4). The individual parameters show that 35.19% for temperature and 20% for pulse retained the daily rhythmicity. Temperature peak early in the morning was 6.79%, in the afternoon and evening it was 28.40%, and the rest showed no daily rhythmicity. BP will not be discussed as it does not show typical chronobiological features. After medication, the daily rhythmical process of temperature and pulse disappeared, and they were synchronised because of the absence of daily rhythmicity.

As the group of ND was heterogeneous the patients were distributed according to their subgroups. We evaluated several subgroups of ND according to ICD-10:

- F40.0 - Phobic anxiety disorder (300.2); n = 48;
- F41.1 - Generalised anxiety disorder (300.02); n = 47;
- F43 - Adjustment disorder with depressed mood (309.0); n = 24;
- F44 - Dissociative disorder (300.11); n = 23;
- F.48.0 - Neurasthenia; n = 48.

The various subgroups before therapy *(see fig. 2-8):*

- The tendency for higher temperature/pulse MESORs remained in all subgroups ND, but the values were not significant because of the small number of studied people.
- Patients with general anxiety disorders did not have an expressed temperature and pulse peak during the day and they were relatively synchronised.

- Phobic anxiety disorders - temperature and pulse peaks were not different from the peaks of the HC, they were in the afternoon and were synchronised.
- Desynchronisation between the two vegetative parameters was typical for Neurasthenia and Dissociative disorders.

Chronograms of the various subgroups after therapy (see fig. 2-8):

- MESORs of temperature and pulse in all groups were not significantly higher for temperature and pulse, with the exception of adjustment disorder with depressed mood, in comparison with the HC.
- Daily rhythmicity disappeared for pulse in all studied groups.
- Temperature peaks in general anxiety and dissociative disorders were in the afternoon near by the hours of the HC. They were desynchronised with the pulse.
- Phobic anxiety disorders, adjustment disorders with depressed mood, and neurasthenia showed no daily rhythmicity of temperature and were relatively synchronised with the pulse.

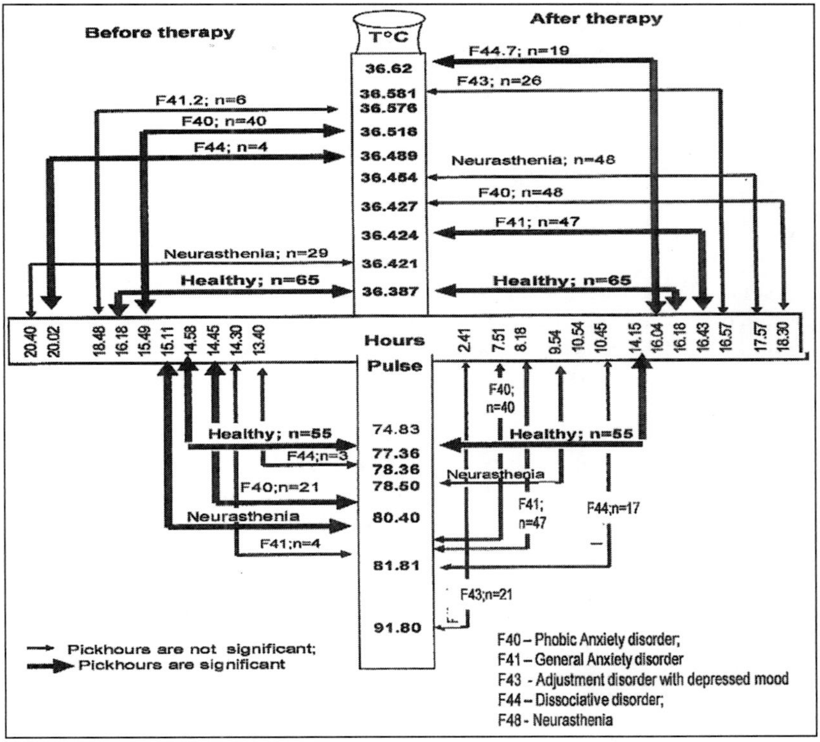

Fig. 2-8 MESORs and peak-hours of temperature and pulse in various subgroups ND

6. How can antidepressants and mood stabilisers change circadian rhythm in patients with ND and AD?

The question whether some psychotropic drugs are capable of altering the circadian rhythm of temperature and pulse is disputable and their viewpoints are quite different.

6.1 Antidepressants

Some authors assume that antidepressants can slow/dissociate the circadian rhythm in depressive patients. Moreas et al. (2013) thought that the changes in chronobiological parameters may be related with the medication of antidepressant treatment used in chronically depressed patients. Montes et al. (1997) established that acrophase was bigger in experimental rats treated with clomipramine in comparison with control group. They also found decreased period length of motor activity circadian rhythm in a rat model ED.

The first studies of antidepressants were done by Wehr et al. (1975), Surgue (1981), Wirz-Justice and Campbell (1982), Wehr and Wirz-Justice (1982), Wehr et al. (1982), Giedke and Pflug (1994), Wirz-Justice and Wehr (1983). They established that antidepressants could delay or accelerate the circadian rhythm. Duncan et al. (1995) and Duncan (1996) established that antidepressants could delay the circadian rhythm of body temperature, without changing its amplitude and MESOR in experimental rats. There were no data about these changes when the drugs were given for a longer period of time.

These results correlate with our data – temperature peak-hour (17.10 h) was later with 1.52 hours in comparison with HC. Kripke et al. (1979) established the effect of Lithium carbonate on the circadian rhythm of sleep in normal people, whereas Le Sauter & Silver (1993) proved that Lithium could lengthen the free-running period of the circadian rhythm (LeSauter & Silver, 1993). Pettegrew et al. (2001) discussed the effect of chronic administration of lithium.

Germain & Kripke (2008) discussed the effect of antidepressant drugs on the circadian rhythm and sleep rhythm: although there is variation between individual drugs, tricyclic antidepressants (TCAs) generally shorten sleep latency and improve sleep continuity in depressed patients and may be associated with daytime drowsiness. Most TCAs (tricyclic antidepressants) increased REM sleep latency and reduced the percentage of REM sleep, normalised the disturbed sleep architecture in the depressed patients. According to Rush et al. (1989) the reduced REM latency at baseline predicts a positive response to TSAs treatment.

A great number of the scientific studies of psychopharmacological drugs are connected with the influence of agomelatine and melatonin on the circadian rhythm of the depressive patients. According to Reeth et al. (2001) melatonin or melatonin agonist corrects age-related changes in circadian response to environmental stimulus. Monk et al. (1997) found relationship between melatonin, temperature, cortisol, and mood.

Antidepressants influenced the circadian rhythm (Brown, Seggie, 1988). An increase in REM sleep latency was found to predict clinical response in patients treated with amitriptyline (Kupfer et al., 1981), and antidepressant activity across different drugs was found to be related to their capacity to suppress REM sleep (Vogel, 1983). REM sleep changes with antidepressant medications may reflect underlying the circadian effect.

Some antidepressants (Agomelatine) can advance the circadian phase (Banasr, et al., 2006; Boer, et al., 2005). Agomelatine can entrain free-running circadian rhythm in rats kept in total darkness in a similar way to melatonin. According to Cajachen et al. in 1997 the administration of agomelatine and melatonin 5 hours before bed established increased REM sleep duration and REM sleep percentage in the first part of the night compared to placebo. In 2005 they found high sensitivity of human melatonin, alertness, thermoregulation, and heart rate to short wavelength light. They followed the effect of long-term desipramine treatment. Many authors reported that the curative effect of melatonin/agomelatonin was connected with the improvement of sleep (Hamon & Boyer, 2005; Fourtillan, 2002; Emsley, 2005; Grassi et al., 1997). According to Krauchi et al. (1997) melatonin influenced the circadian phase of core body temperature and improved the sleep. Most scientists stress on the fact that treatment of BAD provoked advanced circadian phase in mania and delayed circadian phase in mixed depression returned to normal state.

Our idea is to examine the temperature/pulse chronomes of some antidepressant drugs applied to patients with ND and AD. Thus, we can have information on how the various drugs transform the circadian rhythm in AD and ND.

Total number of our examined patients was 451 (243 – AD, 208 – ND) and 181 of them were followed before/after medication and during several hospitalisations. The total number of cases amounted to 1073 patient days. The patients examined before treatment were 181 (81- ND; 100 - AD). The number of patients receiving antidepressant medication was 356. Of these, 21 received Imipramine = Psychoforine = Tofranil, 73 – Amitriptyline, 32 – Imipramine & Amitriptyline, 94 – Clomipramine (30 – Anafranil, and 64 – Hydiphen), 52 – Maprotiline = Ludiomil, 26 – Viloxazine = Emovit, 12 – Trimipramine = Herphonal = Sapilent, 25 - Moclobemid=Aurorix; 21-comedication of CBZ and antidepressant.

The values of temperature/pulse MESORs and their peak-hours of the various antidepressants for the total group (patients with AD & ND) and for the group with AD and ND are given on table. 2-3.

Antidepressant drugs	N of patients	N of days	Temper .mesor	Peak hour	Signi-ficance	N of days	Pulse mesor	Peak hour	Significance	Synch-roniz.
Affectlve di i s o r d e r s (n=243 patient; 530 days)										
Imipramine	11	11	36.462	16.38	No	11	81.61	9.15	No	**Yes**
CBA & antidepr	6	110	36.476	**18.38**	**Yes**	26	77.61	**17.52**	**Yes**	**Yes**
Moclobemid	11	27	36.339	**18.37**	**Yes**	15	69.09	**18.08**	**Yes**	**Yes**
Venlafaxine	5	59	36.423	16.14	No	59	77.71	13.52	No	**Yes**
Fluoxetine	1	3	36.516	**13.07**	**Yes**					
Leponex	1	3	36.317	**12.22**	**Yes**					
Amitriptyline	50	50	36.42	**17.48**	**Yes**	51	86.48	6.45	No	No
Imipr.& Amitr.	32	32	36.356	15.57	No	32	86.06	7.25	No	**Yes**
Anafranil	30	30	36.376	**22.01**	**Yes**	30	81.12	1.34	No	No
Hydiphen	15	15	36.287	16.12	No	10	74.2	9.45	No	**Yes**
Viloxazine	26	26	36.37	**17.26**	**Yes**	22	81.61	16.47	No	No
Fluvoxamine	7	45	36.447	**19.1**	**Yes**	40	79.06	3.03	No	No
Normothymin	1	6	36.458	**17.23**	**Yes**	6	64.98	**18.21**	**Yes**	**Yes**
Clonazepam& antid.	5	16	36.305	**5.50**	**Yes**	16	74.76	15.10	No	No
Trimipramine	6	6	36.323	14.4	No	6	81.72	5.13	No	**Yes**
Maprotiline	27	27	36.409	**15.5**	**Yes**	26	81.12	3.01	No	No
Nomifnsine	3	3	36.060	15.36	No	3	75.0	15.50	No	Yes
Citalopram	4	38	36.148	**15.41**	**Yes**	38	71.04	11.31	No	No
CBZ, Clonazepam, Moclobemid	2	23	36.519	15.28	No	6	93.21	23.46	No	**Yes**
AD-before therapy	100	100	36.416	**16.01**	**Yes**	100	82.91	11.44	No	No
N e u r o t i c d i s o r d e r s (n=208 patients, n=362 patients days)										
Imipramine	10	10	36.63	17.24	No	8	80.55	13.52	No	**Yes**
CBZ & antidepr	15	67	36.41	16.11	No	46	84.31	14.14	No	**Yes**
Clonazepam& antid.	6	41	36.52	20.51	No	11	77.73	12.10	No	**Yes**
Moclobemid	15	82	36.592	**16.02**	**Yes**	58	83.30	**14.58**	**Yes**	**Yes**
Amitriptyline	23	23	36.48	**16.21**	**Yes**	23	82.03	13.05	No	No
Tranquilizers	59	59	36.46	**18.51**	**Yes**	56	78.43	**7.54**	**Yes**	No
Hydiphen	49	49	36.44	**18.1**	**Yes**	40	80.8	7.41	No	No
Maprotiline	25	25	36.51	14.29	No	24	82.27	7.36	No	**Yes**
Trimipramine	6	6	36.57	20.51	No	6	84.19	4.18	No	**Yes**
ND-before therapy	**81**	**81**	**36.48**	**16.19**	**Yes**	**46**	**80.47**	**14.17**	**Yes**	**Yes**
T o t a l Affective disorders & Neurotic dIsorders (n=451; n=653 days)										
Imipramine	21	21	36.54	**16.47**	**Yes**	19	81.53	10.1	No	No
Amitriptyline	73	73	36.46	**18.2**	**Yes**	74	80.03	6.36	No	No
Trimipramine	12	12	36.44	15.16	No	12	81.95	4.38	No	**Yes**
Clomipramine	94	94	36.38	17.51	No	80	79.71	6.4	No	No
Viloxazine	26	26	36.37	17.2	No	22	81.53	16.47	No	**Yes**
Moclobemid	25	109	36.47	**17.17**	**Yes**	73	76.19	**16.35**	**Yes**	**Yes**
Maprotiline	52	52	36.46	**18.20**	**Yes**	44	81.95	4.14	No	No
Clonazepam&antid.	11	57	36.41	15.42	No	27	75.93	14.23	No	No
CBZ & antidepr.	21	177	36.44	18.03	No	72	80.96	**15.10**	**Yes**	No
Healthy persons	65	65	36.387	**16.18**	**Yes**	55	74.83	14.15	Yes	Yes

*Total num*ber of the patients – 451 (243 – AD, 208 – ND) and 181 of them were followed before/after medication. The total number of the patient's days was 1073.

Table 3 Data of temperature and pulse MESORs determined by Halberg's cosinor method in patients with AD and ND treated with different antidepressant drugs.

*All studied patients were hospitalised in the Department of Psychiatry and Medical Psychology at the MU – Plovdiv, Bulgaria for the period 1982-1994. The diagnoses were made on the basis of clinical observation and evaluation; the self-rating depression scale and Tashev's neurotic-depression questionnaire; and a part of the group with the Hamilton Depression scale. The axillary temperature of all of them was taken hourly from 7:00 am to 11:00 pm and additional 2-3 night measurements with a mercury thermometer for 5 min. The pulse rate was measured hourly for 1 minute on a. radialis. In approximately 1/5 of the sample these measurements were taken in the night hours too. The data were analysed with the method of Halberg, for COSINOR analyses (cosinor rhythmometry). In analysing the results, the MESORs and the circadian peaks exhibited the most significant differences and that is why the remaining parameters are not discussed.

The analysis of the data indicates that all antidepressants accelerate the pulse rate, while their effect on temperature is two-way – some raise the temperature, others lower it (fig. 2-9).

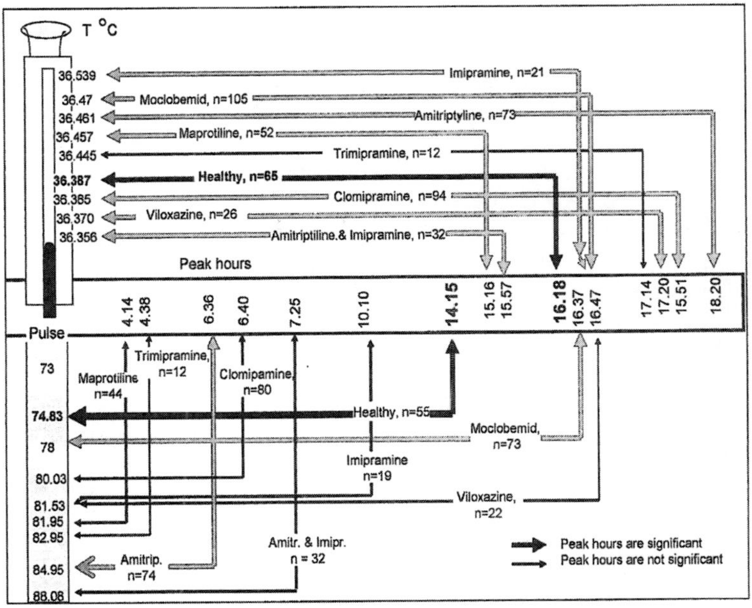

Fig. 2..9. MESORS of temperature and pulse of various antidepressant drugs in patients with ND and AD.

All patients, with the exception of those treated with trimipramine, demonstrated a pronounced circadian peak in the afternoon hours, which was not significantly earlier or later than the peak of the healthy controls. All patients, with the exception of those treated with amitriptyline, did not exhibit a pronounced circadian pulse peak nor a desynchronised temperature peak. Desynchronises between the two vegetative parameters was typical for all groups, with the exception of patients on moclobemid (04.47 pm and 04.37 pm).

The distribution by diagnoses is given on fig. 2-10. Our first visual impression is:

- All temperature MESORs of the antidepressant drugs in ND were higher in comparison with healthy controls, whereas in the group of AD, some of them were higher, others were lower. However, it was typical that when the antidepressant drug was used by a patient with ND its value was higher than if the same antidepressant was given to a patient with AD.
- All pulse mesors, with the exception of Hydiphen*, moclobemide, co-medication of clonazepam, and antidepressant in patients with AD, were higher in comparison with the healthy controls (from 4.4 to 11.65 beats/min.), and their mesors were significantly higher with amitriptyline and co-medication of amitriptiline and imipramine ($p<0.05$).
- Desynchronisation between the vegetative parameters: we see that the temperature peaks were in the afternoon, whereas the pulse peaks showed no daily rhythmicity, but the pulse rate was higher in the morning. So, desynchronisation in ND and AD was typical after medication with antidepressant drugs.

*In the present study an interesting fact is that patients treated with Clomipramine (generic name), but some with the Swiss-made clomipramine under the proprietary name Anafranil and others with the German-made clomipramine under the proprietary name Hydiphen, showed some differences. In patients with AD, Hydiphen exhibited lower temperature and pulse MESORs than Anafranil and did not exhibit circadian rhythm in the two parameters (pulse and temperature). In patients treated with Anafranil, the temperature peak was at 10.01pm, which was desynchronised in relation to the pulse peak (table 2-3; Fig. 10). The established differences between the two trademark drugs which have the same chemical composition and are administered to patients with the same diagnosis, could be explained, to a certain degree, with the different complementary ingredients added to the drug used by each manufacturing company, as well with some idiosyncrasies of the treated patients. As a recommendation it may be said that Hydiphen is more suitable in depressive patients with accelerated pulse rate. Patients treated with Anafranil/ Hydiphen showed different chronograms, so we separate them. Pulse rate and temperature of Hydiphen was the lowest in AD, and for this purpose some of the patients with AD prefer to be on Hydiphen, instead of Anafranil. The differences could be explained with their specific way of reducing the re-uptake of norepinephrine and serotonin in the central nervous system thereby enhancing the effects of these neurotransmitters.

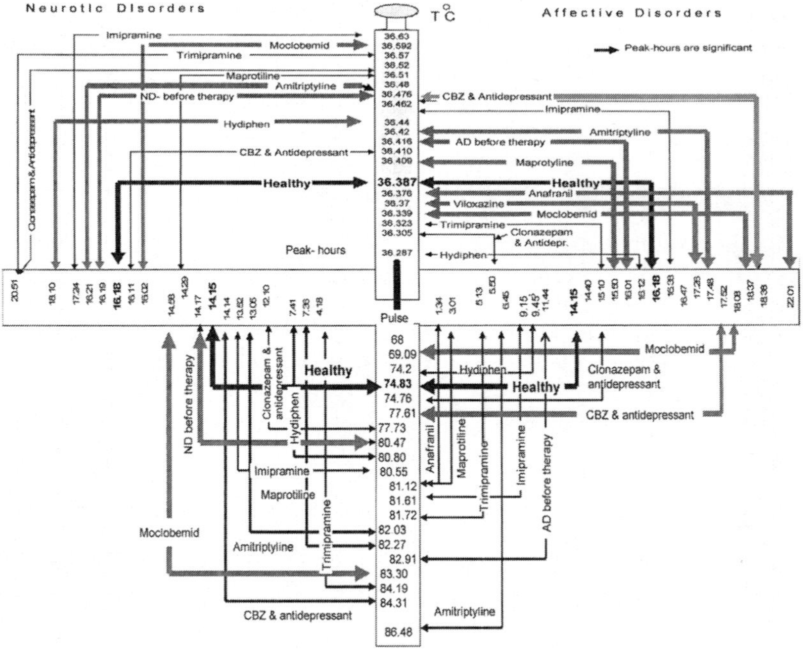

Fig. 2.10. MESORS and peak-hours of temperature and pulse in patients with ND and AD treated with various antidepressants and thymostabilizers.

Our findings show that patients with ND and AD before treatment exhibit higher temperature and pulse MESORs than healthy individuals. Antidepressant medication produces a rising/falling of the temperature MESORs and acceleration of pulse rate. The temperature peaks were in the afternoon hours, while the pulse peaks did not exhibit a marked circadian rhythmicity and showed a trend towards acceleration in the morning hours, which in fact indicated a desynchronises between the two parameters. According to Wirz-Justice and Campbell (1982), prolonged administration of chlorgiline/imipramine to female hamsters caused a dissociation of the circadian activity of rhythm components in them. Wehr and Wirz-Justice (1982), Wirz-Justice (1994) also support the view that antidepressants alter the rhythm in depressive patients. Engelmann and Pflug (1978) had found a shift forward of temperature maximum in patients treated with lithium drugs. Pflug suggested that the anti-depressive effect of sleep deprivation was due to a phase shift by moving forward the wake phase or by slowing down the phase shifted oscillator. *Kuhn (2001)* reported that desynchronies take many physiological systems, including those with circadian timing. He stressed on the negative effect of the disruption of the circadian rhythm in physicians engaged in shift work.

According to Bicacova-Rocher et al. (1996) patients with AD were characterised by a shorter-than-24-hour axillary temperature rhythm, which explains their desynchronies.

The time of antidepressants administrations are also of significance. Demish (1990) findings show that the best chrono pharmacological effect was obtained when the drug was administered after 4:00 pm. These data must focus our attention upon circadian aspects of drug timing and the search for drug administration schedules that optimise treatment efficacy, by determining the time most suitable for antidepressant drugs administration depending on the hours when human organism's absorption capacity is at its best.

6.2. Mood stabilizers

CBZ (Carbamazepine, Finlepsin, Tegretol, Neurotop) - Comedication between CBZ and antidepressants is very important. We followed the daily rhythmicity in 21 patients (6 with AD, 15 with ND), who were on antidepressant and CBZ. For the total group, the vegetative parameters were desynchronised – temperature shows no daily rhythmicity, whereas the pulse peak-hour is at 03:00 pm.

Co-medication of antidepressants and CBZ in AD was characterised with synchronisation between temperature and pulse peak-hours (6:37pm/6.08 pm) and their values were similar to the values of healthy group, whereas for ND temperature and pulse chronograms were relatively synchronised because of the absence of rhythmicity.

Ikonomov and Manji (1999) critically examined the hypothesis that lithium's therapeutic effects in BAD were mediated by alternations in the expression of specific genes in neural circuits. Using "initiation and adaptation paradigm" they appraised the biological effects and underlying molecular and cellular mechanisms of lithium's action. Lithium's acute effects were mediated through inhibition of specific enzymes involved in two distinct but interacting signalling pathways - the protein kinase C and glycogen synthase kinase 3 beta signalling cascades – that coverage at the level of gene transcriptional regulation. The expression of different genes, including transcription factors, was markedly altered by chronic lithium administration. According to them, the chronic lithium also increased the expression of the neuroprotective protein Bcl-2, raising the intriguing possibility that some of lithium's effects are mediated through underappreciated neurotropic/neuroprotective effects. They discussed the validity of the role on specific genes in lithium's therapeutic effects. The combination of sensitive molecular technologies, appropriately designed paradigms, better behavioural analysis, and a chronobiologic approach seems necessary for the future identification of one or more clinically relevant lithium-target genes.

Conclusion

- *The temperature and pulse MESORS in patients with ND before treatment are higher than in healthy individuals, do not exhibit circadian rhythmicity, and are synchronous during the day.*
- *The temperature and pulse MESORS in patients with bad before treatment are close to those of healthy individuals. The pulse MESORs are significantly higher than in healthy persons and desynchronies exists between their peaks.*
- *Various antidepressants and thymostabilizers administered to patients with ND and AD produce desynchronies between temperature and pulse.*
- *The antidepressants can transform in a different way the pulse and temperature circadian rhythms in patients with ND and AD. The average daily temperature' MESOR in patients with ND, treated with antidepressants (imipramine, trimipramine, moclobemide, maprotiline and amitriptyline) are higher than in patients with AD treated with the same antidepressants.*

Our findings indicate that the same antidepressant can transform the pulse/temperature chronome in different ways. This is due, on the one hand, to the different aetiology of the disease process in each patient and on the other hand, to the external agent (drugs).

Recent progress in understanding chronobiological and sleep regulation mechanisms may provide novel insights and avenues into the development of new pharmacological and behavioural treatment strategies for psychiatric disorders.

Conclusion: If we would like to have the perfect circadian rhythm, we must have in mind the endogenous factors (sex, menstruation cycle for females, sleep disturbances, endogenous circadian pacemaker, temperament, genetic predisposition), and exogenous factors (seasons of the year, life events, somatic/psychic disorders, hours of the day, the use of medications, geomagnetic field). Maybe in the future everybody will take their temperature, pulse, and BP chronogram and will follow it periodically as we already do with our ECG, blood, and other parameters. This would provide us with an impression of our premorbid circadian rhythm and allow us to follow its transformation with age and during various somatic/mental diseases.

References

Ankov, V., N. Kolebinov, N., Jelev, M., Shuleva (1970) – Spectrofluorimetic determination of 11-hydrocorticosteroides in plasma in healthy dogs. Sovremenna Medizina, 1970; 11; 23-26.

Aschoff, J., Wever, R. (1980). Uber Reproduzierbarkeit circadianer Rhythmen beim Menschen - Klinische Wochenschrift, Springer - Verlag., 58:323-335.

Aschoff, J. (1981). Annual Rhythm in man. - Handbook of Behavioral Neurobiology, 4:475-487.

Azorin JM, Kaladjian A (2009) - Depression and circadian rhythm - Encephale. *2009* Jan; 35 Suppl 2:S68-71.

Balabanova V. (1981) – Clinical and personality characteristic in depressive patients. – Dissertation for master degree, Sofia.

Banasr M, Soumier A, Hery M, Mocaer E, Daszuta A. (2006). Agomelatine, a new antidepressant, induces regional changes in hippoal neurogenesis. Biol Psychiatry. 2006; 59:1087–1096.

Beersma, D. G., van den Hoofdakker, R. H., Hans, W. B., van Berkestijn (1983). Circadian Rhythm in Affective Disorders. Body Temperature and Sleep Physiology in Endogenous Depressives. - Adv. Biol. Psychiat., 11:114-127.

Beïer EV (2007) Chronobiological similarity of the specific activity of anxiolytic and antidepressant drugs, Eksperimental'naia i klinicheskaia farmakologiia 70(5):52-8, September 2007

Bicakova-Rocher, A., Gorceix, A., Reinberg, A. et al. (1996). Temperature rhythm of patients with major affective disorders: reduced circadian period length - Chronobiol. Int.:13:1:47-57.

Biryukevich, A. A. (1972) – The changes of heart-rate frequency of rhythms in newborn children till 18 years of age. Pediatric, 6: 27-32. (in Russan)

Boer, JA, FJ Bosker, Y Meesters (2005) – Clinical Efficacy of Agomelatine in depression: the evidence. Presented at the Satellite Symposium on the occasion of the 18th ECNP Congres, 22-26=05, Amsrerdam, Eur. Neuropsychophar. J, vol. 153, 660.

Boyce P, Barriball E (2010) - Circadian rhythms and depression. Aust Fam Physician. 2010 May;39(5):307-10.

Bromundt V et al. (2011). Circadian rest-activity cycles - Br J Psychiatry. 2011.9

Buysse, D. (1998) – Psychiatric disorders associated with disturbed sleep and circadian rhythms.
(http:/www.websciences.org/sleepandhealth/buysse.html)

Cahn HA, *Folk* GE Jr, *Huston* PE (*1968*) – Age comparison of human day-night physiological differences. Aerosp Med. *1968* Jun; 39 (6):608-10.

Carr O, Saunders KEA, Bilderbeck AC, Tsanas A, Palmius N, Geddes JR (2018) -*Desynchronization of diurnal rhythms* in bipolar disorder and borderline personality disorder. *2018* Apr 12; 8 (1):79.
Doi: 10.1038/s41398-018-0125-7.

Carroll, B., Schroeder, K., et al. (1980). Plasma dexamethasone Concentration in Patients with Endogenous Depression. - J. Clin. Endocr. & Metabol., 51:3:433-437.

Carrier J, TH Monk, DJ Buysse, DJ Kupfer (1996) – Amplitude reduction of the circadian temperature and sleep rhythm in elderly: Chronobiol. International, 1996; 13; 13; 373-386.

Chong, TVH, Castle, DJ (2004) – Layer upon layer: Thermoregulation in schizophrenia. Schizophr. Res. 2004; 69; 2-3; 1Aug., 149-157;

Cornelissen, G, D. Watson, G. Mitsutake, B. Fiser, J. Siegelova, J. Dusek, I. Volhidalova, H. Svaeinova, and F. Halberg (2015) – Mapping of circaseptan and circadian changes in mood - Scr Med (Brno). 2005; 78(2): 89–98.

Czeisler, CA, JF Duffy, TL Shanahan, EN Brown, JF Mitchell, DW Rimmer, JM Ronda, EJ Silva, JS Allan, JS. Emens, D-J Dijk, RE Kronauehttp://science.sciencemag.org/content/284/5423/2177 (1999) - Stability, Precision, and Near-24-Hour Period of the Human Circadian

Pacemaker. *Science* 25 Jun 1999: Vol. 284, Issue 5423, pp. 2177-2181; DOI: 00.1126/science.284.5423.2177.

Davis, F. (1981). Ontogeny of circadian rhythms. In: Handbook of Behavioural Neurobiology, 4:257-273.

Demish, L, K Gebhart, K Vagal, E Tuksoy, B Pflug, R Reiter (1996) Chronobiological effect of fluvoxamine on rat pineal serotonin and melatonin metabolism. - Chronobiol. Intern. 13:1:22.

Dirlich, G., Kammerloher,A., Schulz,H., Lund,R., Doerr,P., Zerssen,D. von. (1982). Temporal coordi-nation of Rest-Activity Cycle, body temperature, urinary free cortisol, and mood in patients with 48-hour unipolar-depressive cycles in clinical & time - cue - free environments. - Biol. Psychiat., 16:2:163-179.

Duncan, WC, FA Johnson, TA Wehr, (1995) - Clinical Psychobiology Branch. NIMH, NIH, Bethesda, Meryland 20892, USA. – Neuropsychopharmacology (USA), Feb., 1995, 12;1;17-37.

Duncan, CJ (1996) - Circadian rhythms and the pharmacology of affective illness - Pharmacology & Therapeutics Volume 71, Issue 3, 1996, Pages 253-312

Emsley, R (2005) – Efficacy and Safety of Agomelatine (25-50mg), a melatoninergic and specific serotoninergic antidepressant, in the treatment of mayor depressive disorder: a randomized, double – blind, placebo effect. 18th ECNP, 22-26, Oct., 2005, Amsterdam.

Emsley, R. (2005) – The impact sleep disorders on the course of depression. Medicographia, vol. 27;3;273-278.

Engelmann W, B Pflug (1978) - Rhythmische Aspecte der Lithiumwirkung. Rhythmusproblemein der Psychiatrie.- Gustav Fischer Verlag-Stuttgart-New York, 65-67.

Faravelli, C., La Malfa, G., Romano, S. (1985). Circadian Rhythm in Primary Affective Disorder. - Comprehensive Psychiatry, 26:4: 364-369.

Foret J, N Touron, Benoit O, Bouard G. (1985) - Sleep and body temperature in "morning" and "evening" people. Sleep. 1985 Dec; 8 (4): 311-8.

Fourtillan, JB (2002) – Role of melatonin in the induction and maintenance of sleep. Dialogues in clinical neuroscience, 2002:4:4:395-401.

Jablensi, A. (1986) – Schizophrenia – Nosological unity and cultural diversity. PH "Medizina I Fizkultura", Sofia, 1986.

Joung-HoMoon, MS, Chul-HyunCho, Hoon Son, Dongho Geum, Sooyoung Chung et al. (2016) - Advanced Circadian Phase in Mania and Delayed Circadian Phase in Mixed Mania and Depression Returned to Normal after Treatment of Bipolar Disorder. - EBioMedicine, Vol. 11, September 2016, Pages 25-26

Germain A, DJ Kupfer (2008) – Circadian rhythm disturbances in depression. Human Psychopharmacology; Clinical Experimental, Oct. 2008; Vol. 23; 7; 571-585.

Giedke H., B. Pflug (1994) – Diurnal variations of mood in depressed patients in relation to severity of depression. J. Affec. Dis., Vol. 31, 4, 261-273, August..

Gonzalez R, CA Tamminga, M Tohen, T Suppes (2014) - The Relationship Between Affective State and the Rhythmicity of Activity in Bipolar Disorder - J Clin Psychiatry. 2014 Apr; 75 (4): e317–e322.

GORWOOD, PH. (2012). - Anxiety disorders and circadian rhythms. Centre Hospitalier Sainte-Anne (CMME), Paris, and INSERM U894 and University Paris-Descartes, Center of Psych. & Neuroscience, Paris, France. Medicographia.34: 289-294

Goulet G, M. Mongrain, C. Desrosiers, J. Paquet M, Dumont (2007) Daily light exposure in morning-type and evening-type individuals. J Biol Rhythms. 2007 Apr; 22 (2): 151-8.

Grassi ZG, M Semprevivo, F Carandente, E Mocaer, K Kristensson, M Bentivoglio (1997) - Melotonin and S-20098 improve sleep disorder and life expectancy in an animal model of sleeping sickness. - Chronobiol. Intenat., 14: 1: 57 (Abstracts).

Halberg, F. (1953). Some physiological and clinical aspects of 24-hour periodicity. - J. Lancet (USA) 73:20-32.

Halberg, F. (1959). "Physiologic 24-hour periodicity: general and procedural considerations with reference to the adrenal cycle". Zeitschrift für Vitamin- Hormone- und Fermentforschung. 10: 225-296.

Halberg F, Carandente F, Cornelissen G, Katinas GS (1977). "[Glossary of chronobiology (author's transl)]". Chronobiologia. 4 Suppl 1: 1–189.

Halberg F. (1969) – Chronobiology. Ann. Rev. Physiol., 31, 675-725.

Halberg, F., Johnson,, E. A., Nelson, W., Runge, W., Sothern, R. (1972). Autorhythmometry: Procedur for physiologic self measurements and their analysis. - The Physiol. Teacher, 1:4:1-11.

Halberg F. (1986). Chronobiology:Printed in USA.

Halberg, F., Cornelissen, G. (1994). Introduction to Chronobiology. Variability; from foe to friend, mice and men. Printed in USA.

Hamon, M., Boyer, P-A (2005) – New perspectives in the pathophysiology and treatment of affective disorders: the role of melatonin and serotonin. Medicographia, vol. 27; 3; 228-235.

Hampp, H. (1961). Die Tagesrhythmischen Schwankungen der Stimmung und des Atriebestbeim gesunden Menschen. - Arch., fur Psychiatr. Und Zeitschrift f. d. ges Neurologie, 201: 355-377.

Hare, EH, JS Price, (1983). Menthal Disorders and Seasons of Birth. Comparison of Psychoses with Neurosis. - Br. J. Psychiat., 115: 533-540.

Haug, HJ (1989) - Diurnal variations of mood predict sleep deprivation-outcome. - Chronobiology, 16:2:76.

Haug, H. J. (1989). On the frequency of the diurnal variation in psychiatric patients. - Chronobiology, 16: 2: 75.

Haug H.-J, E Fähndrich (1994) - Diurnal variations of mood in depressed patients in relation to severity of depression. J. Affective Dis., Vol. 31, 4, August, 261-273

Hildebrandt, G, I Stratmann (1979) - Circadian system response to night in relation to the individual circadian phase position - Health, 43: 73-83.

Ikonomov O, HK Mandji (1999) – Molecular mechanisms underlying Mood Stabilisation in Manic-Depressive illness: The Phenotype Challenge. – Am. J Psychiatry, 1999; 156;1506-1516

Karatsoreos, I. N. (2014) - Links between Circadian Rhythms and Psychiatric Disease. Front Behav Neurosci. 2014; 8: 162. Published online 2014 May 6. doi: 10.3389/fnbeh.2014.00162

Kirov, K. (1967) – Atipical psychoses. Medizina I phiskultura, Sofia.

Kivelä L, MR Papadopoulos, N Antypa (2018) - Chronotype and Psychiatric Disorders. Sleep and Psychological Disorders - Current Sleep Medicine Reports; June 2018, Volume 4, Issue 2, pp 94–103|

Knorring L von, C Perris, E Strandman (1977) - Diurnal variations in Intensity of Symptoms in Patients of Different Diagnostic Groups. - Arch. Psychiat. Nervenkr, 224: 295-312.

Krauchi, K., Cajochen, C., Wirz-Justice, A. (1997). Melatonin and bright light interactons on circadian phase of core body temperature and on subjective sleepiness. - Chronobiol. International, 14 1: 86 (Abstracts).

Krauchi K, A. Wirz-Justice (1987) - The four seasons: Food intake frequency in Seasonal Affective Disorders in the course of a year. – Psych. Res., 25: 323-338.

Kripke, D. F., Mullaney, D. J., Atkinson, M. L. et al. (1979). Circadian Rhythm Phases in Manic-Depressives illness. - Chronobiol., 6, October-December, 4:365-375.

Kripke DF, LL Judd, B Hubbard, et al. (1979) -The effect of lithium carbonate on the circadian rhythm of sleep in normal human subjects. Biol. Psych. 14 (3): 545–548.

Kronfeld-Schor N., H Einat (2012) - Circadian rhythms and depression: human psychopathology and animal models. Neuropharmacology. 2012 Jan; 62 (1): 101-14.

Kuhn, G. (2001) - Circadian rhythm, shift work, and emergency medicineAnnals of Emergency Medicine, Volume 37, Issue 1, January 2001, Pages 88-98

Kuhs, H., Hermann, W., Kammen, K., Tollr, R. (1989) -The daily course of the symptomatology and the impaired time estimation in endogenous depression (melancholia) – J. Aff. Dis., Vol. 17; 3; November–December; 1989; 285-290

Kupfer D, G Gilin, P Coble, D Spiker, S Show, B Holser (1981) – REM Sleep, Naps, and Depression. Psychiat. Research, 1981, 5, 195-203.

Lack L, M Bailey, N Lovato, H Wright. (2009) - Discover the world's research between morning and evening types and the possible vulnerability of evening types to delayed sleep phase disorder. Nature and Science of Sleep 2009:1; 1–8;

Leibenluft, E. (1996) - Circadian Rhythms Factor in Rapid - Cycling Bipolar Disorder. Psychiatric time, May 1996; Vol. 13; 5;

LeSauter J, R Silver (1993) - Lithium lengthens the free-running period of circadian rhythms in a wide variety. Erratum in Biol Psychiatry *1993* Sep 1; 34 (5): 343.

Linkowski P, Mendlewiz J, Leclercq R, et al. (1985) - The 24-hour profile of adrenocortkotropin and cortisol in major depressive illness. J Clin Endocrinol Metab. 1985; 61(3): 429–438.

Madjirova N (1985) – Circadian rhythm of depressive syndrome and its stability during treatment of depressive patients with antidepressant drugs. Dissertation for MD, Sofia.

Madjirova N. (1987) Pyramem and Cinnarizine - Stability of the circadian rhythm of depressive syndrome at combined antidepressive therapy. - MBI, 3:26-30.

Madjirova N (1987) - Emovit (Viloxazine): Stability of the circadian rhythm of mood in depressed patients - MBI, 3:36-39.

Madjirova N (1987) - A prolonged investigation of the rhythm of mood and sleep in healthy individuals and patients with depression and neuroses. - Folia medica (Bulgaria), 29:1:14-21.

Madjirova N (1987) - Investigation of the circadian rhythm of mood in healthy individuals using our own questionnaire and that of H. Hampp - Folia medica, 29:3:13-20.

Madjirova, N (1990). Der Einfluss verschiedener Psychopharmaca auf die Stabilitat des Rhythmus der Stimmung. In: Aktuelle Aspekte und Trends in der Neuropsychopharmaco-therapie. Jena, Sweden: Universitatsverlag, pp.14-21.

Madjirova N, Tashev, T, Bakalova R (1992). The Interrelationship Between Cortisol Plasma Levels and Stability of the Circadian Rhythms in Depressed Patients - Integr. Psychiatr, 8: 1: 31-36.

Madjirova N. (1995) – Daily rhythmicity of temperature and pulse in patients with schizophrenia, manic-depressive psychosis and neuroses. – Folia medica, XXXVII, 4A/80-81.

Madjirova, N, N Petrova, N Delchev, (1995). Daily Rhythmicity of Temperature, Pulse and Blood Pressure in Schizophrenic Patients. - Schizophr. Res., 14:183.

Madjirova N, T Tashev, N Delchev, R Bakalova (1995) - The Interrelationship between cortisol plasma levels and the circadian rhythm of temperature, pulse and blood pressure in depressed patients with good and disturbed sleep. – Int. J. Psychophys., 20:145-154.

Madjirova N (1995) – Chronobiological Aspects in Psychiatry, Public House "Poligraf", Plovdiv. 208 pages.

Madjirova N (1997) - Temperature and pulse chronomes in patients with neurotic and affective disorders treated with some antidepressants and tranquilizers, Folia Medica (Bul), 39: 2:71-77.

Madjirova, N., Halberg, F., Dimitrov, B., Petrova, N., Kitcheva, L. (1997). Carbamazepine stability of the circadian rhythm of mood, vigor, temperature and pulse during combined anti-depressive therapy in patients with affective disorders. - 3rd International Workshop "Chronobiology and its Roots in the Cosmos", 2-6 Sep., High Tatras, Slovakia. Proceedings. Ed: M. Mikulecky, pp 285-290.

Madjirova, N., Kuysepoashova, Peytchev, L. (1997). Electric-acupuncture can dissociate the stability of the circadian rhythm of mood and vigor in patients with endogenous depression. - Chronobiol. International, 14:1;103 (Abst.), presented at the Inter. Congress on Chronobiology in Paris, 7-11 September, 1997

Madjirova N., BD Dimitrov, M. Semerdjieva, R. Stefanov, N. Petrova (2001) – Chronobiological and biometeorological studies of suicides and attempted suicide. In: Chronobiology and Biometeorology in Bulgariam Medicne, ed. N. Madjirova, Public House "MACROS-2000", 2001, pp 87-98.

Madjirova N, F Halberg, N Petrova (1998) Chronomes of temperature, pulse, mood and vigor in schizophrenic patients treated with Semap. 1st Joint Symposium of the Bulgarian and German Societies of clinical pharmacology and therapy. Today and tomorrow: Sept. 3-4, Plovdiv, Bulgaria. Folia med. 2A/98, p.44 (abst.).

Madjirova N, F Halberg (1998) - Daily rhythmicity of temperature and pulse in schizophrenic patients treated with Leponex (Clozapin). Folia med., 2A/98, 44-45.

Madjirova, N., Atanasov, T., Atanasov K (2005) – Mood Color Test for express evaluation of anxiety and depression. – Scientific Reseachers of the Union of Scientists Plovdiv, 2005; Series Medicine, Pharmacy and Stomatology, vol. VI; 176-177.

Madjirova N. (2006) – The place of chronobiology in the Pathogenesis of some psychiatric states. Dissertation for DMS, Sofia.

Madjirova N, Velkova S. (2011) – Circadian rhythm of temperature and pulse of Moclobemid, Venlafaxine, Fluvoxamine and Citalopram. Bulgarian Medicine; vol.1; No2; 2011; 22-33.

Martin J, DV Jeste, MP Caliguiri, T Paterson, R Heaton, S Ancolilsrael (2001) – Circadian rhythms and sleep-wake in older schizophrenia patients. Sch Res., 44: 77-86.

Mendlewicz J, Linkovski P, Branchey et al. (1979). Abnormal 24 hour pattern of melatonin secretion in depression. - The Lancet, 22-29 December, 1362.

Mendlewicz J. (2009) – Disruption of the circadian timing systems: molecular mechanisms in mood disorders. CNS Drugs, 2009; 23 Suppl. 2; 15-26

Mendlewicz, J, G Hoffmann, P Linkovski et al. (1983). Chronobiology and Manic Depression Neuroendocrine and Sleep EEG Parameters. - Advance in Biol. Psychiat., 11:128-135.

Menninger-Lerhenthal, E. (1960). Periodiciat in der Psychopathologie Neuro- und Allge-meinpathologie), Vien, Bon, Berlin.

Menshikov, V., Bolshakova, T., Berezin, F. (1980) - The effect of climatic and geographic conditions of the Northeast of the USSR, on the catecholamine metabolism in healthy subjects. Catecholamines and Stress - Recent Advances, North Holland, 443-447.

Middelhoff HD (1967) - Tagesrhythmische Schwankungen bei endogenen Depressiver im symptom-freien Interval und wahrend der Phase. - Arch. Fur Psychiattrie und Zeitschrift. f. d. ges Neurologie, 209:315-339.

Milenkov, K (1982) – Epidemiological and clinical and diagnostic examinations of affective disorders., Dissertation for DMS, Sofia.

Mitsutake G, K Otsuka, G Cornélissen, M Herold, R Günthe, C Dawes JB Burch, D Watson, F Halberg (2000) - Circadian and infradian rhythms in mood - Biomedicine & Pharmacotherapy; Vol. 55, Suppl. 1, 11 Nov. 2000, Pages s94-s100;

Monk TH, DJ Buysse, CF Reynolds, DJ Kupfer (1997) - Endogenous circadian performance rhythms. Relationship to temperature, cortisol, melatonin, mood and alertness. - Chronobiol. Intenational, 14; 1; 117 (Abstracts).

Moiseeva NI (1978) – Structura biorhythm as a kriterium for physical adaptation of the organism – Physiol. Journal, SSSR im. "Sechenov", LXIV; 11; 1632-1640.

Montes, J. M., Barrenechea, C., Romero, M., Abraira, V., Saiz, J., Gaztelu, J. M. (1997). Decreased period length of motor activity circadian rhythm in a rat model of endogenous depression. - Chronobiol. Internation., 14; 1; 118

Moreas AC, T Cambas, A Diez-Noguera et al (2013) – A New Chronobiological approach to discriminate between acute and chronic depression using peripheral temperature, rest-activity, and light exposure parameters. BMC Psychiatry, 2013, March, 9, 13, 77.

Murray, G., BAller N., Trinder, J., Burgess H. (2002) - Is weakened circadian rhythmicity a characteristic of neuroticism? (2002) - J. Affective Disorders, Vol. 72; Issue 3; December 2002; 281-289.

Murray G, Harvey A.(2010)- Circadian rhythms and sleep in bipolar disorder. Bipolar Disord 2010: 12: 459–472.

Nadjarov, RA (1988) – Handbook in Psychiatry. Ed. GB Morosov; Moscow, "Medizina", 1988 (Russian).

Nelson W, Y Tong, J.-K Lee, F Halberg (1979) - Method for Cosinor-Rhythmometry. Chronobiologia, 6: 4: 305-322.

Nikolov G, S Solakova (1984) – Rhythms of life and health – DI "Narodna Prosveta", Sofia.

NOVAKOVA M, J PRASKO, K LATANOVA, M SLADEK, A SUMOVA (2015) –THE CIRCADIAN SYSTEM OF PATIENTS WITH BIPOLAR DISORDER DIFFERS IN EPISODES OF MANIA AND DEPRESSION, Bipolar Disord., 17 (2015), pp. 303-314.

Pettegrew JW, K Panchalingam, RJ, S McClure et al. (2001) - Effects of chronic lithium administration on rat brain phosphatidylinositol cycle constituents, membrane phospholipids and amino acids; Bipolar Disorder

Pflug, B., Tolle, R. (1971) - Disturbance of the 24-h rhythm in endogenous depression by sleep deprivation. - Int. Pharmacopsychiatr., 6:187-196.

Pflug B, R Erikson, A Johnsson (1976) Depression and Daily Temperature. A Long-Term study - Acta Psych. Scand. 54:254-266.

Pflug B, W Martin (1980). Analyse circadianer Tepperaturgange bei endogener Depression. - Arch. Psychiatr. Nervenkr. 229: 127-143.

Pflug, B., Johnsson, A., Tweiti Ekse, A. (1981). Manic-depressive states and daily temperature - Acta Psychiatr. Scand. 63:277-289.

Pflug, B. (1987). Rhythmusfragen bei Affektiven Psychosen. In: von K. P. Kisker, H. Lauter, J-E. Meyer, C., Muller, E., Stromgren, (eds) Psychiatrie der Gegenwart 5. Affektiven Psychosen. Springer-Verlag, Berlin Heidelberg, New York, London, Paris, Tokio, pp 241-270.

Pittendrigh CS (1993). "Temporal organization: reflections of a Darwinian clock-watcher". Annual Review of Physiology. 55 (1): 16–54.

Poppei M, K Hecht, M, Airapetjanz (1982) - Biorhythmische prozesse als Kriterium zur berteilung Gestore zeitregulation bei axperimentaller Neurose. - 10 Donausymposium fur Psychiatrie, Magdeburg, DDR, 23-25; Spt., p. 120.

Reeth, O van, Weibel, L., Olovares, E., Maccary, S., Mocaer, E., Turek, FW. (2001) – Melatonin ore Melatonin agonist corrects age-related changes in circadian response to environmental stimulsus. Am.J Psych., 2001, vol.280, 5; R 1582-R1591.

Rose, B, E Wachter, A Kolometsewa et al. (1982) - Gestorte schlaf bei Experimentaller Neurose als Ausdruck Gestorter Biorhythmik - 10 Donausymposium fur Psichiatrie, Magdeburg, DDR, 23-25 Sept., 128.

Rush AJ, DE Giles, RB Jarrett, F Feldman-Koffler, JR Debus, PJ Orsulak, J Weissenburger, HP Roffwarg (1989) - Reduced REM latency predicts response to tricyclic medication in depressed outpatients. Biol Psychiatry. 1989; 26: 61–72.

Saleem, PT (1984). Dexamethasone supression test in depressive illness. Its relation to anxiety states. - Brit. J. Psychiat. 144:2:181-184.

Saunder WA (1970) – Organic or psychogenic stupor. Br. Med. Journal, Febr., 1: (5692); 367.

Shuaib BM, Haq MF. (1977). Electro-acupuncture treatment in psychiatry. Am J Chin Med (Gard City N Y).

Schulz P (2007) – Biological clock and the practice of psychiatry. Dialogues in Clinical neuroscience; 2007; Vol. 9; 3; 237-255.

Shumilina AL et al. (1956) - [Use of hypothermia in experimental neurosis in dogs Zh Nevropatol Psikhiatr Im S S Korsakova. 1956.

Souêtre E, E Salvati, JL Belugou, et al. (1989) - Circadian rhythms in depression and recovery: evidence for blunted amplitude as the main chronobiological abnormality. Psychiatry Res. 1989;28(3):263–278.

Strain F, W. Albert, C. Klicpera (1979) - Antidepressive treatment and mood swing patterns in endogenous depression. Pharmakopsychiat. I2, 432–437.

Srinvasan V, SR Pandi-Perumal, I Trakht et al. (2009) – Pathophysiology of depression & role of sleep and the melatonergic system. Psych. Res., Feb 28; 165 (3): 201-214, Feb 1.

Stoyanov, Dr. (2005) - Prion diseases. Ed. Velchev I., Stoyanov, D. PH "ARSO", 2005, Sofia.

Stoyanov Dr. (2009) - The cross-Validation in the Dialogue of Mental and Neurosciences. - Dialogue in Philosophy, Mental and Neuro-sciences, 2; 1; 24-28.

Stojanov, D. St. (2013) – Neuroscience and psychopathology: The science of translational validation. In: Psychopathology: Theory, Perspectives and Future Approaches. Nova Biomedical, New York. Ed. Dr. Stoyanov, 125-147.

Stoyanov, St. (1980) – Schizophrenia and paraphrenia – Moscow, dissertation for DMS.

Suvisaari JM, JK Haukka, JK Lönnqvist (2001) -Season of birth among patients with schizophrenia and their siblings: evidence for the procreational habits hypothesis. Am J Psychiatry. 2001 May; 158 (5): 754-7.

Swade, G., Coppen, A. (1980). Seasonal variations in biochemical factors related to depressive illness. - J. Affective Disorders, 2:249-255.

Tashev, T. (1979) – Manic-depressive disorders -"Medizina I phizkultura", Sofia.

Tsai, M-T , Y-C Su, Y-H Chen, & C-H Chen (2001)- Lack of evidence to support the association of the human prion gene with schizophrenia. *Molecular Psychiatry* volume6, pages74–78 (2001)

Thommen, George S. (1972) - *"Is This Your Day"*. 1973. ISBN 0-517-00742-8

Tsujimoto, T., Yamada, N., Shimoda, K., Takahashi, S. (2014) - Circadian rhythms in depression: Part II: Circadian rhythms in inpatients with various mental disorders – J. Affec. Dis., Vol.163, 2014, pp. 70-75

Turek F W, S Losee-Olson (1986). A benzodiazepine used in the treatment of insomnia phase - shifts the mammalian circadian clock. Nature, 312, 167-168.

Vogel G, W, Vogel, F, McAbee, RS, Thurmond, AJ. (1980). Improvement of depression by REM sleep deprivation: New findings and theory. - Arch. Gen. Psychiatry, 37:247-253.

Waldmann H (1970) - Zur Psychopathologie der Tagesschwankung beim depressiven Syndrom. Arch. Psychiatr. Nervenkr., 213: 177-199.

Wehr T, A.Wirz-Justice, W Dunkan, F Goodwin, J Gillin (1979) - Phase Advance of the Circadian Sleep-Wake Cycle as an Antidepressant. - Science, 206:9 Nov., 710-713.

Wehr, T., Wirz-Justice, A. (1982). Circadian Rhythm Mechanisms in Affective illness and an Antidepressant Drug Action. - Pharmacopsychiat., 15: 31-39.

Wehr T, M, Sack, DA, Mendelson W, B, Rosenthal, NE, Gillin, JC, Goodwin, FK. (1985). Sleep and circadian rhythm in affective patients isolated from external time cues. - Psychiatry Res., 15, 327-339.

Wehr T, DA Sack, NE Rosenthal, RW Cowdry (1987) - Rapid cycling dffective disorder: contributing factors and treatment responses in fifty-one cases. - Am. J. Psychiatry.

Wehr TA., Goodwin, FK. (1983). Biological rhythms in manic-deprssive illness. In: Wehr TA, Goodwin, FK. (eds). Circadian rhythms in psychiatry. Boxwood Press, Pacific Grove, pp 129-184.

Weiner, D., J. Waterhouse (2006) - The circadian rhythm of core temperature: Effects of physical activity and aging - Physiology & Behavior, Volume 90, Issues 2–3, 28 February 2007, Pages 246-256;

Weitbrecht, HJ (1973) – Psychiatry im Grundriss. – Springer-Verlag Berlin--Heidelberg-New York.

Wever RA, J Polasek, Ch.M Wildgruber (1983) - Bright light affect human circadian rhythm/ Pfluger Arch., 396:1:85-87.

Williams, R. L.; *Karacan*, I.(1985) Recent developments in the diagnosis and treatment of sleep disorders. Hosp Commirniiy Psychiatry *1985;* Sep; 36 (9): 951-7. https://www.ncbi.nlm.nih.gov/m/pubmed/6480567/Wirz-Justice A, IC Campbell (1982) Antidepressant can slow or dissociate circadian rhythm. - Experientia, 38:1301-1309.

Wirz-Justice, A., T Wehr (1983) - Neuropsychopharmacology and Biological Rhythms. - Adv. Biol. Psychiat., 11: 1: 20-34.

Wirz-Justice, A., Terman, M., Terman, J. S., Boulos, et al. (1998). Circadian functions and clinical applications of dawn simulation. In: Biological Clocks and Mechanisms and Applications. Ed. by Y. Touitou, Elsevier, pp. 189-194.

Wirz-Justice, A (2003) – Circadian disturbances in depression: therapeutic perspectives. Medicographia, 2003; 25; 1; 29-36.

Wirz-Justice, A.; Cajochen, C.; Nussbaum, P. (1997) - A schizophrenic patient with an arrhythmic circadian rest-activity cycle. Psychiatry Res. 73: 83-90.,

Wirz-Justice, A. (2005) – Chronobiological strategies for umet needs in the treatment of depression. Medicographia, vol. 27; 3; 223-227.

Witting W, M Mirmiran, N Bos, DF Swaab (1994). The effect of old age on the free-running period of circadian rhythms in rat. - Chronobiol. Int. 11: 2: 103-112.

Wood J, B Birmaher, D Axelson, et al. (2009) - Replicable differences in preferred circadian phase between bipolar disorder patients and control individuals. Psychiatry Res. 2009;166(2-3):201–209

Wu, JC, Potkin, SG, Gullin, JC, Bunney JN, Schahar, CG, Darnall, L. (2004) – Antidepressant effects of a Chronibiological combined with SSRIs and Mood Mood Stabilizers in depression. – Int. J. Neuropsychopharmacology, Suppl.1, Vol. 7, 345.

Wulff K. , Derk-Jan Dijk, B. Middleton, R. G. Foster (2018) Sleep and circadian rhythm disruption in schizophrenia; Volume 20, Issue 4 April 2012 , pp. 308-316 Published online: 02 January 2018 https://doi.org/10.1192/bjp.bp.111.096321

Wulff K, Dijk DJ, Middleton B, Foster RG, Joyce EM. (2012) Sleep and circadian rhythm disruption in schizophrenia. Br J Psychiatry. 2012 Apr;200(4):308-16. doi: 10.1192/bjp.bp.111.096321. Epub 2011 Dec 22.

Yates NJ.(2016) Schizophrenia: the role of sleep and circadian rhythms in regulating dopamine and psychosis. Oct 1;27(7):669-687. doi: 10.1515/revneuro-2016-2030.

Zanghi Brian M, Gardner,C. Araujo J., W.Milgram, N. (2016) - Diurnal changes in core body temperature, day/night locomotor activity patterns, and actigraphy-generated behavioral sleep in aged canines with varying levels of cognitive dysfunction; Neurobiology of Sleep and Circadian Rhythms; Volume 1, Issue 1, October 2016, Pages 8-18;

Zarizinskii VP (1984) – The treatment of paranoid schizophrenia and their daily biological rhythm – Jurnal Nevrologii I Psichiatrii, 1984; 1; 92-98.

CHAPTER SEVEN

STRESS-RELATED ALTERATIONS IN ADULT NEUROGENESIS: RELEVANCE TO PSYCHOPATHOLOGY

BOGOMIL PESHEV[1] AND VIHRA MILANOVA[2]

[1]INSTITUTE OF NEUROBIOLOGY,
BULGARIAN ACADEMY OF SCIENCE, SOFIA
[2] PSYCHIATRIC CLINIC, ALEXANDROVSKA UNIVERSITY
HOSPITAL, SOFIA, BULGARIA

Abstract

Stress is a term used to describe the changes in the normal homeostasis of the organism caused by internal factors (physical stressors) or external, unpredictable stimuli (psychological stressors), interpreted in accordance with the individual's prior experience. Mild stress could be beneficial as it could lead to adaptation and lack of future homeostatic disturbance. However chronic or very acute stress could lead to long-lasting alterations in the regulation of behaviour obtained through adult neurogenesis and sleep. An exciting hypothesis in behavioural neuroscience considers the possibility that the overgeneralisation of fear observed in stress-related disorders such as posttraumatic stress disorder (PTSD) may be due to the inability to disambiguate similar sensory input and store them as discrete memory traces, a process that is known as pattern separation. It has been demonstrated that hippocampal adult-born granule cells are particularly important for this process and changes induced in the levels or quality of adult neurogenesis by stress may therefore lead to maladaptive behaviour. Therefore, by analysing the current literature, this review paper aims to explore the neurobiology of stress-induced alteration in adult neurogenesis. The main objective here is to link these alterations to maladaptive behaviours observed in anxiety, affective, and traumatic disorders, and by doing so, to bridge basic research in model animals to the field of psychiatry

Keywords: neurogenesis, stress, hippocampus, psychopathology

Introduction

Stress is a word associated with many connotations, most of which carry negative meaning. In the context of our daily routine, stress has been linked to the mental load we experience when facing problematic situations in our professional, family, or social life. In terms of biology, neuroscience, and medicine, the concept of stress encompasses a number of physiological processes existing to adapt our organisms to the ever-changing environment we live in. Indeed, moderate stress can be beneficial, as the interaction between the nervous and the endocrine systems that characterises it, serves to signal to the rest of the body in cases of unexpected occurrence of external threatening stimulus (psychological stress) or internal atypical change in homeostasis (physical stress). Walter Cannon was the first physiologist to notice the interaction between the sympathetic nervous system and medulla of the adrenal gland during moments of intense emotional arousal or pain (Cannon, 1914). Since then, the scientific definition of stress has gone a long way from the original "nonspecific response of the body to any demand made upon it", an interpretation provided by one of the pioneers of stress research, Hans Selye. Selye himself focused on the elucidation of the primary physiological responses to internal or external demands, which he named "general adaptation syndrome", but never really considered how the nature of these demands influences organismic adaptation (Mason, 1971). Later on, another prominent figure in the field, Jason W. Mason, further expanded the concept of stress by introducing the notion that the interpretation of external stimuli may trigger neuroendocrine responses (Mason, 1968). By outlining novelty, uncertainty, and unpredictability as factors of the external milieu that could cause functional changes in the organism, Mason established the foundations upon which the modern psychobiological framework of stress will emerge. To further objectify the scientific effort to understand how the social and physical environment could modulate physiological processes in the body, Sterling and Eyer (1988) proposed the concept of allostasis. Allostasis subsumes all the different systemic responses and interactions - endocrine, automatic, immune, and metabolic- that are activated upon registration of environmental change (the presence of a stressor) and that function to restore and maintain the stability in body functioning (homeostasis). These adaptive interactions are mediated by chemical messengers such as catecholamines - adrenalin, norepinephrine - and cortisol. The secretion of these "stress molecules" in the body is regulated by two independent pathways: the sympatho-adrenomedullary system increases the levels of catecholamines, and the hypothalamic-pituitary-adrenocortical (HPA) axis controls the levels of circulating cortisol. Both pathways are governed by limbic and cortical structures, like the hippocampus, the amygdala, and the medial prefrontal cortex (mPFC) (for review Ulrich-Lai and Herman, 2009). Moreover, in the brain, the main source of norepinephrine, locus coeruleus, is activated by situations characterised by their novelty and unpredictability (Ross and Van Bockstaele, 2021). This leads to greater release of the neurotransmitter and the activation of a large-scale brain network known as the salience network (Hermans et al, 2011; Sara and Bouret, 2012). The salience network is a group of cortical (e.g., anterior insula, anterior cingulate cortex) and subcortical structures (e.g., amygdala, ventral striatum) which upon activation redirects attention to the most significant and emotionally relevant stimuli (Seeley, 2019). However, since systemically high levels of catecholamines and glucocorticoids could lead to malfunctions of different body systems, (for example, chronically high levels of adrenaline increase the risk of cardiovascular diseases), McEwen and Stellar (1993) advanced the concept of allostasis by putting forward the idea of the allostatic load. Allostatic load was defined as the "wear and tear" of tissues, organs, and systems due to either too much stress or the dysfunction of the pathways controlling allostasis.

The advance of cognitive, systems and molecular neuroscience in the last several decades has provided clinical psychiatry with a more in-depth understanding of the pathological changes in brain functioning and architecture related to the development and progression of mental disorders. Behavioural testing in laboratory animals in combination with the utilisation of modern research methods like optogenetics, pharmacogenetics, and calcium imaging is a reliable strategy for the elucidation of the molecular, cellular, and circuit mechanisms of normal and pathological cognitive, affective, and motor processes (Shen et al., 2022). These approaches coupled with the progress in human neuroimaging are powerful sources of information for clinicians and could advance the development of more sophisticated therapies in psychiatry (Linden, 2012; Gordon, 2016; Xia and Kheirbek, 2020). It is safe to say that these fields are essential for the process of redefining the main clinical characteristics associated with major psychiatric diagnoses. In this regard, it is now becoming more evident that affective, anxiety and trauma-related disorders are merely pathologies of disturbed emotional states and behaviour. Evidence showcasing abnormalities in cognitive domains such as learning and memory, attention and social cognition in these disorders are accumulating (Weightman, Air and Baune, 2014; Dillon and Pizzagalli, 2018; Keller et al. 2019;). This is happening during a moment of a slow, but stable, paradigm shift in neuroscience, where emotion and cognition are starting to be viewed as functions of interacting brain systems, composed of overlapping structural networks and not as behaviourally separated entities (Pessoa, 2022). A captivating feature of the different cortical and subcortical structures composing these networks is their ability to undergo physical changes in order to maintain their capacities to process and store information regarding the encountered environmental stimuli. These structural alterations commonly known as neuroplasticity encompass a number of cellular processes - experience-dependent changes in synaptic strength, synaptogenesis, synaptic pruning, dendritic remodelling - leading to morphological rearrangements in the neuronal assemblies building up particular brain circuits. Unsurprisingly, unravelling the mechanisms and dynamics of the neuroplastic processes and their role for behaviour is of great value to psychiatry as it will allow for better understanding of the effects of current pharmacological and non-pharmacological therapies used in everyday practice and open the doors for the development of novel treatments (Kays et al., 2012).

Decades of neuroendocrinological investigation have shown that prolonged stress leads to serious disturbance in neuroplasticity (Radley et al., 2015). Hence, chronic stress-associated changes in brain architecture affect cognitive functions and lead to maladaptive behaviours. For instance, stress has profound effects on social behaviour, with chronic stress reducing social motivation and interactions in adulthood, and early stress during the periods of development leading to increased aggressiveness (Sandi and Haller, 2015). Chronic stress also influences reward processing, where it affects reward sensitivity and induces anhedonic behaviours (Ironside et al., 2018). This is in accordance with the "excitatory synapse hypothesis" of depression, which proposed that the hyperactivity of the HPA axis, combined with genetic susceptibility, causes weakening of excitatory synapses in the mesolimbic reward circuitry (Thompson et al., 2015). Animal model research further demonstrated that the effect of chronic stress is particularly strong in brain areas involved in the control of stress responses. Structural reorganisation caused by chronic stress has been particularly well studied in three regions – the aforementioned hippocampus, amygdala, and mPFC (Radley et al., 2015; McEwen et al., 2016). Not only are those regions part of a corticolimbic circuit regulating the HPA axis, but also they are part of the neural circuits responsible for the generation of fear and anxiety-related behaviours (Jankord and Herman, 2008; Shin and Liberzon, 2010). Furthermore, there is now substantial evidence coming from both research in rodents and humans, showing that these brain areas are strongly interconnected, and that deficiencies in their coupled work may be related to the development of mood and anxiety disorders (Godsil et al., 2013; Liu et al., 2020; Xia and Kheirbek, 2020).

The elucidation of stress effects on brain plasticity and functioning began with one ground-breaking study. McEwen, Weiss and Schwartz (1968) discovered for the first time the uptake of corticosterone (the animal analog of cortisol) by limbic structures. This was particularly prominent in the hippocampus. The hippocampus is located in the medial temporal lobe of the brain. The structure is composed of several different subfields – the dentate gyrus (DG), the cornu ammonis regions 1, 2 and 3 (CA1, CA2, CA3) and the subiculum. Each of these sections has its own cytoarchitecture and unique role in the processes executed by the hippocampus. The entorhinal cortex provides the main sensory input to the hippocampus. Furthermore, the hippocampus could be functionally divided into dorsal (posterior in humans) and ventral (anterior in humans). Because these subdivisions are part of a larger functional circuit, they have their own specific connections with other cortical and subcortical regions (Fanselow and Dong, 2010; Strange et al., 2014). The dorsal hippocampus has been linked to such functions like formation of episodic memories and navigation and through the projections of the dorsal CA1 and the dorsal subiculum is well connected to cortical areas like the retrosplenial cortex and anterior cingulate cortex. These cortices are also involved in various cognitive and mnemonic functions. On the other side, the ventral hippocampus is involved in emotional behaviour, reward processing, and stress responses, processes that are dependent on the direct and indirect projections of the ventral CA1 and the ventral subiculum to the amygdala, nucleus accumbens, and bed nucleus of stria terminalis (Fanselow and Dong, 2010; Strange et al., 2014). The hippocampus is very vulnerable to chronic stress. Perhaps the clearest example for this is hippocampal subfield CA3. Experiments using laboratory rodents have revealed that chronic stress will lead to retraction of the apical dendrites of the pyramidal neurons there. Moreover, this structural damage is associated with impaired performance during spatial tasks (for review Conrad,Ortiz and Judd, 2016; Ortiz and Conrad, 2018). Of course, CA3 is not the only affected hippocampal subfield, with a recent publication reporting that multimodal stress (exposure to a combination of hours-long bright light, loud noise, jostling, and restraint) reduced the number of synapses in dorsal CA1 area in mice (Maras et al., 2014). The same study also demonstrated that this effect was specific to the dorsal hippocampus, giving rise to functional deficiencies during the execution of a novel object recognition memory task.. Finally, the researchers compared the effect of multimodal stress to the one caused by unimodal stress (restraint or unexpected loud noise) and were able to find out that while the former affected synapses in both dorsal CA1 and CA3, the latter affected only those in dorsal CA3. This is pure evidence that the intensity of the stressors has different effects on the hippocampal circuitry and that some fields are more affected than others.

There are two types of receptors activated by glucocorticoids, both of which are found in the hippocampus - high affinity mineralocorticoid receptors (MRs) and low affinity glucocorticoid receptors (GRs). Even though the exact molecular mechanisms of hippocampal dysfunction caused by chronic stress are far from understood, an exciting proposal is that elevated levels of cortisol/corticosterone and dysregulation of the intracellular signal pathways governed by the GRs may lead to disruption of the expression of brain-derived neurotrophic factor (BDNF), a molecule important for synaptic plasticity and memory consolidation (for riview Finsterwald and Alberini, 2013). This idea is in unison with earlier hypotheses like the "neurotrophic hypothesis" of stress-related mood disorders (Duman and Monteggia 2006).

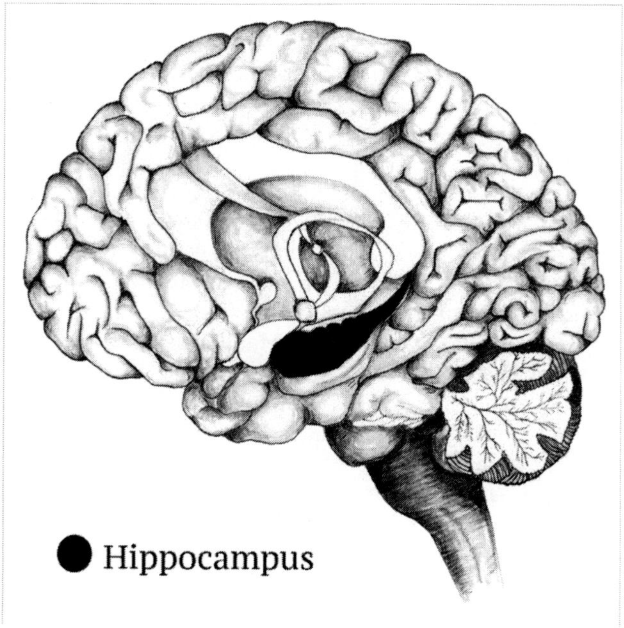

Fig.1: Relative location of the hippocampus

The effect of chronic stress is not limited only to structural changes in existing neurons and their synaptic connection but could also affect other forms of hippocampal neuroplasticity. In 1965 Altman and Das presented the first histological evidence that new granule cells are being generated postnatally in the DG of the hippocampus of an adult rat. This phenomenon, now known as adult hippocampal neurogenesis (AHN), was later confirmed to occur in the DG of old-world monkeys like marmosets and macaques (Gould et al., 1999) and most importantly, humans (Eriksson et al., 1998). AHN is an umbrella term that encompasses all the neurodevelopmental processes required for generation of new neurons in adult animals. All adult-born neurons originate from a pool of precursor cells located in the subgranular zone of the DG. AHN can be subdivided into four developmental stages - precursor cell phase, early survival phase, postmitotic maturation phase, and late survival phase (Kempermann, Song and Gage, 2015). Modern neuroscience is now starting to recognise AHN as an important modulator of various cognitive processes. For instance, adult-born neurons have been shown to facilitate remodelling of the hippocampal circuit leading to forgetting of already established memories (Frankland et al., 2013). Moreover, adult-born neurons have been reported to participate in pattern separation, the process of encoding highly similar experiences into distinct memory traces, limiting interference, and enhancing differentiation of environmental stimuli (Clelland et al., 2009; Nakashiba et al., 2012). Finally, Kumar et al. (2020) revealed the role of adult-born neurons in memory consolidation during REM sleep.

However, stress affects cell proliferation, differentiation, and survival and leads to reduced levels of AHC (Schoenfeld and Gould, 2012). This could harm the mnemonic functions of the hippocampus, leading to the formation of maladaptive memories and disturbed interpretation of emotionally charged stimuli (Besnard and Sahay, 2016). To the contrary, elevated levels of neurogenesis may have protective capacities, increasing resilience to the effect of future stressful events and improving the control over the activation on the HPA axis imposed by the hippocampus (Surget and Belzung, 2022). These adaptive properties of the AHN have been linked to ventral hippocampus, since this portion of the structure is connected to emotional behaviour and stress (Levone, Cryan and O'Leary, 2014). Furthermore, classic antidepressant drugs like the selective serotonin reuptake inhibitors (SSRIs) enhance AHN in animal models (Planchez, Surgery and Belzung, 2020). The idea that stress-related alterations in AHN levels cause deficits in information processing and behaviour that can be reversed with antidepressants, led to the neurogenic theory of depression (Jacobs, van Praag and Gage, 2000; Miller and Hen, 2016).

Trying to establish stress as a risk factor in anxiety and mood disorders, we have outlined some of its effects on brain plasticity, particularly in the hippocampus. Neuroimaging studies report reduced hippocampal volume in patients suffering from depression and PTSD (MacQueen and Frodl 2011; Logue et al., 2018). Furthermore, these patients are showing marked deficits in their hippocampal-dependent memory processes that could further intensify their symptoms (Dillon and Pizzagali, 2018; Barry et al., 2018). Both disorders are associated with sleep disturbances (Richard, Kanady and Neylan, 2019; Riemann et al, 2020;), which may impact hippocampal plasticity additionally. The hippocampal reduction and the changes in neuroplastic mechanisms associated with it cannot be solely caused by stress. Recently, using diffusion-weighted imaging, van Dijk et al. (2021) established alteration in the DG of people with high familial risk of depression as a risk factor. This suggests the presence of structural predispositions before the onset of the disorder. However, it is important to understand how adversities could further augment existing abnormalities in the brain. AHN is a unique form of neuroplasticity, with a profound modulatory role in memory, adaptivity, and emotional behaviour. AHN is greatly influenced by both environmental conditions and internal states. Currently, it is not possible to examine the functional contributions or the stages of AHN in humans. Nevertheless, animal models have played an immense part in advancing the knowledge of AHN-dependent enhancement of information processing and the therapeutic potential of these processes. Therefore, by further reviewing how stress affects AHN and its role for cognition, we intend to demonstrate the connection between these alterations and the general pathophysiology of depression, PTSD, and anxiety disorders. In doing so, we hope to outline the value of basic neurobiological research to clinical psychiatry.

Adult neurogenesis in the hippocampus - functional significance and the effect of chronic stress

The role of AHN in mood and stress-related disorders can be approached in several different ways. First, AHN is an important modulator of memory processes and facilitates flexible behaviour. Thus, stress-induced changes in the rates of AHN may have a negative effect on memory formation and could lead to cognitive distortions which will affect the generation of appropriate behavioural responses. Second, AHN may boost the resilience towards chronic stress. Increased rates of AHN, especially in ventral DG of the HPC, could increase the adaptive capacities of the brain and limit the consequences associated with allostatic load. And third, AHN may have important therapeutic implications. One of the effects of antidepressants on neuroplasticity may be to increase the rates of AHN and to improve the processing of information related to emotionally salient stimuli. Research using animal models of chronic stress and different depressive traits has provided evidence for three outlined scenarios.

Regarding the mnemonic role of AHN, it has been proposed that the new-born cells may be particularly active in the process of pattern separation (Miller and Sahay, 2019). Pattern separation is a hypothetical process that was proposed by the British neurophysiologist David Marr, which functions to store the information about similar environmental events into non-overlapping cellular ensembles. This results in the formation of separate representation of these memories, limiting interference, and increasing memory discrimination upon recall (Sahay, Wilson and Hen, 2011). Studies have shown that pattern separation may be one of the affected cognitive processes in individuals displaying depressive symptoms and some scholars have suggested that this could be interpreted as a marker for damaged AHN (Fujii et al., 2014; Leal et 2014; Gandy et al., 2017; Leal and Yassa, 2018). Interestingly enough, researchers have observed increased discrimination of negative stimuli in the group of depressed participants, suggesting the existence of affective bias (Leal, Tighe and Yassa, 2014). Moreover, Kheirbek and colleagues (2012) put forward an intriguing model, linking decreased neurogenesis and pattern separation to the overgeneralisation of fear associated with trauma-related disorders like PTSD and anxiety disorders like panic disorder. According to the authors, stressful conditions will limit AHN rates, which decreases the ability to discriminate between similar contextual information associated with different emotional valence. These pathophysiological changes will affect behaviour, leading to maladaptive defensive responses during non-threatening situations. Animal research confirms the positive correlation between neurogenesis and improved pattern separation. These studies have used strategies to increase or reduce neurogenesis in combination with multiple behavioural paradigms. For example, Sahay et al. (2011) used a genetic manipulation to enhance the survival of adult-born neurons in mice. By ablating the pro-apoptotic gene *Bax* the researchers expanded the population of the new-born cells in DG. Using a contextual fear-discrimination task, they demonstrated that the genetically modified animals were better that the control group in distinguishing to similar contexts, one of which was associated with a mild foot shock.

A different study (Niibori et al., 2016), applied the opposite approach, chemically or genetically suppressing neurogenesis in mice in order to investigate possible deficits in contextual discrimination. Using a fear conditioning task, the group found that both manipulations led to the same outcomes. Animals were unable to discriminate in which context they received a foot shock, and this was marked by altered populational coding in the neighbouring CA3 field. This alteration was observed thanks to the utilisation of a cellular imaging approach that localises the induction of *Arc mRNA* - a marker for experience-dependent neuronal activation. The obtained results showed a greater number of neurons in CA3 have been co-activated by both contexts, indicating a greater overlap between separate memory representations. This study nicely illustrates how neurogenesis in DG can influence information processing in downstream regions and therefore to influence their behavioural function. The impact of AN on memory is not only limited to pattern separation modulation. A great number of studies have explored the capacity of adult-born cells to regulate memory clearance and transformation (Akerset al.,2014; Gao et al., 2018; Scott et al., 2021; Evans et al., 2022). As time passes, memories become less dependent on the hippocampus for their retrieval and different cortical structures become more involved in their expression. Some theoretical accounts argue that this structural reorganisation of mnemonic representation, commonly referred to as systems consolidation, leads to gradual transformation of memories, making them less detailed and more gist-like in nature (Sekeres, Wincour and Moscovich, 2018; Gilboa and Moscovitch, 2021). Using the contextual fear conditioning task, Kitamura et al. (2009) have verified the role of AN in regulating the hippocampal dependency of memories. The authors examined memory-related hippocampal activity in mice, in which the incorporation of new-born cells in DG was suppressed either through X-ray irradiation or by genetic overexpression of follistatin. They found out that these manipulations maintained retrieval-associated activity in the hippocampus at a remote time point, evident by their ability to block memory expression through intrahippocampal infusion of tetrodotoxin (TTX) 28 days after training. To the contrary, running wheel exercise increased neurogenesis levels and accelerated the disengagement of the hippocampus, since the researchers were unable to disrupt retrieval by TTX application at day 7. Nevertheless, taking advantage of the of the same behavioural task, Ishikawa et al. (2016) discovered that following prolonged exposure to contextual remainders (context re-exposure), hippocampal dependency of the memory was restored. The authors of the study then stimulated neurogenesis either by using the pharmacological agent memantine or by submitting the animals to voluntary exercise (running). They discovered that the renewed involvement of the hippocampus made the memory susceptible to forgetting, dictated by elevated rates of neurogenesis. Memories that do not rely on the hippocampus are resistant to changes produced by neurogenesis. Continuing this line of research, Ishikawa et al. (2019), studied neurogenesis-induced forgetting in the context of social aversive experience. Because avoidance behaviours are a prominent feature of PTSD that could be driven by the existing memory for the traumatic event, the researchers used the social defeat stress paradigm to examine if neurogenesis-induced forgetting could suppress maladaptive memory and the social avoidance associated with it. Male mice were exposed to other aggressive mice for 10 days and were then evaluated for the presence of social avoidance memory - represented by time spent in interactive or avoidance zones within the open field where the encaged aggressor mice were placed - and anxiety-associated behaviours using elevated zero maze task. To enhance the levels of neurogenesis in the mice subjected to social defeat stress, the team again used systemic injections of memantine once a week for 4 weeks. Since no reinstatement of the social avoidance memory was observed and anxiety-associated behaviour was diminished, the obtained results were interpreted as related to forgetting due to uplifted neurogenesis. Epp and colleagues (2016) revealed a crucial role of AN for the regulation of proactive interference through forgetting. Their study compared the effect of reduced or increased levels of AN on encoding conflicting information. They discovered that post-learning increase of neurogenesis in mice through voluntary exercise improved learning of new information in a familiar context by degrading previously formed memories. Thus neurogenesis-induced forgetting may limit the chance of overlap between the representation of past and more recent events and adapt the animals to the present state of the environment. This effect was not observed when a running-induced boost of neurogenesis was suppressed by a genetic manipulation. Taking into consideration the accumulated evidence linking AN and forgetting, recently Ko and Frankland (2021) suggested a theoretical framework of how the continuous integration of adult-born granule cells into the hippocampal circuitry may determine the fate of memories. They outlined the competition between new and mature neurons at both the synaptic and cellular levels as a mark of ongoing structural reorganisation of the DG-CA3 microcircuit that leads to slow elimination of the existing synaptic connections. This results in the gradual loss of specificity of the hippocampal-dependent memories (as proposed by some theories of systems consolidation) and culminates with the complete silencing of the memory trace in the hippocampus, making it impossible to be reactivated by external reminders. According to this view, the forgetting of contextual attributes of particular stimuli supports the ability of animals to generalise and to adapt faster to the changes taking part in the external world. Previously, other researchers have made similar propositions regarding the connection between neurogenesis and memory generalisation (Terranova, Ogawa and Kitamura, 2019), so future work in this direction promises to bring important advances that could be pivotal for the development of more sophisticated therapies for traumatic memories and the behavioural consequences.

Many of the existing studies portraying the functional significance of AN, including the ones discussed here, use genetic or pharmacological strategies to elevate the production of granule cells. A question then arises regarding the impact of different environmental conditions on the cellular processes composing neurogenesis and thereafter on functions of the hippocampus. As it was mentioned already, physical exercise enhances neurogenesis. Environmental enrichment, defined as the manipulation of the environment to include a greater variety of stimuli, also has beneficial effects on AHN. Both of these conditions may upregulate the levels of growth factors like brain-derived neurotrophic factor (BDNF) and vascular endothelial growth factor (VEGF) which influence the proliferation of neural progenitor cells (van Praag, 2008; Clemenson, Deng and Gage, 2015). On the other hand, research employing various animal chronic stress protocols reported that the accumulation of aversive experiences impacts the stages of neurogenesis differently. Most of these studies report that chronic stress affects mainly cell proliferation and cell survival (Lee et al., 2006; Mineur, Belzung and Crusio, 2007; Schoenfeld and Gould, 2012). However, is important to keep in mind that the results of these studies are equivocal, since the effect of stress may be multifactorial - encompassing intensity of the stressor, sex differences, and the strain of the laboratory animals (Jones, Zhou and Jhaveri, 2022). Dagyte et al. (2009) compared the effect of acute and chronic stress on cell proliferation in the DG of male Wistar rats using foot shock stress protocol. The chronic stress experiment consisted of daily foot shock sessions for 21 consecutive days. The team did not observe any changes in the animals subjected to the acute stress conditions.

Conversely, a transient decrease in cell proliferation and neurons expressing doublecortin - protein used as a marker for neurogenesis - was noted in animals exposed to chronic stress. No changes in the rates of cell survival for cells generated before stress exposure was observed. Even if the marked suppression in cell proliferation was temporary (lasting 2 horse after stress), the authors speculate that in the long-term this may have greater impact on the pool of adult-born neurons. Lagace et al. (2010), decided to use chronic social defeat stress paradigm to establish the behavioural consequences of stress-induced AHN impairment. First, they divided mice into two groups - "susceptible" and "unsusceptible" to stress. The "susceptible group" was marked by prolonged social avoidance behaviour and depressive-like phenotypes (anhedonia, social anxiety, circadian changes, etc.), while the "resilient group" had responses identical to the control group. Interestingly, it was discovered that both groups suffered from transient reduction of cell proliferation (24 hours post-stress) but unexpectedly, the vulnerable mice had increased rates in cell survival of new-born cells after exposure to stress conditions. Regarding the rates of cell survival for cells generated before stress exposure, there was no marked difference in any of the studied group. Ablating AHN via x-ray irradiation 4 weeks before social defeat stress, decreased the social avoidance associated with it. This study demonstrates that compensatory increase in neurogenesis after social stress may have negative consequences, maintaining stress-induced behaviours. Taking a different approach, De Miguel et al. (2017), explored the structural and functional characteristics of cells generated at the end of chronic stress protocol. Male CD1 mice were subjected to chronic social stress protocol for 14 days. The team labelled the cells born during the last 5 days of stress exposure. Similar to the study of Lagace and associates (2010), the researchers observed an increase in the levels of survival and incorporation of new-born cells during the 10 weeks recovery from social stress. In one of their experiments, mice underwent a second session of chronic stress for 2 weeks, 8 weeks after the first. After the end of the second chronic stress session, the animals were trained in water maze spatial learning tasks. Subsequent analysis showed that cells generated near the end of first chronic stress exposure were negatively affected by the second one, which was manifested by their low density of dendritic spines, and decreased number of dendritic branches. Furthermore, these cells were not activated by the spatial learning task which may directly link to their morphological changes.

The studies by Lagace (2010) and De Miguel et al. (2017) open the doors to a different plausible explanation of the chronic stress - neurogenesis connection. Rather than decreased rates in the long-term (changes in quantity after stress termination), chronic stress may impact the structure and responsiveness to subsequent stimuli of the adult-born cells, thus decreasing the effectiveness of their integration into the hippocampal circuitry once they are mature enough. This notion could be further reinforced by other results of the studies outlined above. First, both Dagyte et al. (2009) and Legace et al. (2010) observed only a transient decrease in cell proliferation. Second, both studies did not find reduction in the survival rates of new-born neurons generated before the onset of stress. However,

Lagace and colleagues (2010) reported an increase in survival rate for cells generated after the termination of stress, while Dagyte revealed a decrease in the doublecortin-positive cells born during stress periods. Thereafter, hypothetically, chronic stress may affect mainly the survival rates of these cells that are born during the actual course of accumulating adversities. Increased levels of AHN during the post-stress period or repeated exposure to a familiar stressor could be viewed as a compensatory mechanism, but these cells may express deficits in their information processing properties and further strengthen maladaptive behavioural responses.

Conclusion

We begin our paper by mentioning the common belief - stress is a dangerous phenomenon. However, much as every other biological entity that survived the test of evolution, stress has an apparent adaptive purpose. The union of cognitive, psychoendocrinological, metabolic, and immunological processes that stress is, exists to make us alert in the cases of unexpected environmental change and to prepare us for similar future events. One of the giants in stress biology, Bruce McEwen, endorsed the view of stress as a mechanism of adaptation throughout his spectacular career (2005). Moreover, his work has also been the driving force behind the now well-established perspective of the deleterious accumulating effect of persistent stress (Mcewen, 2017). Once corticosterone-binding receptors were discovered in the brain, it became apparent that they can influence glutamate transmission, synaptic plasticity, and dendritic remodelling, with high glucocorticoid levels associated with chronic stress leading to dendritic atrophy, retraction, and decreased levels of dendritic spines (Popoli et al., 2011). When brain areas involved in the generation of cognitive and affective states are damaged, the risk for the occurrence of stress-driven mood pathologies increases (McEwen and Akil, 2020).

Throughout our review, we have tried to establish chronic stress as a major risk factor for the development of mood, anxiety, and trauma-related disorders. We decided to focus our attention particularly on the effects of chronic stress on AHN, because of its functional implication and because we believe that future teraphytical approaches targeting this form of neuroplasticity may bring great progress in the treatment of the disorders that are part of the abovementioned diagnostic clusters. This view of ours is reinforced by the hub-like properties of the hippocampus, a structure with wide projections to other cortical and subcortical areas, important for both memory formation and behavioural regulation (Fanselow and Dong, 2010).

The question regarding the presence of neurogenesis in the adult human hippocampus remains a controversial one (Kempermann, 2018). Reports providing evidence for the two opposing positions have been published (Tobin et al., 2019; Franjic et al., 2022). Resolving this issue is beyond the scope of this review, but our opinion is that animal research on AHN will advance our understanding of the general properties of neuroplasticity, regardless of the answers that the future holds.

Here we fulfilled two important goals. We described the role of neurogenesis in memory modulation and proposed a different hypothetical framework for the effect of chronic stress on AHN. It is important to note that we have outlined only a small number of the existing literature on the topic of stress and neurogenesis. However, the studies that we have mentioned perfectly illustrate the maladaptive consequences of chronic stress. It is possible that chronic stress affects both the processes on which neurogenesis depends (cell proliferation and survival) during the time of adversity and the synaptic integration of the cells born during recovery. The fact that some studies report an increase in AHN during recovery suggests there may be some kind of compensatory reaction that replaces the cells that died during stress. However, these post-stress cells may "suffer" from decreased responsivity to environmental stimuli and may be unable to fully integrate into DG-CA3 circuit.

References

Akers, K.G., Martinez-Canabal, A., Restivo, L., Yiu, A.P., De Cristofaro, A., Hsiang, H.-L. (Liz), Wheeler, A.L., Guskjolen, A., Niibori, Y., Shoji, H., Ohira, K., Richards, B.A., Miyakawa, T., Josselyn, S.A., Frankland, P.W., 2014. Hippocampal Neurogenesis Regulates Forgetting During Adulthood and Infancy. Science 344, 598–602. https://doi.org/10.1126/science.1248903

Altman, J., Das, G.D., 1965. Autoradiographic and histological evidence of postnatal hippocampal neurogenesis in rats. J. Comp. Neurol. 124, 319–335. https://doi.org/10.1002/cne.901240303

Barry, T.J., Chiu, C.P.Y., Raes, F., Ricarte, J., Lau, H., 2018. The Neurobiology of Reduced Autobiographical Memory Specificity. Trends in Cognitive Sciences 22, 1038–1049. https://doi.org/10.1016/j.tics.2018.09.001

Besnard, A., Sahay, A., 2016. Adult Hippocampal Neurogenesis, Fear Generalization, and Stress. Neuropsychopharmacol 41, 24–44. https://doi.org/10.1038/npp.2015.167

Cannon, W.B., 1914. THE EMERGENCY FUNCTION OF THE ADRENAL MEDULLA IN PAIN AND THE MAJOR EMOTIONS. American Journal of Physiology-Legacy Content 33, 356–372. https://doi.org/10.1152/ajplegacy.1914.33.2.356

Clelland, C.D., Choi, M., Romberg, C., Clemenson, G.D., Fragniere, A., Tyers, P., Jessberger, S., Saksida, L.M., Barker, R.A., Gage, F.H., Bussey, T.J., 2009. A Functional Role for Adult Hippocampal Neurogenesis in Spatial Pattern Separation. Science 325, 210–213. https://doi.org/10.1126/science.1173215

Clemenson, G.D., Deng, W., Gage, F.H., 2015. Environmental enrichment and neurogenesis: from mice to humans. Current Opinion in Behavioral Sciences 4, 56–62. https://doi.org/10.1016/j.cobeha.2015.02.005

Conrad, C.D., Ortiz, J.B., Judd, J.M., 2017. Chronic stress and hippocampal dendritic complexity: Methodological and functional considerations. Physiology & Behavior 178, 66–81. https://doi.org/10.1016/j.physbeh.2016.11.017

Dagytė, G., Van der Zee, E.A., Postema, F., Luiten, P.G.M., Den Boer, J.A., Trentani, A., Meerlo, P., 2009. Chronic but not acute foot-shock stress leads to temporary suppression of cell proliferation in rat hippocampus. Neuroscience 162, 904–913. https://doi.org/10.1016/j.neuroscience.2009.05.053

De Miguel, Z., Haditsch, U., Palmer, T.D., Azpiroz, A., Sapolsky, R.M., 2019. Adult-generated neurons born during chronic social stress are uniquely adapted to respond to subsequent chronic social stress. Mol Psychiatry 24, 1178–1188. https://doi.org/10.1038/s41380-017-0013-1

Duman, R.S., Monteggia, L.M., 2006. A Neurotrophic Model for Stress-Related Mood Disorders. Biological Psychiatry 59, 1116–1127. https://doi.org/10.1016/j.biopsych.2006.02.013

Epp, J.R., Silva Mera, R., Köhler, S., Josselyn, S.A., Frankland, P.W., 2016. Neurogenesis-mediated forgetting minimizes proactive interference. Nat Commun 7, 10838. https://doi.org/10.1038/ncomms10838

Eriksson, P.S., Perfilieva, E., Björk-Eriksson, T., Alborn, A.-M., Nordborg, C., Peterson, D.A., Gage, F.H., 1998. Neurogenesis in the adult human hippocampus. Nat Med 4, 1313–1317. https://doi.org/10.1038/3305

Evans, A., Terstege, D.J., Scott, G.A., Tsutsui, M., Epp, J.R., 2022. Neurogenesis mediated plasticity is associated with reduced neuronal activity in CA1 during context fear memory retrieval. Sci Rep 12, 7016. https://doi.org/10.1038/s41598-022-10947-w

Fanselow, M.S., Dong, H.-W., 2010. Are the Dorsal and Ventral Hippocampus Functionally Distinct Structures? Neuron 65, 7–19. https://doi.org/10.1016/j.neuron.2009.11.031

Finsterwald, C., Alberini, C.M., 2014. Stress and glucocorticoid receptor-dependent mechanisms in long-term memory: From adaptive responses to psychopathologies. Neurobiology of Learning and Memory 112, 17–29. https://doi.org/10.1016/j.nlm.2013.09.017

Franjic, D., Skarica, M., Ma, S., Arellano, J.I., Tebbenkamp, A.T.N., Choi, J., Xu, C., Li, Q., Morozov, Y.M., Andrijevic, D., Vrselja, Z., Spajic, A., Santpere, G., Li, M., Zhang, S., Liu, Y., Spurrier, J., Zhang, L., Gudelj, I., Rapan, L., Takahashi, H., Huttner, A., Fan, R., Strittmatter, S.M., Sousa, A.M.M., Rakic, P., Sestan, N., 2022. Transcriptomic taxonomy and neurogenic trajectories of adult human, macaque, and pig hippocampal and entorhinal cells. Neuron 110, 452-469.e14. https://doi.org/10.1016/j.neuron.2021.10.036

Frankland, P.W., Köhler, S., Josselyn, S.A., 2013. Hippocampal neurogenesis and forgetting. Trends in Neurosciences 36, 497–503. https://doi.org/10.1016/j.tins.2013.05.002

Fujii, T., Saito, D.N., Yanaka, H.T., Kosaka, H., Okazawa, H., 2014. Depressive mood modulates the anterior lateral CA1 and DG/CA3 during a pattern separation task in cognitively intact individuals: A functional MRI study: Depressive Mood Modulates CA1 and DG/CA3. Hippocampus 24, 214–224. https://doi.org/10.1002/hipo.22216

Gandy, K., Kim, S., Sharp, C., Dindo, L., Maletic-Savatic, M., Calarge, C., 2017. Pattern Separation: A Potential Marker of Impaired Hippocampal Adult Neurogenesis in Major Depressive Disorder. Front. Neurosci. 11, 571. https://doi.org/10.3389/fnins.2017.00571

Gao, A., Xia, F., Guskjolen, A.J., Ramsaran, A.I., Santoro, A., Josselyn, S.A., Frankland, P.W., 2018. Elevation of Hippocampal Neurogenesis Induces a Temporally Graded Pattern of Forgetting of Contextual Fear Memories. J. Neurosci. 38, 3190–3198. https://doi.org/10.1523/JNEUROSCI.3126-17.2018

Gilboa, A., Moscovitch, M., 2021. No consolidation without representation: Correspondence between neural and psychological representations in recent and remote memory. Neuron 109, 2239–2255. https://doi.org/10.1016/j.neuron.2021.04.025

Godsil, B.P., Kiss, J.P., Spedding, M., Jay, T.M., 2013. The hippocampal–prefrontal pathway: The weak link in psychiatric disorders? European Neuropsychopharmacology 23, 1165–1181. https://doi.org/10.1016/j.euroneuro.2012.10.018

Gordon, J.A., 2016. On being a circuit psychiatrist. Nat Neurosci 19, 1385–1386. https://doi.org/10.1038/nn.4419

Gould, E., Reeves, A.J., Fallah, M., Tanapat, P., Gross, C.G., Fuchs, E., 1999. Hippocampal neurogenesis in adult Old World primates. Proc. Natl. Acad. Sci. U.S.A. 96, 5263–5267. https://doi.org/10.1073/pnas.96.9.5263

Hermans, E.J., van Marle, H.J.F., Ossewaarde, L., Henckens, M.J.A.G., Qin, S., van Kesteren, M.T.R., Schoots, V.C., Cousijn, H., Rijpkema, M., Oostenveld, R., Fernández, G., 2011. Stress-Related Noradrenergic Activity Prompts Large-Scale Neural Network Reconfiguration. Science 334, 1151–1153. https://doi.org/10.1126/science.1209603

Ironside, M., Kumar, P., Kang, M.-S., Pizzagalli, D.A., 2018. Brain mechanisms mediating effects of stress on reward sensitivity. Current Opinion in Behavioral Sciences 22, 106–113. https://doi.org/10.1016/j.cobeha.2018.01.016

Ishikawa, R., Fukushima, H., Frankland, P.W., Kida, S., 2016. Hippocampal neurogenesis enhancers promote forgetting of remote fear memory after hippocampal reactivation by retrieval. eLife 5, e17464. https://doi.org/10.7554/eLife.17464

Ishikawa, R., Uchida, C., Kitaoka, S., Furuyashiki, T., Kida, S., 2019. Improvement of PTSD-like behavior by the forgetting effect of hippocampal neurogenesis enhancer memantine in a social defeat stress paradigm. Mol Brain 12, 68. https://doi.org/10.1186/s13041-019-0488-6

Jacobs, B.L., van Praag, H., Gage, F.H., 2000. Adult brain neurogenesis and psychiatry: a novel theory of depression. Mol Psychiatry 5, 262–269. https://doi.org/10.1038/sj.mp.4000712

Jankord, R., Herman, J.P., 2008. Limbic Regulation of Hypothalamo-Pituitary-Adrenocortical Function during Acute and Chronic Stress. Annals of the New York Academy of Sciences 1148, 64–73. https://doi.org/10.1196/annals.1410.012

Jones, K.L., Zhou, M., Jhaveri, D.J., 2022. Dissecting the role of adult hippocampal neurogenesis towards resilience versus susceptibility to stress-related mood disorders. npj Sci. Learn. 7, 16. https://doi.org/10.1038/s41539-022-00133-y

Kays, J.L., Hurley, R.A., Taber, K.H., 2012. The Dynamic Brain: Neuroplasticity and Mental Health. JNP 24, 118–124. https://doi.org/10.1176/appi.neuropsych.12050109

Keller, A.S., Leikauf, J.E., Holt-Gosselin, B., Staveland, B.R., Williams, L.M., 2019. Paying attention to attention in depression. Transl Psychiatry 9, 279. https://doi.org/10.1038/s41398-019-0616-1

Kempermann, G., Gage, F.H., Aigner, L., Song, H., Curtis, M.A., Thuret, S., Kuhn, H.G., Jessberger, S., Frankland, P.W., Cameron, H.A., Gould, E., Hen, R., Abrous, D.N., Toni, N., Schinder, A.F., Zhao, X., Lucassen,

P.J., Frisén, J., 2018. Human Adult Neurogenesis: Evidence and Remaining Questions. Cell Stem Cell 23, 25–30. https://doi.org/10.1016/j.stem.2018.04.004

Kempermann, G., Song, H., Gage, F.H., 2015. Neurogenesis in the Adult Hippocampus. Cold Spring Harb Perspect Biol 7, a018812. https://doi.org/10.1101/cshperspect.a018812

Kheirbek, M.A., Klemenhagen, K.C., Sahay, A., Hen, R., 2012. Neurogenesis and generalization: a new approach to stratify and treat anxiety disorders. Nat Neurosci 15, 1613–1620. https://doi.org/10.1038/nn.3262

Kitamura, T., Saitoh, Y., Takashima, N., Murayama, A., Niibori, Y., Ageta, H., Sekiguchi, M., Sugiyama, H., Inokuchi, K., 2009. Adult Neurogenesis Modulates the Hippocampus-Dependent Period of Associative Fear Memory. Cell 139, 814–827. https://doi.org/10.1016/j.cell.2009.10.020

Ko, S.Y., Frankland, P.W., 2021. Neurogenesis-dependent transformation of hippocampal engrams. Neuroscience Letters 762, 136176. https://doi.org/10.1016/j.neulet.2021.136176

Kumar, D., Koyanagi, I., Carrier-Ruiz, A., Vergara, P., Srinivasan, S., Sugaya, Y., Kasuya, M., Yu, T.-S., Vogt, K.E., Muratani, M., Ohnishi, T., Singh, S., Teixeira, C.M., Chérasse, Y., Naoi, T., Wang, S.-H., Nondhalee, P., Osman, B.A.H., Kaneko, N., Sawamoto, K., Kernie, S.G., Sakurai, T., McHugh, T.J., Kano, M., Yanagisawa, M., Sakaguchi, M., 2020. Sparse Activity of Hippocampal Adult-Born Neurons during REM Sleep Is Necessary for Memory Consolidation. Neuron 107, 552-565.e10. https://doi.org/10.1016/j.neuron.2020.05.008

Lagace, D.C., Donovan, M.H., DeCarolis, N.A., Farnbauch, L.A., Malhotra, S., Berton, O., Nestler, E.J., Krishnan, V., Eisch, A.J., 2010. Adult hippocampal neurogenesis is functionally important for stress-induced social avoidance. Proc. Natl. Acad. Sci. U.S.A. 107, 4436–4441. https://doi.org/10.1073/pnas.0910072107

Leal, S.L., Tighe, S.K., Jones, C.K., Yassa, M.A., 2014a. Pattern separation of emotional information in hippocampal dentate and CA3: Emotional Pattern Separation in Dentate Gyrus/Ca3. Hippocampus 24, 1146–1155. https://doi.org/10.1002/hipo.22298

Leal, S.L., Tighe, S.K., Yassa, M.A., 2014b. Asymmetric effects of emotion on mnemonic interference. Neurobiology of Learning and Memory 111, 41–48. https://doi.org/10.1016/j.nlm.2014.02.013

Lee, K.-J., Kim, S.-J., Kim, S.-W., Choi, Song-Hyen, Shin, Y.-C., Park, S.-H., Moon, B.-H., Cho, E., Lee, M.-S., Choi, Sang-Hyun, Chun, B.-G., Shin, K.-H., 2006. Chronic mild stress decreases survival, but not proliferation, of new-born cells in adult rat hippocampus. Exp Mol Med 38, 44–54. https://doi.org/10.1038/emm.2006.6

Levone, B.R., Cryan, J.F., O'Leary, O.F., 2015. Role of adult hippocampal neurogenesis in stress resilience. Neurobiology of Stress 1, 147–155. https://doi.org/10.1016/j.ynstr.2014.11.003

Linden, D.E.J., 2012. The Challenges and Promise of Neuroimaging in Psychiatry. Neuron 73, 8–22. https://doi.org/10.1016/j.neuron.2011.12.014

Liu, W.-Z., Zhang, W.-H., Zheng, Z.-H., Zou, J.-X., Liu, X.-X., Huang, S.-H., You, W.-J., He, Y., Zhang, J.-Y., Wang, X.-D., Pan, B.-X., 2020. Identification of a prefrontal cortex-to-amygdala pathway for chronic stress-induced anxiety. Nat Commun 11, 2221. https://doi.org/10.1038/s41467-020-15920-7

Logue, M.W., van Rooij, S.J.H., Dennis, E.L., Davis, S.L., Hayes, J.P., Stevens, J.S., Densmore, M., Haswell, C.C., Ipser, J., Koch, S.B.J., Korgaonkar, M., Lebois, L.A.M., Peverill, M., Baker, J.T., Boedhoe, P.S.W., Frijling, J.L., Gruber, S.A., Harpaz-Rotem, I., Jahanshad, N., Koopowitz, S., Levy, I., Nawijn, L., O'Connor, L., Olff, M., Salat, D.H., Sheridan, M.A., Spielberg, J.M., van Zuiden, M., Winternitz, S.R., Wolff, J.D., Wolf, E.J., Wang, X., Wrocklage, K., Abdallah, C.G., Bryant, R.A., Geuze, E., Jovanovic, T., Kaufman, M.L., King, A.P., Krystal, J.H., Lagopoulos, J., Bennett, M., Lanius, R., Liberzon, I., McGlinchey, R.E., McLaughlin, K.A., Milberg, W.P., Miller, M.W., Ressler, K.J., Veltman, D.J., Stein, D.J., Thomaes, K., Thompson, P.M., Morey, R.A., 2018. Smaller Hippocampal Volume in Posttraumatic Stress Disorder: A Multisite ENIGMA-PGC Study: Subcortical Volumetry Results from Posttraumatic Stress Disorder Consortia. Biological Psychiatry 83, 244–253. https://doi.org/10.1016/j.biopsych.2017.09.006

MacQueen, G., Frodl, T., 2011. The hippocampus in major depression: evidence for the convergence of the bench and bedside in psychiatric research? Mol Psychiatry 16, 252–264. https://doi.org/10.1038/mp.2010.80

Maras, P.M., Molet, J., Chen, Y., Rice, C., Ji, S.G., Solodkin, A., Baram, T.Z., 2014. Preferential loss of dorsal-hippocampus synapses underlies memory impairments provoked by short, multimodal stress. Mol Psychiatry 19, 811–822. https://doi.org/10.1038/mp.2014.12

Mason J. W., 1968. A review of psychoendocrine research on the pituitary-adrenal cortical system 30, 576–607.

Mason, J.W., 1971. A re-evaluation of the concept of 'non-specificity' in stress theory. Journal of Psychiatric Research 8, 323–333.

https://doi.org/10.1016/0022-3956(71)90028-8
McEwen, B.S., 2017. Neurobiological and Systemic Effects of Chronic Stress. Chronic Stress 1, 247054701769232. https://doi.org/10.1177/2470547017692328
McEwen, B.S., 2005. Stressed or stressed out: what is the difference? J Psychiatry Neurosci 30, 315–318.
McEwen, B.S., 1993. Stress and the Individual: Mechanisms Leading to Disease. Arch Intern Med 153, 2093. https://doi.org/10.1001/archinte.1993.00410180039004
McEwen, B.S., Akil, H., 2020. Revisiting the Stress Concept: Implications for Affective Disorders. J. Neurosci. 40, 12–21. https://doi.org/10.1523/JNEUROSCI.0733-19.2019
McEwen, B.S., Nasca, C., Gray, J.D., 2016. Stress Effects on Neuronal Structure: Hippocampus, Amygdala, and Prefrontal Cortex. Neuropsychopharmacol 41, 3–23. https://doi.org/10.1038/npp.2015.171
McEwen, B.S., Stellar, E., 1993. Stress and the individual. Mechanisms leading to disease. Arch Intern Med 153, 2093–2101.
Mcewen, B.S., Weiss, J.M., Schwartz, L.S., 1968. Selective Retention of Corticosterone by Limbic Structures in Rat Brain. Nature 220, 911–912. https://doi.org/10.1038/220911a0
Miller, B.R., Hen, R., 2015. The current state of the neurogenic theory of depression and anxiety. Current Opinion in Neurobiology 30, 51–58. https://doi.org/10.1016/j.conb.2014.08.012
Miller, S.M., Sahay, A., 2019. Functions of adult-born neurons in hippocampal memory interference and indexing. Nat Neurosci 22, 1565–1575. https://doi.org/10.1038/s41593-019-0484-2
Mineur, Y.S., Belzung, C., Crusio, W.E., 2007. Functional implications of decreases in neurogenesis following chronic mild stress in mice. Neuroscience 150, 251–259. https://doi.org/10.1016/j.neuroscience.2007.09.045
Nakashiba, T., Cushman, J.D., Pelkey, K.A., Renaudineau, S., Buhl, D.L., McHugh, T.J., Barrera, V.R., Chittajallu, R., Iwamoto, K.S., McBain, C.J., Fanselow, M.S., Tonegawa, S., 2012. Young Dentate Granule Cells Mediate Pattern Separation, whereas Old Granule Cells Facilitate Pattern Completion. Cell 149, 188–201. https://doi.org/10.1016/j.cell.2012.01.046
Niibori, Y., Yu, T.-S., Epp, J.R., Akers, K.G., Josselyn, S.A., Frankland, P.W., 2012. Suppression of adult neurogenesis impairs population coding of similar contexts in hippocampal CA3 region. Nat Commun 3, 1253. https://doi.org/10.1038/ncomms2261

Ortiz, J.B., Conrad, C.D., 2018. The impact from the aftermath of chronic stress on hippocampal structure and function: Is there a recovery? Frontiers in Neuroendocrinology 49, 114–123. https://doi.org/10.1016/j.yfrne.2018.02.005

Pessoa, L., 2010. Emergent processes in cognitive-emotional interactions. Dialogues in Clinical Neuroscience 12, 433–448. https://doi.org/10.31887/DCNS.2010.12.4/lpessoa

Planchez, B., Surget, A., Belzung, C., 2020. Adult hippocampal neurogenesis and antidepressants effects. Current Opinion in Pharmacology 50, 88–95. https://doi.org/10.1016/j.coph.2019.11.009

Popoli, M., Yan, Z., McEwen, B.S., Sanacora, G., 2012. The stressed synapse: the impact of stress and glucocorticoids on glutamate transmission. Nat Rev Neurosci 13, 22–37. https://doi.org/10.1038/nrn3138

Radley, J., Morilak, D., Viau, V., Campeau, S., 2015. Chronic stress and brain plasticity: Mechanisms underlying adaptive and maladaptive changes and implications for stress-related CNS disorders. Neuroscience & Biobehavioral Reviews 58, 79–91. https://doi.org/10.1016/j.neubiorev.2015.06.018

Richards, A., Kanady, J.C., Neylan, T.C., 2020. Sleep disturbance in PTSD and other anxiety-related disorders: an updated review of clinical features, physiological characteristics, and psychological and neurobiological mechanisms. Neuropsychopharmacol. 45, 55–73. https://doi.org/10.1038/s41386-019-0486-5

Riemann, D., Krone, L.B., Wulff, K., Nissen, C., 2020. Sleep, insomnia, and depression. Neuropsychopharmacol. 45, 74–89. https://doi.org/10.1038/s41386-019-0411-y

Ross, J.A., Van Bockstaele, E.J., 2021. The Locus Coeruleus-Norepinephrine System in Stress and Arousal: Unraveling Historical, Current, and Future Perspectives. Front. Psychiatry 11, 601519. https://doi.org/10.3389/fpsyt.2020.601519

Sahay, A., Scobie, K.N., Hill, A.S., O'Carroll, C.M., Kheirbek, M.A., Burghardt, N.S., Fenton, A.A., Dranovsky, A., Hen, R., 2011a. Increasing adult hippocampal neurogenesis is sufficient to improve pattern separation. Nature 472, 466–470. https://doi.org/10.1038/nature09817

Sahay, A., Wilson, D.A., Hen, R., 2011b. Pattern Separation: A Common Function for New Neurons in Hippocampus and Olfactory Bulb. Neuron 70, 582–588. https://doi.org/10.1016/j.neuron.2011.05.012

Sandi, C., Haller, J., 2015. Stress and the social brain: behavioural effects and neurobiological mechanisms. Nat Rev Neurosci 16, 290–304.

https://doi.org/10.1038/nrn3918
Sara, S.J., Bouret, S., 2012. Orienting and Reorienting: The Locus Coeruleus Mediates Cognition through Arousal. Neuron 76, 130–141. https://doi.org/10.1016/j.neuron.2012.09.011
Schoenfeld, T.J., Gould, E., 2012. Stress, stress hormones, and adult neurogenesis. Experimental Neurology 233, 12–21. https://doi.org/10.1016/j.expneurol.2011.01.008
Scott, G.A., Terstege, D.J., Roebuck, A.J., Gorzo, K.A., Vu, A.P., Howland, J.G., Epp, J.R., 2021. Adult neurogenesis mediates forgetting of multiple types of memory in the rat. Mol Brain 14, 97. https://doi.org/10.1186/s13041-021-00808-4
Seeley, W.W., 2019. The Salience Network: A Neural System for Perceiving and Responding to Homeostatic Demands. J. Neurosci. 39, 9878–9882. https://doi.org/10.1523/JNEUROSCI.1138-17.2019
Sekeres, M.J., Winocur, G., Moscovitch, M., 2018. The hippocampus and related neocortical structures in memory transformation. Neuroscience Letters 680, 39–53. https://doi.org/10.1016/j.neulet.2018.05.006
Selye, H., 1936. A Syndrome produced by Diverse Nocuous Agents. Nature 138, 32–32. https://doi.org/10.1038/138032a0
Shen, Y., Luchetti, A., Fernandes, G., Do Heo, W., Silva, A.J., 2022. The emergence of molecular systems neuroscience. Mol Brain 15, 7. https://doi.org/10.1186/s13041-021-00885-5
Shin, L.M., Liberzon, I., 2010. The Neurocircuitry of Fear, Stress, and Anxiety Disorders. Neuropsychopharmacol 35, 169–191. https://doi.org/10.1038/npp.2009.83
Sterling P., Eyer J., n.d. allostasis: A New Paradigm to Explain Arousal Pathology, in: Handbook of Life Stress, Cognition and Health. John Wiley & Sons, Ltd.
Strange, B.A., Witter, M.P., Lein, E.S., Moser, E.I., 2014. Functional organization of the hippocampal longitudinal axis. Nat Rev Neurosci 15, 655–669. https://doi.org/10.1038/nrn3785
Surget, A., Belzung, C., 2022. Adult hippocampal neurogenesis shapes adaptation and improves stress response: a mechanistic and integrative perspective. Mol Psychiatry 27, 403–421. https://doi.org/10.1038/s41380-021-01136-8
Terranova, J.I., Ogawa, S.K., Kitamura, T., 2019. Adult hippocampal neurogenesis for systems consolidation of memory. Behavioural Brain Research 372, 112035. https://doi.org/10.1016/j.bbr.2019.112035
Thompson, S.M., Kallarackal, A.J., Kvarta, M.D., Van Dyke, A.M., LeGates, T.A., Cai, X., 2015. An excitatory synapse hypothesis of depression. Trends in Neurosciences 38, 279–294.

https://doi.org/10.1016/j.tins.2015.03.003
Tobin, M.K., Musaraca, K., Disouky, A., Shetti, A., Bheri, A., Honer, W.G., Kim, N., Dawe, R.J., Bennett, D.A., Arfanakis, K., Lazarov, O., 2019. Human Hippocampal Neurogenesis Persists in Aged Adults and Alzheimer's Disease Patients. Cell Stem Cell 24, 974-982.e3. https://doi.org/10.1016/j.stem.2019.05.003
Ulrich-Lai, Y.M., Herman, J.P., 2009. Neural regulation of endocrine and autonomic stress responses. Nat Rev Neurosci 10, 397–409. https://doi.org/10.1038/nrn2647
van Dijk, M.T., Cha, J., Semanek, D., Aw, N., Gameroff, M.J., Abraham, E., Wickramaratne, P.J., Weissman, M.M., Posner, J., Talati, A., 2021. Altered Dentate Gyrus Microstructure in Individuals at High Familial Risk for Depression Predicts Future Symptoms. Biological Psychiatry: Cognitive Neuroscience and Neuroimaging 6, 50–58. https://doi.org/10.1016/j.bpsc.2020.06.006
van Praag, H., 2008. Neurogenesis and Exercise: Past and Future Directions. Neuromol Med 10, 128–140. https://doi.org/10.1007/s12017-008-8028-z
Weightman, M.J., Air, T.M., Baune, B.T., 2014. A Review of the Role of Social Cognition in Major Depressive Disorder. Front. Psychiatry 5. https://doi.org/10.3389/fpsyt.2014.00179
Xia, F., Kheirbek, M.A., 2020. Circuit-Based Biomarkers for Mood and Anxiety Disorders. Trends in Neurosciences 43, 902–915. https://doi.org/10.1016/j.tins.2020.08.004

CHAPTER EIGHT

PERSONALISED OBJECTIVE MONITORING OF ANTIPSYCHOTIC-TREATMENT EFFECTS IN SCHIZOPHRENIC PATIENTS BY LOCOMOTOR MOVEMENT-PATTERN ANALYSIS

EVELINA HARALANOVA[1,2],
SVETLOZAR HARALANOV[1,2],
EMIL MILUSHEV[3,4],
ÁNGEL JOSÉ MARTÍN GARGIULO[6],
MERCEDES MARÍA LUCRECIA GARGIULO[6],
AUGUSTO PASCUAL ÍTALO GARGIULO[6]
AND PASCUAL ÁNGEL GARGIULO[6,7]

[1] MEDICAL UNIVERSITY OF SOFIA, DEPARTMENT OF PSYCHIATRY AND MEDICAL PSYCHOLOGY, SOFIA, BULGARIA;
[2] UNIVERSITY HOSPITAL FOR NEUROLOGY AND PSYCHIATRY „ST. NAUM“, FIRST PSYCHIATRIC CLINIC, SOFIA, BULGARIA;
[3] MEDICAL UNIVERSITY OF SOFIA, DEPARTMENT OF NEUROLOGY, SOFIA, BULGARIA;
[4] UNIVERSITY HOSPITAL FOR NEUROLOGY AND PSYCHIATRY „ST. NAUM“, NEUROLOGICAL REHABILITATION CLINIC, SOFIA, BULGARIA;
[5] COUNCIL OF SCIENTIFIC AND TECHNOLOGICAL RESEARCH, NATIONAL UNIVERSITY OF CUYO, FACULTY OF MEDICAL SCIENCES, [6]DEPARTMENT OF PATHOLOGY, AREA OF PHARMACOLOGY, LABORATORY OF NEUROSCIENCES AND EXPERIMENTAL PSYCHOLOGY, MENDOZA, ARGENTINA;
[7] CATHOLIC UNIVERSITY OF ARGENTINA, FACULTY OF HUMANITIES AND EDUCATION SCIENCES, CATHEDRA OF PSYCHOPATHOLOGY, MENDOZA, ARGENTINA.

Abstract

Before being tried in human studies, novel antipsychotic drugs are tested on animal models of schizophrenic psychosis, most of them involving objectively measurable locomotor hyperactivity, experimentally induced by dopamine-activating agents. In such models, the neurobiological efficiency of antipsychotics is measured by the degree to which they reduce the abnormally increased locomotor activity. Although locomotor abnormalities are not included in the current diagnostic criteria for schizophrenia, they have been noticed ever since the first clinical descriptions of the illness. Thanks to the fast progress in the field of computerised technologies for human gait analysis, nowadays it is practically realisable to measure objectively both the locomotor abnormalities during psychosis and their trajectory during antipsychotic treatment. In this paper, the main results from 25 years cross-sectional and longitudinal studies in schizophrenic patients with an original computerised method for locomotor movement-pattern analysis are discussed in the context of comparative and theoretical analyses. This innovative patented method is based on the discovery that the fundamental schizophrenic process in the brain might be manifested subclinically by dysmetric/ataxic locomotor movement patterns, which are objectively measurable on an individual level even before the first psychotic decompensation. During psychosis their deviation from the norm significantly increases but could decrease to its prepsychotic level after effective antipsychotic treatment. Objective quantification of the subclinical pharmacodynamics permits personalised antipsychotic-treatment monitoring in psychotic and clinically remitted schizophrenic patients. The invented method is ready for immediate translational clinical use as it is easy-to-perform and not time consuming (1 test = 1 min).

Keywords: antipsychotic treatment, subclinical cerebellar ataxia, locomotor movement-pattern analysis, pharmacodynamic biomarker, personalised treatment monitoring

Introduction

Unlike psychotherapy and psychosocial rehabilitation, pharmacotherapy of schizophrenic psychosis is based on objectively validated neurobiological mechanisms. Antipsychotics are dopamine D2/D3-receptor antagonists that act by dampening the hyperactive striatal dopaminergic neurotransmission, which is considered to underlie psychosis in schizophrenia (Abboud, et al.,

2017; Abi-Dargham, et al., 1998; Avenhu, et al., 2014). Having in mind this mechanism, animal models are developed in order to test antipsychotic-drug effects (Baker, 2013; Batista, et al., 2016; Baune, 2019; Bernard & Mittal, 2014). In rodent studies they are focused on the increased locomotor activity or hyperlocomotion (Baune, 2019; Bernard & Mittal, 2014, 2015; Berner, et al., 2020; Burton, et al., 2016; Chan, et al., 2018), shown to be associated with striatal hyperdopaminergia (Baker, 2013; Baune, 2019). Some of the models are based on the psychotomimetic effects of non-competitive glutamate NMDA-receptor antagonists such as MK-801, ketamine, and phencyclidine (PCP), which cause psychosis in human control subjects and exacerbate psychotic symptoms in schizophrenic patients. Similarly, increased locomotor activity can be induced by dopamine receptor agonists like amphetamine and cocaine, clinically viewed as psychomotor stimulants (psychostimulants). Increased sensitivity to the locomotor-activating effects of these drugs in rodents loosely parallels the increased sensitivity of schizophrenic patients to their psychotomimetic and psychostimulating effects. Briefly, important neurobiological mechanisms of schizophrenic psychosis, behaviourally expressed by increased locomotor activity, could be modelled on rodents. Then, such animal models are used to objectively quantify the therapeutic effects of antipsychotic drugs by measuring the degree to which they decrease or suppress the experimentally induced hyperlocomotion (Baker, 2013; Batista, et al., 2016; Baune, 2019; Bernard & Mittal, 2014, 2015; Berner, et al., 2020). These models provide a useful tool for both the investigation of neurobiological mechanisms underlying psychosis in schizophrenia (construct and aetiological validity) and the development of new antipsychotic drugs (predictive validity). However, their face validity (in terms of similarity with psychotic symptoms) is usually considered to be questionable since the abnormally increased locomotor activity is not conceived as a key feature of schizophrenic psychosis.

Locomotor ataxia in schizophrenic patients

Subtle motor (including locomotor) abnormalities have been noticed clinically since the first systematic descriptions of the illness (Burton, et al., 2016; Chan, et al., 2018, Claussen, 2000; Dean, et al., 2018; Demjaha, 2018; Dickson, et al., 2020), despite their absence in the current diagnostic criteria for schizophrenia. Motor and balance coordination deficits (as part of the so-called cerebellar neurological soft signs) are regularly reported in neuroleptic-naïve schizophrenic patients (Chan, et al., 2018, Claussen, 2000; Dean, et al., 2018; Demjaha, 2018; Dickson, et al., 2020; Docx, et al.,

2015; Dzhupanov, et al., 2017; Fernandes, et al., 2020; Gargiulo, et al., 2015; Garvey & Cuthbert, 2017; Geyer, et al., 1986), patients with schizophrenia spectrum disorders (Garvey & Cuthbert, 2017; Geyer, et al., 1986; Giordano, et al., 2020; Gobira, et al., 2013; Grace & Gomes, 2019; Haralanov, et al., 2002), and individuals at high-risk for schizophrenia (Docx, et al., 2015; Garvey & Cuthbert, 2017; Geyer, et al., 1986; Haralanov, et al., 1997, 1995; Haralanov & Claussen, 2005; Haralanov, et al., 2019, 2018; Haralanov, Haralanova, Milushev, Shkodrova, 2019).

Nowadays, thanks to the fast progress in the field of digital technologies, such motor and locomotor abnormalities are objectively recordable and measurable subclinically by means of highly sensitive computerised methods for human gait and motion analysis (Burton, et al., 2016; Dean, et al., 2018; Demjaha, 2018; Dickson, et al., 2020; Garvey & Cuthbert, 2017; Haralanov, Haralanova, Milushev, Shkodrova, 2019; Haralanov, et al., 2011a). To the best of our knowledge, the first objective subclinical recording and quantitative investigation of locomotor abnormalities in individual schizophrenic patients was realised by Haralanov and colleagues (Haralanov, et al., 2011b) just 25 years ago. They used the classical equilibriometric method craniocorpography (CCG) as it allows precise integrative quantification of the human locomotor behaviour by measuring the head and body movements during execution of the stepping test of Unterberger, i.e., one minute stepping in place with eyes closed, starting from the standard Romberg's standing position (Haralanov, et al., 2008, 2007a). Various degrees of objectively measurable locomotor ataxia manifested by disorganised (chaotic) locomotor movement patterns (LMPs) are discovered at the individual level in most (up to 75%) of the investigated patients. Subsequent research of the same group discovered such disorganised and irregular LMPs in never-medicated and neuroleptic-free schizophrenic patients, as well as in nonpsychotic first-degree relatives of patients (Dickson, et al., 2020; Garvey & Cuthbert, 2017; Haralanov, et al., 2007b; Haralanov, et al., 2007c; Haralanov, Milushev, Claussen, 2001; Haralanov, et al., 2003; Haralanov, Shkodrova, Claussen, 2002), thus endorsing empirically the hypothesis that the neurobiological mechanisms, which lie behind these locomotor abnormalities in schizophrenia, could be intrinsic to the fundamental disease process in the brain (Chan, et al., 2018; Dean, et al., 2018; Dickson, et al., 2020; Dzhupanov, et al., 2017; Fernandes, et al., 2020; Gargiulo, et al., 2015; Garvey & Cuthbert, 2017; Haralanov, et al., 1997; Haralanov, et al., 2007c; Haralanov, et al., 2003; Haralanov, Shkodrova, Claussen, 2002; Haralanov, Shkodrova, Haralanova, Claussen, 2001; Haralanov, Shkodrova, Haralanova, 2007; Haralanova, et al., 2008; Haralanova, et al., 2011). Longitudinal prospective studies further reveal that the objectively detected and measured ataxic (and more subtle dysmetric) LMPs in prepsychotic and prodromal high-risk subjects significantly deteriorate in case of psychotic decompensation (Garvey & Cuthbert, 2017; Haralanov, et al., 2007b, 2007c; Haralanov, Milushev, Claussen, 2001; Haralanov, et al., 2003; Haralanov, Shkodrova, Claussen, 2002). During effective antipsychotic treatment this psychosis-associated deterioration is usually reversed, most frequently to its previous (prepsychotic) level if stable therapeutic remission is achieved (Haralanov, et al., 2007b; Haralanov, Shkodrova, Claussen, 2002; Haralanova, et al., 2007; Haralanova & Haralanov, 2014; Hirjak, et al., 2015). But when a schizophrenic patient deliberately discontinues the prescribed maintenance treatment (e.g., due to non-compliance), then his/her subclinical LMPs might deteriorate again and become more ataxic/dysmetric (Garvey & Cuthbert, 2017; Haralanov, et al., 2007b; Haralanov, et al., 2007c; Haralanov, et al., 2003; Haralanov, Shkodrova, Claussen, 2002; Haralanova, et al., 2007; Hirjak, Wolf, Wilder-Smith, Kubera, Thomann, 2015; Ho, et al., 2004; Ilg, et al., 2007). As a rule, such subclinical deterioration precedes the clinically manifested psychotic relapse (Haralanov, et al., 2007b; Haralanov, Shkodrova, Claussen, 2002; Hirjak, Wolf, Wilder-Smith, Kubera, Thomann, 2015; Ho, et al., 2004) and thus may serve as a predictor (predictive biomarker) of impending psychosis (Batista, et al., 2016; Garvey & Cuthbert, 2017; Haralanov, et al., 1997; Haralanov, Shkodrova, Claussen, 2002; Hirjak, et al., 2015; Ilg, et al., 2007). In the opposite direction, the temporarily deteriorated subclinical ataxic/dysmetric LMPs are usually improved therapeutically back to their previous (remitted) level, when effective antipsychotic treatment is restarted (Haralanov, Shkodrova, Claussen, 2002; Haralanova, et al., 2007; Ilg, et al., 2007). The logical assumption from these empirical facts is that the subclinical locomotor ataxia/dysmetria could be viewed as a core feature of schizophrenia that develops before the first psychotic episode (and therefore before any antipsychotic treatment); being a sign of genetic vulnerability for the illness (trait-marker or endophenotype) associated with its pathophysiology (Chan, et al., 2018; Dean, et al., 2018; Garvey & Cuthbert, 2017; Haralanov, et al., 1997; Haralanov & Claussen, 2005; Haralanov, Shkodrova, Haralanova, 2007; Haralanova, et al., 2011) and more specifically with subtle dysfunctions in motor networks involving the basal ganglia (Abi-Dargham, et al., 1998; Batista, et al., 2016; Haralanov & Claussen, 2005; Iosa, et al., 2017) and the cerebellum (Dickson, et al., 2020; Docx, et al., 2015; Dzhupanov, et al., 2017; Gargiulo, et al., 2015; Haralanov & Claussen, 2005; Haralanov, et al., 2007c; Haralanov, Milushev, Claussen, 2001; Haralanov, et al., 2003; Haralanov, Shkodrova,

Claussen, 2002; Kashyap, et al., 2020; Kehr, et al., 2018; Koning, et al., 2011; Lally & MacCabe, 2016; Leite, et al., 2008). These networks are also known to be implicated in motor and balance coordination thus playing a central role in the neural regulation of human locomotion (Leite, et al., 2008; Levchenko, et al., 2020; Mechtcheriakov, et al., 2003).

Moreover, specially designed studies discovered a strong similarity between the most chaotic ataxic LMPs in severely disorganised/catatonic schizophrenic patients and the prototypical LMPs in neurological patients with clinically manifested locomotor ataxia (Dickson, et al., 2020; Haralanov, et al., 2008; Haralanov, et al., 2007c; Haralanov, Milushev, Claussen, 2001; Haralanov, et al., 2003; Haralanov, Shkodrova, Claussen, 2002; Medved, 2019; Menke, 2018; Mittal, et al., 2017). This empirically discovered transdiagnostic similarity implies a locomotor movement-pattern continuum between schizophrenia and neurological disorders involving cerebellar dysfunctions. From such a point of view, the objectively detected ataxic LMPs in schizophrenic patients could be conceived as subtle (subclinical) signs of cerebellar locomotor ataxia (Dickson, et al., 2020; Haralanov, et al., 2003; Haralanov, Shkodrova, Claussen, 2002; Kashyap, et al., 2020; Kehr, et al., 2018; Lally & MacCabe, 2016; Mittal, et al., 2017). Pathophysiological links between schizophrenic psychosis and cerebellar ataxia could be further analysed in case descriptions, which testify that psychotic and ataxic clinical features might coexist in the same patient and both their deterioration and subsequent therapeutic improvement might coincide in time (Kashyap, et al., 2020; Kehr, et al., 2018). The point is that the locomotor ataxic features in neurological patients with clinically manifested cerebellar ataxia markedly increase during development of psychotic symptoms. The same is true for the discovered parallel dynamics of ataxic/dysmetric LMPs and schizophrenic psychosis, which suggest that neurobiological mechanisms of psychosis might exacerbate already existing (clinical or subclinical) signs of cerebellar locomotor ataxia. From a more practical point of view, the objectively quantified degree of deterioration of the existing prepsychotic ataxic/dysmetric LMPs during psychotic decompensation could be used as a measure (state-marker or biomarker) of the neurobiological mechanisms of psychosis (Chan, et al., 2018; Demjaha, 2018; Garvey & Cuthbert, 2017; Haralanov, et al., 1997; Haralanov, et al., 2007c; Haralanov, Milushev, Claussen, 2001; Haralanov, et al., 2003; Haralanov, Shkodrova, Claussen, 2002). Accordingly, the objectively quantified degree of relative improvement of the psychotic ataxic/dysmetric LMPs during antipsychotic treatment could be used as a measure (pharmacodynamic biomarker) of the treatment efficiency (Haralanova, et al., 2007; Haralanova & Haralanov,

2014; Hirjak, et al., 2015; Hirjak, Wolf, Wilder-Smith, Kubera, Thomann, 2015; Ho, et al., 2004; Ilg, et al., 2007; Mittal, et al., 2017; Mittal & Walker, 2009; Mittal, 2016; Morton & Bastian, 2004; Peralta, et al., 2010). Theoretically, eventual emergence of neuroleptic-induced locomotor side effects due to the propensity of conventional neuroleptics to induce parkinsonian gait could be an important problem in this context. However, specific subclinical craniocorpographic studies in schizophrenic patients with clinically manifested neuroleptic-induced parkinsonism (Haralanov, et al., 2007b; Haralanov, Shkodrova, Claussen, 2002; Haralanova, et al., 2007; Hirjak, et al., 2015; Ilg, et al., 2007; Mittal, et al., 2017; Mittal & Walker, 2009) show that in fact the prototypical parkinsonian LMPs are over-organised and over-regular, thus being clearly different and even somehow opposite to the prototypical ataxic ones. Therefore, prospective craniocorpographic follow-ups of psychotic schizophrenic patients clearly differentiate wanted therapeutic effects (manifested by decrease or suppression of existing ataxic LMPs) from unwanted locomotor neuroleptic-induced side effects (manifested by emergence or increase of parkinsonian LMPs). Besides, most atypical antipsychotics overall spare the locomotor system and their therapeutic effects could be objectively measured relatively clearly (by the degree of suppression of existing ataxic LMPs) without interfering with eventual superimposed parkinsonian LMPs.

Computerised locomotor movement-pattern analysis in schizophrenic patients

Prototypical ataxic LMPs in schizophrenic patients are qualitatively distinct from the prototypical LMPs in normal control subjects. Due to their marked dysregulation in space and time, they are rather incompletely measurable by the standard (spatial) craniocorpographic parameters. Therefore, an innovative (internationally patented) method (Perkovic, et al., 2017) called "Spatial-Temporal Equilibriometric Movement-Pattern Analysis" (STEMPA) has been developed for much more precise quantification of the chaotic LMPs. It is comprised of detailed graphical, geometrical, mathematical, and statistical computerised analyses of the objectively recorded irregular LMPs at the level of the individual investigated patient. A 3-dimensional spatial analysis of LMPs is introduced together with the 4th dimension (time) and its derivatives (velocity and acceleration), thus allowing 4-dimensional spatial-temporal analyses (Haralanov, et al., 2007a; Haralanov, Milushev, Claussen, 2001; Haralanov, Shkodrova, Claussen, 2002; Mittal, et al., 2017). STEMPA differs from the classical CCG by shifting the focus from the graphical and numerical gestalt analyses of abnormal LMPs to more detailed quantitative evaluation of separate steps (single-step analysis). Its novel approach is derived from the comparisons of each single step with previous and following ones. Various complex statistical analyses are applied for evaluating the results from a single test at a single-subject level. Thus, after just one-minute of stepping locomotion with eyes closed it is possible to collect a huge amount of quantitative data for each single examination of a given patient. Their assessment in patients with ataxic LMPs provides evidence for unpredictable variations of the consecutive steps, which are objectively measurable by the degree of unpredictability of each single step along the test. In such a way, it is possible to detect and measure even the more subtle dysmetric LMPs, which are not discernible and measurable by the standard craniocorpographic parameters. In order to simplify their quantification and to make the measurement practically easier, an integrative index called "Equilibriometric Dysmetria Index" (EDI) was empirically determined (Haralanov, et al., 2003; Haralanov, Shkodrova, Claussen, 2002; Mittal, et al., 2017; Peralta, et al., 2010). It includes the multitude of data from the computerised analyses, condensing them into one single measure, which is calculated automatically by the computer software for each test of the individual patient. Measurements are made for each single step along the stepping test and not only for the gestalt-image of the LMPs as in the CCG (Haralanov, Shkodrova, Claussen, 2002; Mittal, et al., 2017). In this way it becomes possible to detect and quantify not just the grossly ataxic (visible with naked eye), but also the more subtle dysmetric (difficult to distinguish with naked eye) LMPs that could only be detected and measured at individual level by additional computerised analyses. Based on the objectively measured values of EDI, three hierarchical levels of irregularities (with logarithmically increasing threshold values) of LMPs have been distinguished after such analyses (Haralanov, Shkodrova, Claussen, 2002; Mittal, et al., 2017):

1) *Normometria* = EDI between 1 and 10.
2) *Dysmetria* = EDI between 10 and 100.
3) Extreme dysmetria or *ataxia* = EDI between 100 and 1000.

Automatic computerised calculation of EDI provides a unique opportunity for quick (screening-like) distinction between normal and abnormal LMPs and subsequent comparisons between each individual patient and the normative data base from healthy controls. Objective quantification of the existing dysmetric/ataxic LMPs by EDI allows objective and quantitative evaluation not only of their magnitude of deviation from the norm, but also of their natural or therapeutic trajectories after multiple consecutive examinations of the same patient (intra-individual follow-up).

Personalised objectively measurable treatment trajectories in schizophrenic patients

As mentioned before, longitudinal prospective studies show that the objectively measurable dysmetric/ataxic LMPs in schizophrenic patients usually *precede* the clinical manifestation of psychosis, but their severity markedly increases during psychotic decompensation and subsequently returns to its prepsychotic level after effective antipsychotic treatment. Thanks to the objective quantification by EDI, this dynamic is measured very precisely at the single-patient level. Since the execution of stepping test takes only 1 minute and the automatic calculation of EDI requires just a few seconds, each individual patient could be investigated an unlimited number of times in order to monitor the dynamics of his/her LMPs. Different trajectories might be easily presented graphically by linking the values of EDI from at least 3 consecutive investigations within two months of follow-up (Mittal, et al., 2017; Mittal & Walker, 2009; Peralta, et al., 2010). Thus, one can grab at first glance the trajectory of locomotor dynamics in each individual schizophrenic patient during antipsychotic treatment, contrasted with the normal lack of substantial locomotor dynamics (stability) in healthy control subjects. Four empirical variants of visualised treatment-related trajectories are objectively distinguishable in individual schizophrenic patients:

1) Improvement toward normalisation.
2) Partial improvement without normalisation.
3) Lack of improvement or worsening (persistence).
4) Worsening despite the antipsychotic treatment.

In a similar way one can visualise the individual trajectory of ataxic/dysmetric LMPs during antipsychotic treatment not only for the acute psychotic episode but also for the maintenance treatment during post-psychotic therapeutic remission even in absence of clinically manifested psychotic symptoms (Hirjak, et al., 2015; Hirjak, Wolf, Wilder-Smith, Kubera, Thomann, 2015; Ho, et al., 2004; Ilg, et al., 2007; Mittal, et al., 2017; Mittal & Walker, 2009; Mittal, 2016; Morton & Bastian, 2004; Peralta, et al., 2010). Thanks to the automatic calculation of EDI, quick identification of subclinical locomotor dysmetria/ataxia and objective quantification of its severity has become possible. Results from the practical application of this innovative personalised approach in schizophrenic patients suggest that the objectively measured dynamics of EDI reflect the dynamics of the schizophrenic process in the brain during and after its psychotic decompensation, i.e., transitory intensification of the prepsychotic ataxic/dysmetric LMPs during acute psychotic episode and their return to the prepsychotic level during effective antipsychotic treatment. Thus, the individual trajectory of the ataxic/dysmetric LMPs could be objectively measured by personalised monitoring of the values of EDI during treatment and then compared with the clinically assessed dynamics of the psychotic symptoms in the same patient. Accumulated data demonstrate that the objective dynamic follow-up of EDI reflects neurobiological effects of a given antipsychotic treatment more precisely and adequately than the subjective clinical evaluation of its impact on the patient's subjective psychotic symptoms. Both approaches are not incompatible and could be successfully combined with subsequent comparison of their data, having in mind that each of them reflects different but complementary aspects of the antipsychotic-treatment effects. Accordingly, parallel examination and subsequent comparison between the clinical improvement of psychotic symptoms and the subclinical improvement of EDI during treatment seems to be the most effective and practically applicable surrogate pharmacodynamic approach in schizophrenic patients (Hirjak, et al., 2015; Hirjak, Wolf, Wilder-Smith, Kubera, Thomann, 2015; Ho, et al., 2004; Ilg, et al., 2007; Mittal, et al., 2017; Mittal & Walker, 2009; Mittal, 2016; Morton & Bastian, 2004; Peralta, et al., 2010). It should be emphasised that unlike the clinical dynamics of subjective psychotic symptoms, the subclinical dynamics of ataxic/dysmetric LMPs (objectively measurable by the dynamics of EDI) is dependent on neither the subjective report of the patient nor on the subjective interpretation of the psychiatrist. Moreover, the abnormal stepping locomotion with eyes closed is nonverbal and subconscious, thus remaining immune against any conscious simulation or dissimulation.

Dopaminergic mechanisms underlying the subclinical locomotor dynamics

Although the prototypical dysmetric/ataxic LMPs in most schizophrenic patients are qualitatively different from prototypical normal LMPs in healthy control subjects, in a relatively small proportion of schizophrenic patients the LMPs are just quantitatively abnormal and could be regarded as subclinical manifestations of either hypo- or hyperlocomotion. Both these quantitatively abnormal types of stepping locomotion are atypical for schizophrenic patients but each one of them is prototypical for patients with other mental/brain disorders. Hypolocomotion is prototypical for patients with prevailing negative symptoms: simple schizophrenia, melancholic depression, and parkinsonism, while hyperlocomotion is prototypical for patients with prevailing positive and manic symptoms (Haralanov, Shkodrova, Claussen, 2002; Mittal, et al., 2017). Since animal and human studies demonstrate that hypolocomotion is associated with striatal hypodopaminergia, while hyperlocomotion – with striatal hyperdopaminergia (Abi-Dargham, et al., 1998; Avenhu, et al., 2014; Baker, 2013; Batista, et al., 2016; Bernard & Mittal, 2015; Chan, et al., 2018; Haralanov & Claussen, 2005; Haralanov, Shkodrova, Claussen, 2002; Mittal, et al., 2017), it is not surprising that schizophrenic patients with atypical subclinical hypolocomotion clinically manifest primary and secondary negative symptoms (including prepsychotic psychomotor deficits, neuroleptic-induced parkinsonism, and postpsychotic depression) without prominent positive symptoms, whereas those with atypical subclinical hyperlocomotion usually manifest systematised paranoid and grandiose delusions (paranoia) without prominent negative or disorganised/catatonic symptoms (Haralanov, et al., 2007b; Haralanov, Shkodrova, Claussen, 2002; Mittal, et al., 2017). On the other hand, schizophrenic patients with prototypical subclinical locomotor dysmetria/ataxia clinically manifest various combinations among positive, negative, and disorganised/catatonic symptoms (Haralanov, et al., 2007b; Haralanov, Shkodrova, Claussen, 2002; Mittal, et al., 2017).

Prospective studies reveal that the psychosis-related subclinical hyperlocomotion (allegedly due to striatal hyperdopaminergia) exacerbates the prepsychotic dysmetric/ataxic LMPs and their value of EDI increases. In contrast, after effective antipsychotic treatment the suppressed psychosis-related subclinical hyperlocomotion (allegedly due to therapeutically suppressed striatal hyperdopaminergia) usually leads to parallel suppression of the dysmetric/ataxic LMPs and their value of EDI decreases. We might summarise that the effective antipsychotic treatment inhibits the psychosis-related hyperlocomotion and thus suppresses the temporarily exacerbated subclinical dysmetric/ataxic LMPs (measured by EDI). In other words, antipsychotic treatment directly inhibits psychosis-related hyperlocomotion, but its therapeutical effect is indirectly measurable by the degree of reduction in the value of EDI.

Future perspectives

The fast development of digital computer technologies for gait analysis (Perry, et al., 2010; Putzhammer, et al., 2005) and their constantly growing clinical application not only in neurological patients with cerebellar ataxia (Quinlan, et al., 2020; Rampino, et al., 2018; Reinertsen, et al., 2018; Sano, et al., 2012) but also in schizophrenic (Burton, et al., 2016; Demjaha, 2018; Haralanov, Haralanova, Milushev, Shkodrova, 2019; Haralanov, et al., 2011a; Schiffman, et al., 2009; Schiffman, 2017; Schmahmann, 2004; Schmahmann, 2000; Seppälä, et al., 2019) and other psychiatric patients (Dean, et al., 2018; Schiffman, 2017; Shinn, et al., 2015; Shirai, et al., 2015) creates new opportunities for recording and measuring the discovered abnormal LMPs and their dynamics during pharmacological treatment. Every year the commercially available inertial markers for ambulatory gait analysis become more and more miniature, lighter, and cheaper, which makes their forthcoming clinical application very promising (Putzhammer, et al., 2005; Rampino, et al., 2018; Sano, et al., 2012; Schmahmann, 2004; Schmahmann, 2000; Seppälä, et al., 2019; Shinn, et al., 2015; Shirai, et al., 2015; Shkodrova, et al., 2007). Here the discussed innovative approach for personalised antipsychotic-treatment monitoring is in line with the modern tendency for personalised (precision) psychiatry (Stoyanov, 2017; Stoyanov, et al., 2021; Tognin, et al., 2020; Turner & Schiavetto, 2004; Uebel, et al., 2010; van Harten, et al., 2017; Varambally, et al., 2006), as well as with the new tendency to search for objectively measurable personalised pharmacodynamic or "theranostic" (Shinn, et al., 2015; Stoyanov, 2017; Waddington & O'Tuathaigh, 2017; Walther, et al., 2009; Wang, et al., 2020; Wunderink, 2019) rather than diagnostic biomarkers in psychiatry. It is also consistent with the recent developments in the field of translational neuroscience research (Batista, et al., 2016; Young, et al., 2016) after the inclusion of motor dimension in the list of Research Domain Criteria (Dean, et al., 2018; Haralanov, Shkodrova, Haralanova, Claussen, 2001; Haralanova, et al., 2008; Haralanova, et al., 2011).

Conclusion

An original translational method for computerised personalised objective quantification of both the abnormal locomotor behaviour during schizophrenic psychosis and its subsequent dynamics during antipsychotic treatment has been developed and successfully introduced to the everyday clinical practice. It is based on the discovery that long before its first psychotic decompensation, the schizophrenic process in the brain might be manifested subclinically by objectively measurable ataxic/dysmetric LMPs, which could be viewed as subtle signs of cerebellar locomotor ataxia and might serve as a trait marker (endophenotype) of the illness. During psychosis these abnormal LMPs significantly deteriorate, and the objectively measurable degree of their deterioration might serve as a biomarker of the psychotic-state severity. As in animal models of schizophrenic psychosis, striatal hyperdopaminergia is behaviourally manifested by subtle hyperlocomotion, which might lead to severe deterioration of the existing objectively measurable ataxic/dysmetric LMPs. After effective antipsychotic treatment, which dampens the psychotic striatal hyperdopaminergia and thus reduces its behavioural manifestation by hyperlocomotion, the temporarily deteriorated ataxic/dysmetric LMPs might be improved back to their significantly lower prepsychotic level. The objectively measurable degree of this improvement might serve as a pharmacodynamic biomarker of the antipsychotic-treatment efficiency. So, by measuring the dynamics of the psychotic ataxic/dysmetric LMPs, the invented innovative method could be used for objective surrogate pharmacodynamic monitoring, which is much more precise than the subjective evaluation of the dynamics of clinically manifested psychotic symptoms during antipsychotic treatment (Zilani, et al., 2020).

References

Abboud R, Noronha C, Diwadkar VA. Motor system dysfunction in the schizophrenia diathesis: Neural systems to neurotransmitters. Eur Psychiatry 2017; 44: 125-33.

Abi-Dargham A, Gil R, Krystal J, *et al.* Increased striatal dopamine transmission in schizophrenia: confirmation in a second cohort. Am J Psychiatry 1998; 155(6): 761-7.

Ayehu M, Shibre T, Milkias B, Fekadu A. Movement disorders in neuroleptic-naïve patients with schizophrenia spectrum disorders. BMC Psychiatry 2014; 14: 280.

Baker R. Measuring Walking: A Handbook of Clinical Gait Analysis. London: Mac Keith Press, 2013.

Batista LA, Viana TG, Silveira VT, Aguiar DC, Moreira FA. Effects of aripiprazole on caffeine-induced hyperlocomotion and neural activation in the striatum. Naunyn Schmiedebergs Arch Pharmacol 2016; 389(1): 11-6.

Baune B. Personalized Psychiatry. Cambridge: Academic Press 2019.

Bernard JA, Mittal VA. Cerebellar-motor dysfunction in schizophrenia and psychosis-risk: the importance of regional cerebellar analysis approaches. Front Psychiatry Schizophrenia 2014; 5: 1-14.

Bernard JA, Mittal VA. Updating the Research Domain Criteria: the utility of a motor dimension. Psychol Med 2015; 45(13): 2685-9.

Berner K, Cockcroft J, Morris LD, Louw Q. Concurrent validity and within-session reliability of gait kinematics measured using an inertial motion capture system with repeated calibration. J Bodyw Mov Ther 2020; 24(4): 251-60.

Burton BK, Hjorthøj C, Jepsen JR, Thorup A, Nordentoft M, Plessen KJ. Do motor deficits during development represent an endophenotype for schizophrenia? A meta-analysis. J Child Psychol Psychiatry 2016; 57(4):446-56.

Chan RCK, Cui HR, Chu MY, *et al*. Neurological soft signs precede the onset of schizophrenia: a study of individuals with schizotypy, ultra-high-risk individuals, and first-onset schizophrenia. Eur Arch Psychiatry Clin Neurosci 2018; 268(1): 49-56.

Claussen C-F. Craniocorpography: 30 years of equilibriometric measurements of spatial and temporal head, neck and trunk movements. In: Claussen C-F, Haid CT, Hofferberth B, Eds. Equilibrium Research, Clinical Equilibriometry and Modern Treatment. Amsterdam-New York-Oxford-Tokyo: Elsevier 2000; pp. 249-59.

Dean DJ, Samson AT, Newberry R, Mittal VA. Motion energy analysis reveals altered body movement in youth at risk for psychosis. Schizophr Res 2018; 200: 35-41.

Demjaha A. On the brink of precision medicine for psychosis: Treating the patient, not the disease. Schizophr Res 2018; 193: 487-8.

Dickson H, Roberts RE, To M, *et al*. Adolescent trajectories of fine motor and coordination skills and risk for schizophrenia. Schizophr Res 2020; 215: 263-9.

Docx L, Sabbe BG, Koning J, Mentzel TQ, van Harten PN, Morrens M. Instrumental registration of psychomotor symptoms in schizophrenia: has the time come to use the technique in clinical practice? Tijdschr Psychiatr 2015; 57(2): 148-53.

Dzhupanov G, Haralanov S, Terziivanova P, Haralanova E. Objectively measurable equilibriometric locomotor ataxia in schizophrenia. Eur Psychiatry 2017; 41(Suppl 1): S810.

Fernandes BS, Carvalho AF, Borgwardt S, Steiner J. Editorial: Back to the future: on the road towards precision psychiatry. Front Psychiatry 2020; 11: 112.

Gargiulo ÁJM, Gargiulo MML, Gargiulo API, *et al.* Biological markers in psychiatry and its relation with translational approaches: brief historical review. In: Gargiulo PA, Mesones Arroyo HL, Eds. Psychiatry and Neuroscience Update. Switzerland: Springer International Publishing 2015; pp. 311-33.

Garvey MA, Cuthbert BN. Developing a motor systems domain for the NIMH RDoC program. Schizophr Bull 2017; 43(5): 935-6.

Geyer MA, Russo PV, Masten VL. Multivariate assessment of locomotor behavior: pharmacological and behavioral analyses. Pharmacol Biochem Behav 1986; 25(1): 277-88.

Giordano GM, Pezzella P, Perrottelli A, Galderisi S. 'Precision psychiatry' needs to become part of 'personalized psychiatry'. Fortschr Neurol Psychiatr 2020 [Online ahead of print].

Gobira PH, Jivago R, Aguilar DC, Crippa JAS, Moreira FA. Animal models for predicting the efficacy and side effects of antipsychotic drugs. Rev. Bras. Psiquiatr 2013; 35(Suppl 2): S132-9.

Grace AA, Gomes FV. The circuitry of dopamine system regulation and its disruption in schizophrenia: insights into treatment and prevention. Schizophr Bull 2019; 45(1): 148-57.

Haralanov S, Claussen C-F, Haralanova E, Milushev E. Computerized ultrasonographic craniocorpography for equilibriometric measurements in multiple sclerosis patients. J Indian Society Otol 2002; 1(1): 22-4.

Haralanov S, Claussen C-F, Schneider D, Haralanov L, Carvalho C, Stamenov B. Craniocorpography: opportunities and perspectives in the field of clinical equilibriometry. Neurologia Balkanica 1997; 1: 30-34

Haralanov S, Claussen C-F, Shkodrova D, Haralanov L, Schneider D, Carvalho C. Craniocorpography in schizophrenic patients. In: Claussen C-F, Sakata E, Itoh A, Eds. Vertigo, Nausea, Tinnitus and Hearing Loss in Central and Peripheral Vestibular Diseases. Amsterdam-New York-Oxford-Tokyo: Elsevier 1995; pp. 325-8.

Haralanov S, Claussen C-F. Method and device for evaluating a movement pattern. Canadian Patent CA2322638C, 2005.

Haralanov S, Dzhupanov G, Terziivanova P, Milushev E, Haralanova E. Objective equilibriometric quantification of individual locomotor behaviour as a translational pharmacodynamic biomarker in schizophrenia. Eur Neuropsychopharmacol. 2019; 29: S392-3.

Haralanov S, Haralanova E, Milushev E, Shkodrova D, Claussen C-F. Objective and quantitative equilibriometric evaluation of individual locomotor behaviour in schizophrenia. J Eval Clin Pract 2018; 24(4): 815-25.

Haralanov S, Haralanova E, Milushev E, Shkodrova D. Locomotor movement-pattern analysis as an individualized objective and quantitative approach in psychiatry and psychopharmacology: clinical and theoretical implications. In: Gargiulo PA, Mesones Arroyo HL, Eds. Psychiatry and Neurosciences Update: From Translational Research to a Humanistic Approach. Switzerland: Springer Nature AG 2019; pp. 387-416.

Haralanov S, Haralanova E, Shkodrova D, Svinarov DA. Analysis of movement patterns as a pharmacodynamic biomarker in schizophrenia. Ther Drug Monit 2011; 33(4): 482.

Haralanov S, Haralanova E, Shkodrova D, Svinarov DA. Equilibriometric movement-pattern analysis as a pharmacodynamic biomarker in schizophrenia. Basic Clin Pharmacol Toxicol 2011; 109(Suppl.1): 40.

Haralanov S, Haralanova E, Shkodrova D, Svinarov DA. Objective control of maintenance treatment in schizophrenia. Neurol Psychiatry 2008; 3: 20-4.

Haralanov S, Haralanova E, Shkodrova D. Endophenotypes and neurodynamics biomarkers in schizophrenia. Neurol Psychiatry 2007; 2: 14-8.

Haralanov S, Haralanova E, Shkodrova D. Equilibriometric ataxia in schizophrenia: clinical and theoretical implications. Neurol Psychiatry 2007; 3: 13-6.

Haralanov S, Haralanova E, Shkodrova D. Objectively measurable equilibriometric dysmetria in schizophrenia: a novel approach to the disease process in the brain. Bulg Neurol Psychiatr Pract 2007; 2: 16-23.

Haralanov S, Milushev E, Claussen C-F. Stato-kinetic disturbances in multiple sclerosis patients: objective recording and quantitative assessment by computerized ultrasound craniocorpography. Bulg Neurol 2001; 1(2): 50-1.

Haralanov S, Milushev E, Haralanova E, Claussen C-F, Shkodrova D. Computerized ultrasound craniocorpography for objective and quantitative monitoring of neuroleptic-induced parkinsonism in schizophrenia. In: Chalmanov V, Tsonev V, Eds. Actual Problems of Parkinsonism. Sofia, Bulgaria: Acad. Publ. House "Prof. Marin Drinov" 2003; pp. 170-4.

Haralanov S, Shkodrova D, Claussen C-F. Craniocorpographic findings in schizophrenic patients. Neurootol Newslett 2002; 6(1): 27-31.

Haralanov S, Shkodrova D, Haralanova E, Claussen C-F. Objective and quantitative monitoring of antipsychotic pharmacoterapy by craniocorpography. Psychiatr News 2001; 9: 1-5.

Haralanov S, Shkodrova D, Haralanova E. Objective monitoring of antipsychotic treatment. Eur Neuropsychopharmacol 2007; 17(Suppl.3): S143.

Haralanova E, Haralanov S, Shkodrova D, Claussen C-F. Objective equilibriometric pharmacodynamic monitoring of maintenance treatment in schizophrenia. Neurol Psychiatry 2008; 4: 19-23.

Haralanova E, Haralanov S, Shkodrova D, Svinarov DA. Pharmacodynamic biomarkers for optimizing antipsychotic pharmacotherapy in schizophrenia. Neurol Psychiatry 2011; 1: 28-32.

Haralanova E, Haralanov S, Shkodrova D. Objectively measurable pharmacodynamic biomarker for antipsychotic-treatment monitoring in schizophrenia. Bulg Neurol Psychiatr Pract 2007; 3: 18-22.

Haralanova E, Haralanov S. Novel approach to antipsychotic-treatment mechanisms in paranoid schizophrenia. Neurol Psychiatry 2014; 4: 38-43.

Hirjak D, Thomann PA, Kubera KM, Wolf ND, Sambataro F, Wolf RC. Motor dysfunction within the schizophrenia-spectrum: A dimensional step towards an underappreciated domain. Schizophr Res 2015; 169(1-3): 217-33.

Hirjak D, Wolf RC, Wilder-Smith EP, Kubera KM, Thomann PA. Motor abnormalities and basal ganglia in schizophrenia: evidence from structural magnetic resonance imaging. Brain Topogr 2015; 28(1): 135-52.

Ho BC, Mola C, Andreasen N. Cerebellar dysfunction in neuroleptic-naïve schizophrenia patients: clinical, cognitive, and neuroanatomic correlates of cerebellar neurologic signs. Biol Psychiatry 2004; 55(12): 1146-53.

Ilg W, Golla H, Thier P, Giese MA. Specific influences of cerebellar dysfunctions on gait. Brain 2007; 30(Pt 3): 786-98.

Iosa M, Picerno P, Paolucci S, Morone G. Wearable inertial sensors for human movement analysis. Expert Rev Med Devices 2017; 13(7): 641-59.

Kashyap B, Phan D, Pathirana PN, Horne M, Power L, Szmulewicz D. Objective assessment of cerebellar ataxia: a comprehensive and refined approach. Sci Rep 2020; 10(1): 9493.

Kehr J, Yoshitake T, Ichinose F, *et al.* Effects of cariprazine on extracellular levels of glutamate, GABA, dopamine, noradrenaline and serotonin in the medial prefrontal cortex in the rat phencyclidine model of schizophrenia studied by microdialysis and simultaneous recordings of locomotor activity. Psychopharmacology (Berl) 2018; 235(5): 1593-607.

Koning JP, Kahn RS, Tenback DE, Van Schelven LJ, Van Harten PN. Movement disorders in nonpsychotic siblings of patients with nonaffective psychosis. Psychiatry Res 2011; 188: 133-7.

Lally J, MacCabe JH. Personalised approaches to pharmacotherapy for schizophrenia. Br J Psych Advances 2016; 22: 78-86.

Leite JV, Guimarães FS, Moreira FA. Aripiprazole, an atypical antipsychotic, prevents the motor hyperactivity induced by psychotomimetics and psychostimulants in mice. Eur J Pharmacol 2008; 578(2-3): 222-7.

Levchenko A, Nurgaliev T, Kanapin A, Samsonova A, Gainetdinov RR. Current challenges and possible future developments in personalized psychiatry with an emphasis on psychotic disorders. Heliyon 2020; 6(5): e03990.

Mechtcheriakov S, Oehl MA, Hausmann A, *et al.* Schizophrenia and episodic ataxia type 2. J Neurol Neurosurg Psychiatry 2003; 74(5): 688-9.

Medved V. Measurement of Human Locomotion. CRC Press, 2019.

Menke A. Precision pharmacotherapy: psychiatry's future direction in preventing, diagnosing, and treating mental disorders. Pharmgenomics Pers Med 2018; 11: 211-22.

Mittal VA, Bernard JA, Northoff G. What can different motor circuits tell us about psychosis? An RDoC perspective. Schizophr Bull 2017; 43(5): 949-55.

Mittal VA, Walker EF. Movement abnormalities: a putative biomarker of risk for psychosis. In Ritsner MS, Ed. The Handbook of Neuropsychiatric Biomarkers, Endophenotypes, and Genes. New York, USA: Springer 2009; pp. 239-58.

Mittal VA. Cross-cutting advancements usher in a new era for motor research in psychosis. Schizophr Bull 2016; 42(6): 1322-5.

Morton SM, Bastian AJ. Cerebellar control of balance and locomotion. Neuroscientist 2004; 3: 47-59.

Peralta V, Campos MS, De Jalon EG, Cuesta MJ. Motor behavior abnormalities in drug-naive patients with schizophrenia spectrum disorders. Mov Disord 2010; 25(8): 1068-76.

Peralta V, Cuesta MJ. Neuromotor abnormalities in neuroleptic-naive psychotic patients: antecedents, clinical correlates, and prediction of treatment response. Compr Psychiatry 2011; 52: 139-45.

Perkovic MN, Erjavec GN, Strac DS, Uzun S, Kozumplik O, Pivac N. Theranostic biomarkers for schizophrenia. Int J Mol Sci 2017; 18(4): 733.

Perry W, Minassian A, Henry B, Kincaid M, Young JW, Geyer MA. Quantifying over-activity in bipolar and schizophrenia patients in a human open field paradigm. Psychiatry Res 2010; 178(1): 84-91.

Putzhammer A, Perfahl M, Pfeiff L, Müller JL. Three-dimensional ultrasonic movement analysis of gait and hand-movements in schizophrenic patients. Psychiatr Prax 2005; 32(Suppl 1): S38-42.

Quinlan EB, Banaschewski T, Barker GJ, *et al.* Identifying biological markers for improved precision medicine in psychiatry. Mol Psychiatry 2020; 25(2): 243-53.

Rampino A, Marakhovskaia A, Soares-Silva T, Torretta S, Veneziani F, Beaulieu JM. Antipsychotic drug responsiveness and dopamine receptor signaling; old players and new prospects. Front. Psychiatry 2018; 9: 702.

Reinertsen E, Shashikumar SP, Shah AJ, Nemati S, Clifford GD. Multiscale network dynamics between heart rate and locomotor activity are altered in schizophrenia. Physiol Meas 2018; 39(11): 115001.

Sano W, Nakamura T, Yoshiuchi K, *et al.* Enhanced persistency of resting and active periods of locomotor activity in schizophrenia. PLoS One 2012; 7(8): e43539.

Schiffman J, Sorensen HJ, Maeda J, et al. Childhood motor coordination and adult schizophrenia spectrum disorders. Am J Psychiatry 2009; 166(9): 1041-7

Schiffman J. Motor issues in the clinical high risk phase of psychosis. Schizophr Bull 2017; 43(5): 937-8.

Schmahmann JD. Disorders of the cerebellum: ataxia, dysmetria of thought, and the cerebellar cognitive affective syndrome. J Neuropsychiatry Clin Neurosci 2004; 16(3): 367-78.

Schmahmann JD. The role of cerebellum in affect and psychosis. J Neurolinguistics 2000; 13: 189-214.

Seppälä J, De Vita I, Jämsä T, *et al.* Mobile phone and wearable sensor-based mhealth approaches for psychiatric disorders and symptoms: systematic review. JMIR Ment Health 2019; 6(2): e9819.

Shinn AK, Baker JT, Lewandowski KE, Öngür D, Cohen BM. Aberrant cerebellar connectivity in motor and association networks in schizophrenia. Front Hum Neurosci 2015; 9: 134.

Shirai S, Yabe I, Matsushima M, Ito YM, Yoneyama M, Sasaki H. Quantitative evaluation of gait ataxia by accelerometers. J Neurol Sci 2015; 58(1-2): 53-8.

Shkodrova D, Haralanova E, Haralanov S. Objective cerebellar signs in schizophrenia: motor and balance coordination deficits. Bulg Neurol Psychiatr Pract 2007; 4: 18-24.

Stoyanov DS. Key developments in translational neuroscience: an update. Balkan Med J 2017; 34: 485-6.

Stoyanov, D., Kandilarova, S., Aryutova, K., Paunova, R., Todeva-Radneva, A., Latypova, A., & Kherif, F. (2021). Multivariate Analysis of Structural and Functional Neuroimaging Can Inform Psychiatric Differential Diagnosis. *Diagnostics*, *11*(1), 19.

Tognin S, van Hell HH, Merritt K, *et al*. Towards precision medicine in psychosis: benefits and challenges of multimodal multicenter studies-PSYSCAN: translating neuroimaging findings from research into clinical practice. Schizophr Bull. 2020; 46(2): 432-41.

Turner R, Schiavetto A. The cerebellum in schizophrenia: a case of intermittent ataxia and psychosis – clinical, cognitive, and neuroanatomical correlates. J Neuropsychiatry Clin Neurosci 2004; 16: 400-8.

Uebel H, Albrecht B, Kirov R, *et al*. What can actigraphy add to the concept of labschool design in clinical trials? Curr Pharm Des 2010; 16(22): 2434-42.

van Harten PN, Walther S, Kent JS, Sponheim SR, Mittal VA. The clinical and prognostic value of motor abnormalities in psychosis, and the importance of instrumental assessment. Neurosci Biobehav Rev 2017; 80: 476-87.

Varambally S, Venkatasubramanian G, Thirthalli J. Janakiramaiah N, Gangadhar BN. Cerebellar and other neurological soft signs in antipsychotic-naive schizophrenia. Acta Psychiatr Scand 2006; 114(5): 352-6.

Waddington JL, O'Tuathaigh CM. Modelling the neuromotor abnormalities of psychotic illness: Putative mechanisms and systems dysfunction. Schizophr Res 2017; 200: 12-9.

Walther S, Koschorke P, Horn H, Strik W. Objectively measured motor activity in schizophrenia challenges the validity of expert ratings. Psychiatry Res 2009; 169: 187-90.

Wang SM, Ouyang WC, Wu MY, Kuo LC. Relationship between motor function and psychotic symptomatology in young-adult patients with schizophrenia. Eur Arch Psychiatry Clin Neurosci 2020; 270(3): 373-82.

Wunderink L. Personalizing antipsychotic treatment: evidence and thoughts on individualized tailoring of antipsychotic dosage in the treatment of psychotic disorders. Ther Adv Psychopharmacol 2019; 9: 1-16.

Young JW, Minassian A, Geyer MA. Locomotor profiling from rodents to the clinic and back again. Curr Top Behav Neurosci 2016; 28: 287-303.

Zilani TA, Al-Turjman F, Khan MB, Zhao N, Yang X. Monitoring movements of ataxia patient by using UWB technology. Sensors (Basel) 2020; 20(3): 931.

CHAPTER NINE

ALZHEIMER'S DISEASE AND THERAPEUTIC STRATEGIES

ABDELKADER BASLI* AND JIHANE BOUNAAS
LABORATORY OF INTERACTION RESEARCH, BIODIVERSITY, ECOSYSTEMS AND BIOTECHNOLOGY. FACULTY OF SCIENCES, UNIVERSITY OF SKIKDA, SKIKDA, ALGERIA.

Abstract

Alzheimer's disease (AD) is characterised by the presence of two types of protein deposits in the brain, amyloid plaques and neurofibrillary tangles. The first, are dense deposits of beta amyloid protein, and the second, are dense deposits of the protein tau. These proteins are present in all of our brains, but in AD they act unusually, leading to neuronal degeneration. This review will provide an overview of AD, including the role of amyloid beta and tau, and mechanisms that lead to the formation of plaques and tangles. The review will also cover the existing research that have focused on the inhibition of amyloid beta formation, cholinesterase, tau hyperphosphorylation, the pathogenic mechanisms of apoE4, and GSK-3 as a solution that could be used to slow or prevent the disease.

Keywords: Alzheimer's disease, Amyloid beta, Tau protein, Novel therapies, Amyloid, β-Amyloid Precursor Protein, Aβ, oligomer, fibril

Introduction

The brain is the command centre for the entire body; it receives information from our senses and controls our thoughts and movements. It is made up of different cell types. The most common brain cells are glia and neurons. There are in total more than 100 billion neurons **(Koechlin, 2006)**. Each of these neurons has two specialised thin branches, a dendrite where neurons receive nerve signals from other neurons and axons, specialised structures through which nerve impulses are transmitted. When the electrical signal reaches the axon terminal, a neurotransmitter is released at the presynaptic terminal. The released neurotransmitter travels to the synapse then binds to receptors to excite or inhibit the postsynaptic neuron **(Lovinger, 2008)**. That's how healthy neurons communicate with each other and when these cells become damaged in an individual, it can lead to the development of dementia.

Dementia is a term used to describe a group of symptoms that begins with memory problems, complex attention issues followed by language problems, social skills, and recognition **(Lyketsos et al., 2006)**. Alzheimer's disease (AD) is the most common type of dementia. It was described for the first time in 1907 by psychiatrist Alois Alzheimer. He was performing a histopathologic study of the brain of his patient Auguste D. who was suffering from dementia. He described two types of lesions in the brain, senile plaque and neurofibrillary tangles (NFTs) which are the two most important markers of AD **(Möller & Graeber, 1998; Robert D. Terry & Peter Davies, 1980)**.

The main parts of this work are summarised as follows:

1) A literature review on tau protein and amyloid beta, their toxicity, and the reasons behind their unusual function.
2) Also, we will deal with studies that tackled this problem and suggested that the inhibition of Aβ, cholinesterase, tau hyperphosphorylation, toxic effects of apoE4, and GSK-3, as a solution to be used against the disease. A review of studies that have suggested inhibition as a treatment for the disease.

1. Tau protein and neurofibrillary tangle

Tau protein is part of the microtubule-associated protein family (MAP) that is present in axons, neurons, and glial cells especially in pathological conditions **(Buée et al., 2000)**. In the human brain, 6 tau isoforms are expressed, distinguished by the presence of 4 or 3 repeat domains, that are in combination with exon 2 only, or with exon 2 and 3, or none of these exons (Table 1; **Cox et al., 2016**). Tau protein is arranged in three distinct regions: a carboxyl terminus region (repeat region), that has the ability to bind microtubules and proteins such as protein phosphatase 2A and presenilin 1; a very acidic amino terminal region that interacts with other cytoskeletal elements and proteins such as PLC-γ and Src-kinases; and a proline rich region containing target sites for multiple kinases **(Buée et al., 2000; Paglini et al., 2000)**.

Isoforms MAPT gene is located on chromosome 17q21.3		Number of amino acids
2N4R (htau40)	N- -C	441
1N4R (htau34)	N- -C	412
0N4R (htau24)	N- -C	383
0N3R (htau23)	N- -C	352
1N3R (htau37)	N- -C	381
2N3R (htau39)	N- -C	410

Table 1: Table represents the human tau isoforms.

Numerous post-translational modifications have been identified in tau protein such as phosphorylation, glycosylation, ubiquitination glycation, polyamination, truncation, oxidation, aggregation, and nitration. These modifications appear to be a common occurrence in physiological as well as pathophysiological conditions **(Mietelska-Porowska et al., 2014)**. We will give a brief summary of some post-translational modifications.

Ubiquitination

Ubiquitination is the process in which misfolded proteins are tagged by chemicals called ubiquitin. It plays an effective role in providing them with the ability to interact with the proteasome, which in turn allows them to be degraded in an ATP-dependent manner. Ubiquitination is considered to be a detoxification process. It is able to form ghost tangles from neurofibrillary tangles (NFTs) in order to stabilise them. Moreover, tau intermediates are harmful to neurons, therefore, their ubiquitination is a way to dispose of them **(F. Chen et al., 2004; Heinisch & Brandt, 2016)**.

Glycation

Glycation is the chemical reaction that occurs when a reducing sugar combines with the amino group of the lysine in proteins, without the participation of an enzyme. This leads to the creation of a chemical called advanced glycation end products (AGEs). Glycation of tau protein might play a role in the disruption of microtubule binding and promote the aggregation of paired helical filaments (PHF) via receptors known as RAGE (receptor for advanced glycation end products), which are found on subsets of neurons and microglial cells **(Mathew et al., 2011)**. It is also known that Glycated tau is able to induce oxidative stress **(Buée et al., 2000)**.

Glycosylation

Glycosylation is a modification that involves enzymes that bind oligosaccharides to polypeptides. There are two types of glycosylation: N-linked (N-glycosylation) and O-linked (O-glycosylation) **(Gong et al., 2005)**. O-glycosylation is a process in which a chemical group known as O-linked N-acetylglucosamine (O-GlcNAc) is added to serine and threonine residues. O-glycosylation is reciprocal to phosphorylation, the two modifications were found to have opposite effects **(Buée et al., 2000)**. It was found that the group of mice that had been starved of glucose (that mimicked those seen in AD) developed a condition in which there was a diminution in O-GlcNAcylation and hyperphosphorylation of tau protein. According to this result, it appears that abnormal hyperphosphorylation of tau may be associated with deficiencies in O-GlcNAcylation **(F. Liu et al., 2004)**. N-glycosylation is the process of adding N-glycan to proteins. The most common N-glycan structure that is attached to asparagine is N-acetyl glucosamine (GlcNAcβ1-Asn) **(Stanley et al., 2009)**. While O-GlcNAcylation occurs to protect against abnormal phosphorylation, N-glycosylation does not. It was found that abnormal N-glycosylation of tau appeared in AD only and increased tau susceptibility to phosphorylation **(Schedin-Weiss et al., 2014)**.

Phosphorylation

This modification is characterised by the addition of a phosphate group at: serine, threonine, and tyrosine. 53% of the phosphorylation sites on tau are serines. The other 41% are threonines and remaining 6% are tyrosines (Table 2; **Martin et al., 2011**).

Tau phosphorylation sites exist in healthy brains	Tau phosphorylation sites exist in AD brains	Tau phosphorylation sites exist in healthy and AD brains
T17, Y29, T39, T50, T52, S56, T95, T101, T102, T111, S131, T135, T149, T169, S195, T220, S241, T245, T263, S285, S293, S305, S316, S320, S324, S341, S352, T361, T373, T386, T414.	Y18, S68, T69, T71, S113, T123, T153, T175, T184, S185, S191, Y197, S208, S210, S214, S237, S238, S258, S262, S289, S356, Y394, T403, S409, S422, T427, S433, S435.	S46, T81, S198, S199, S202, T205, T212, T217, T231, S235, S396, S400, S404, S412, S413, S416.

Table 2: Table illustrates tau phosphorylation sites in healthy and AD brains. S, serine; T, threonine; Y, tyrosine.

Tau phosphorylation is a process in which specific kinases and phosphatases are involved. Kinases induce tau phosphorylation, while phosphatases dephosphorylate the protein. The proper functioning of these two enzymes ensures that interactions between microtubules and tau are tightly regulated **(Stoothoff & Johnson, 2005)**.

Kinases are divided into three categories:

A) proline-directed protein kinases (PDPKs), including mitogen-activated protein kinases, glycogen synthase kinase 3, cyclin-dependent kinases.
B) Non-proline-directed protein kinases (non-PDPKs) including tau-tubulin kinase 1/2, dual-specificity tyrosine phosphorylation and regulated kinase 1A, casein kinase 1a/1d/1e/2, protein kinase cAMP-dependent/B/C/N, microtubule affinity-regulating kinases, and Ca2+ /Calmodulin-dependent protein kinase II.

C) Protein kinases specific for tyrosines **(Martin et al., 2011)**.

The dephosphorylation of tau is provided by protein phosphatases PPs (phosphoserine/ phosphothreonine 1, 2A, 2B and 5). Liu et al. showed that protein phosphatases (PP2A) accounted for as much as 70% of the total tau phosphatase activity compared to the other PPs, which had lower activity (≤ 10%). It has been found that the affinity to tau, enzymatic specificity, and abundance all play important roles in determining PPs activity in the regulation of tau phosphorylation **(F. Liu et al., 2005)**.

In healthy neurons, tau normally stabilises the microtubules and prevents their shortening, decreasing the critical level of tubulin polymerisation, an essential step for microtubule assembly **(Kadavath et al., 2015)**. Although, tau protein is involved in cell signalling by modulating the activity of PSD95 protein and Src and Fyn kinases **(Mietelska-Porowska et al., 2014)**. In addition to that, studies *in vivo* showed that tau protein plays an important role in the maturation of newborn hippocampal granule neurons **(Pallas-Bazarra et al., 2016)**.

However, hyperphosphorylation of tau protein will increase depolymerisation of microtubules (the depolymerisation results in the dissociation of tau protein from microtubules), and then generate the tau oligomers in which turn accumulate to produce protomers that will turn around each other to form paired helical filaments and eventually create neurofibrillary tangles **(Mamun et al., 2020)**. Hyperphosphorylation of tau protein either by activation of GSK3β or by inhibition of PP2A, causes instability of microtubules, perturbs axonal transport, harms the synaptic communication between neurons, and eventually causes the death of the neuron **(Kadavath et al., 2015; Martin et al., 2011)**. In addition to this, studies found that overexpression of glycogen synthase kinase 3 (GSK3) not only increases tau phosphorylation, but also promotes the production of Aβ by facilitating the proteolysis of APP **(G. V. W. Johnson & Stoothoff, 2004)**.

3. Amyloid precursor protein

Amyloid precursor protein (APP) is a transmembrane precursor protein with a unique membrane-spanning domain, a long extracellular glycosylated N-terminus, and a short cytoplasmic C-terminus **(Nguyen, 2015)**. APP is expressed in many tissues in the central nervous system, in the liver, myotubes and adipose tissue **(Guo et al., 2021)**. APP helps the neuron to grow and repair itself, provides intracellular transport, and promotes synaptogenesis, neuronal adhesion, and axonogenesis, etc. **(Baumkotter et al., 2014; G. Chen et al., 2017).** Normally, it gets split by two enzymes α and γ secretase. The cleavage is initiated by α- secretase resulting in the formation of APPsα and CTFα (C83), while the CTFα is then cleaved by γ-secretase (complex made up of: PSEN, NCT, PSEN2 and Aph1) to produce the short peptide P3 and ICD. This is the non-canonical pathway (non-amyloidogenic) **(Walsh et al., 2007)**. In the canonical pathway (amyloidogenic) and in the case of AD, the cleavage by β-secretase will produce APPsβ and CTFβ (C99). CTFβ is subsequently sectioned by γ-secretase leading to the generation of ICD and to the formation of protein called amyloid beta (Aβ) peptides of 36–43 amino acids, they are produced in various isoforms especially $A\beta_{40}$ and $A\beta_{42}$ **(S. J. C. Lee et al., 2017; Tabaton & Tamagno, 2007)**. $A\beta_{40}$ is the major species rather than $A\beta_{42}$. However, $A\beta_{42}$ is the more amyloidogenic species **(Iwatsubo et al., 1994)**. The ICD secreted by γ-secretase (in both pathways) is translocated to the nucleus where it affects the regulation of gene transcription **(Kienlen-Campard et al., 2008)**.

4. Amyloid beta (Aβ)

Aβ monomers initially transformed to a nucleus followed by addition of monomers to the nucleus via the elongation process to form oligomers that are soluble. The oligomers themselves elongate into fibrils, which are insoluble, and they may form amyloid plaques **(G. Chen et al., 2017; Pagano et al., 2020)**. The hippocampus and entorhinal cortex, which control the memory, are the first affected by amyloid plaques **(Grøntvedt et al., 2018)**.

Abnormal accumulations of Aβ are known to contribute to neurodegeneration by several mechanisms, including the production of reactive species, the disruption of synaptic function, calcium ion imbalance, and the phosphorylation of tau protein, etc. **(Nguyen, 2015)**.

ROS production

Aβ stimulates microglia and astrocytes to produce pro-inflammatory cytokines and chemokines such as TNF- α, IFNγ and Il-1β **(Rossi & Bianchini, 1996)**. After cytokine exposure, glial cells expressed inducible nitric oxide synthase (iNOS Ca^{2+}-independent). This enzyme catalyses the transformation of L-arginine into nitric oxide (NO) and L-citrulline.

Knowing that the production of NO is also done by these two isoforms eNOS and nNOS, both are Ca^{2+}-dependent **(Saha & Pahan, 2006)**. NO is neuroprotective, but overproduction of it can be harmful. It induces the production of other reactive species like peroxynitrite ($ONOO^-$), which is formed by the interaction of NO with $O_2^{\bullet-}$ **(Beckman et al., 1990)**. $ONOO^-$ induces lipid peroxidation and as a result, alters membrane fluidity and permeability **(Durand et al., 2013; Szabó, 2003)**. Peroxynitrite induces introducing a carbonyl group into the protein, promoting tyrosine nitration, etc. yielding modification of the protein structure **(Ischiropoulos & Al-Mehdi, 1995)**. $ONOO^-$ interacts with DNA and causes the oxidation and nitration of guanine, which leads respectively to the formation of 8-oxoguanine and 8-nitro-guanine. Mutagenesis, carcinogenesis, and DNA strand breakage are considered a consequence of guanine oxidation and nitration **(PACHER et al., 2007)**.

Furthermore, $A\beta_{42}$ through the NMDA receptor stimulates NADPH oxidase to produce ROS. The latter activates extracellular signal-regulated kinase (ERK1/2), releases arachidonic acid (AA), and induces phosphorylation of cytosolic phospholipase A(2)α [cPLA(2)α] **(Shelat et al., 2008)**.

Transition metals such as Fe^{+2}, Cu^{+2} must be considered as pro-oxidant species **(Vamecq et al., 2004)**. Aβ has the capacity to reduce Cu^{2+} to Cu^{+}. The molecular oxygen interacts with Cu^{+} to generate superoxide anion ($O_2^{\bullet-}$), which is a precursor to other more toxic radical species. Aβ may act as free-radical ($A\beta^{\bullet}$), removing protons from lipids and proteins of their entourage to produce respectively hydroxy-2-nonenal and carbonyls **(Smith et al., 2007)**.

Mitochondria dysfunction

Studies have shown that exposure to Aβ induces oxidative injury of mitochondrial membranes, releases cytochrome c due to increased membrane permeability, disrupts protein mobility, and negatively affects the lipid polarity of mitochondrial membrane **(Rodrigues et al., 2001)**. Moreover, Aβ can reduce the activities of key mitochondrial enzymes such as cytochrome oxidase, pyruvate dehydrogenase, and α-ketoglutarate dehydrogenase **(Casley et al., 2002)**. Aβ and the activation of some enzymes such as NADPH oxidase, xanthine oxidase, and A2 phospholipases induce ROS production and mitochondrial dysfunction **(Carrillo-Mora et al., 2014)**.

Interaction of beta amyloid with receptors

We will review a few of the receptors in which A*β* is interacting.

- MGlu5 receptors

Metabotropic glutamate receptors 5 (MGluR5) are expressed in the central nervous system. They mainly regulate intracellular calcium and participate in synaptic transmission **(Li et al., 2017)**. The interaction between Aβ and mGluR5 receptors elevates intracellular calcium mobilisation and causes synaptotoxicity **(Renner et al., 2010)**.

- NMDA and AMPA receptors

The heterotetramers N-methyl-D-aspartate (NMDA)-type of ionotropic glutamate receptors are permeable to Na^+, K^+ and Ca^{2+}, activated by glutamate and glycine and blocked by Mg^{2+}. NMDA receptors play a fundamental role in controlling synaptic plasticity **(Monyer et al., 1992)**. They induce Ca^{2+} influx and augment the appearance of AMPA receptors; this is an essential step for inducing long-term potentiation (LTP), which represents an enhancement of synaptic transmission. When the input of calcium ions is reduced, the level of AMPA receptors is reduced too, which leads to the production of a long-term depression (LTD) and causes a decrease in synaptic transmission **(Kessels & Malinow, 2009)**. Accumulation of Aβ will cause several anomalies by decreasing the number of AMPA receptors, inhibiting LTP, and stimulating LTD. Moreover, Aβ has a negative impact on NMDA receptor, causing their endocytosis, which affects Ca^{2+} homeostasis, reduces learning and memory, and impairs synaptic plasticity **(Hsieh et al., 2006; Shankar et al., 2008; Snyder et al., 2005)**.

- α7 nACh receptors

The α7 nicotinic acetylcholine receptors (α7 nAChRs) are a type of ligand-gated ion channel that are involved in synaptic plasticity. α7 nAChRs, if properly stimulated, may exert regulation over many physiological functions of the adult and developing brain by modulating Ca^{+2} levels **(Broide & Leslie, 1999)**. The endocytosis of NMDA receptors by Aβ oligomers involves the activation of α7 nAChRs **(Snyder et al., 2005)**. The α7 nAChRs may play a role in neuroprotection by preventing $A\beta_{1\text{–}42}$ – induced toxicity. However, disrupted expression of the CHRNA7 gene that encodes for α7 nAChRs may be involved with numerous neuropsychiatric disorders **(Ma & Qian, 2019)**. Furthermore, α7 nAChRs enhance activation of ERK and JNK by $A\beta_{42}$. This process is induced tau phosphorylation **(H.-Y. Wang et al., 2003)**.

- Insulin receptors

The insulin receptors (IRs) are a class of receptor tyrosine kinase, and they are activated by insulin, a hormone used by the body to control blood glucose levels. In recent years, the role of insulin in the central nervous system (CNS) has become clearer. It has been found to play a key role including regulating metabolic reactions, stimulating energy homeostasis, and neuronal processes **(Plum et al., 2005)**. Zhao et al., by using mature hippocampal neurons cultures, showed that the addition of soluble Aβ oligomers, or ADDLs, significantly and rapidly decreased the expression of IRs on the dendritic surface, increased somatic IRs, inhibited the responses of neurons to insulin, and suggested that ADDLs may cause insulin resistance in AD **(W.-Q. Zhao et al., 2008)**.

Aβ facilitates neurofibrillary tangle (NFT) formation

Aβ stimulates the phosphorylation of tau protein by activating a number of kinases, among which CDK5, MARK, GSK-3, and Fyn kinase, which caused the destabilisation of microtubules and damaged axonal transport **(Busciglio et al., 1995; Rajmohan & Reddy, 2017)**. Three pathways are proposed to show by which Aβ can facilitate NFT formation:

1) Aβ leads to the formation of NFT by activating tau kinases, an enzyme known to phosphorylate tau.
2) Aβ promotes proteasome dysfunction, which decreases tau degradation.
3) Aβ increases the expression of caspase-3, which induces the truncation of tau, and alters tau aggregation and ultimately leads to the formation of NFTs **(Sadigh-Eteghad et al., 2015)**.

Haemorrhage

Amyloid plaque can also deposit around blood vessels in the brain in a process known as amyloid angiopathy, which increases the risk of intracerebral haemorrhage **(Weber et al., 2018)**. Aβ can stimulate haemorrhage by influencing multiple proteolytic systems in the cerebral vasculature. Elevated amyloid β-protein precursor (AβPP) levels can lower thrombosis, promote a haemorrhagic setting, and increase Aβ production. Furthermore, in cerebrovascular cells, Aβ is associated with the activation of certain matrix metalloproteinases (MMPs) and plasminogen that in turn degrade a wide array of extracellular matrix, contributing to loss of vessel wall integrity and haemorrhage **(Van Nostrand, 2016)**.

Positive effect of Aβ

Conversely, Aβ may play an important role against infection. Recently, multiple studies have shown that Aβ displays antiviral activity, in particular against HSV-1, antimicrobial activity against gram-positive and gram-negative bacteria such as *Staphylococcus epidermidis*, *Streptococcus agalactiae*, *Salmonella typhimurium*, and antifungal activity **(Gosztyla et al., 2018; White et al., 2014)**.

5. Factors driving Aβ accumulation and induce AD

AD is divided into two forms, sporadic form or the late onset of AD (LOAD, after 60-65 years of age) representing >95% of cases, and familial form or the early onset of AD (EOAD, before 60-65 years of age), representing <5% of cases **(Bird, 2008)**.

Sporadic form

Genetics

Apolipoprotein E (ApoE) is synthesised by the liver and in the brain by astrocyte, microglia, and oligodendrocytes. Neurons can also express apoE, especially in response to injury **(Q. Xu, 2006)**. ApoE is located on chromosome 19 and present in chylomicron, ILD, VLDL, and certain subclasses of HDL **(Boyles et al., 1985)**. ApoE exists in 3 common isoforms, ApoE2, E3, and E4. The three isoforms vary in terms of amino acid position: apoE2 has cysteines at positions 112 and 158, apoE3 is characterised by the presence of cysteine at position 112, and arginine at position 158, while ApoE4 differs from apoE3 by the substitution of cysteine by arginine at site 112 **(R. W. Mahley & Rall, 2000)**. ApoE plays an important role in the transport of triglyceride, cholesterol redistribution, and facility of the fixation of lipoproteins on LDL receptors. ApoE carries lipids in CSF, when nerve cells are impaired, apoE redistributes lipids to axons and Schwann cells to repair this damage **(Y. Huang & Mahley, 2014; R. Mahley, 1988)**. However, apoE (especially apoE4) is the most important risk factor for the sporadic form of AD **(Strittmatter et al., 1993)**. ApoE4 may be linked to a number of harmful effects, including inhibition of certain proteases activity, resulting in Aβ being unable to be eliminated **(Theendakara et al., 2018)**. Additionally, apoE4 could stimulate hyperphosphorylation of tau protein **(Tesseur et al., 2000)**, cerebral amyloid angiopathy (CAA) formation, and cause mitochondrial dysfunction **(Q. Xu, 2006)**. Researchers have recently shown that an ApoE-ApoE receptor complex is involved in the activation of APP transcription and increased Aβ synthesis transcription via MAP Kinase pathway (Figure 1; **Huang et al., 2017**).

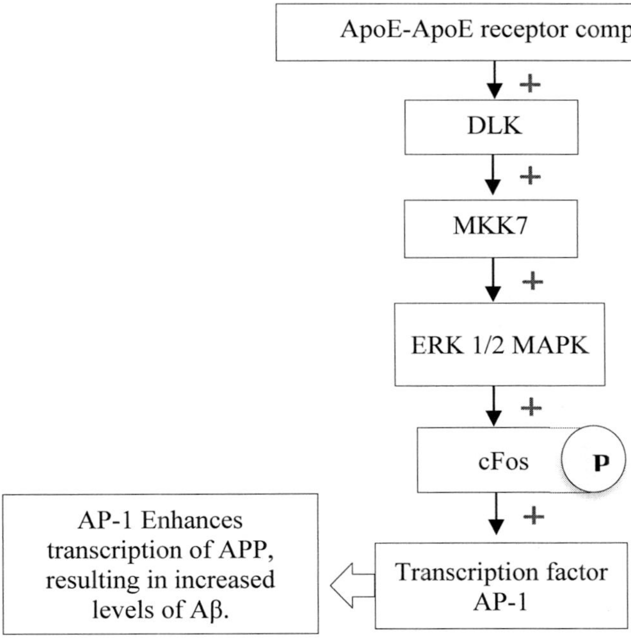

Figure 1: Schema shows how the fixation of ApoE on its receptor increases Aβ transcription via MAPK pathway. DLK, dual leucine-zipper kinase; MKK7, mitogen-activated protein kinase kinase 7; ERK 1/2, extracellular signal-regulated protein kinases 1 and 2; AP-1, Activator protein 1.

Another study *in vivo* showed that ApoE4 could bind to IR and trap them within the endosomes, which prevented insulin fixation in its receptors and harmed cerebral insulin signalling **(N. Zhao et al., 2017)**.

Environments

Certain diseases such as hyperglycaemia obstruct the degradation (not the production) of the APP, which increases Aβ production **(H. J. Lee et al., 2018)**. Hypertension (high blood pressure) may also play an important role in the pathological development of AD. Hypertension can lead to changes in the brain's vessels' walls, which causes ischaemia, decreases blood flow (hypoperfusion), and reduces oxygen flow (hypoxia). Studies have shown that ischaemia brings about the build-up of APP and Aβ in the brain **(Skoog & Gustafson, 2006)**.

Ageing has a role in the development of mitochondrial dysfunction; as a result, many problems could occur, such as reactive oxygen species (ROS) and reactive nitrogen species (RNS) production. ROS may increase Aβ production by affecting the processing of APP. Furthermore, research shows that H_2O_2 increases the expression of β-site APP cleaving enzyme 1 (BACE-1), which in turn causes an increase in the production of $A\beta_{40}$ and $A\beta_{42}$. The RNS, including $ONOO^-$, induces the nitrotyrosination of PSEN1, produces $A\beta_{42}$, and augments the $A\beta_{42}/A\beta_{40}$ ratio **(Guix et al., 2012; Swerdlow et al., 2014)**.

Certain habits such as smoking and alcohol abuse can lead to AD. Studies have demonstrated that excessive consumption of ethanol, the form of alcohol that is consumed, can incite the development of AD by altering APP processing, increasing the levels of BACE-1, stimulating the production of Aβ, and promoting the formation of neuritic plaques **(D. Huang et al., 2018)**.

Pesticides are neurotoxins. They can participate in the development of AD by damaging the mitochondrial function, inducing oxidative stress, increasing levels of AβPP and BACE1, and preventing Aβ degradation and clearance **(Yan et al., 2016)**.

Familial form

Three mutated genes have been identified: Presenilin (PSEN-1 chromosome 14 /PSEN-2 chromosome 1) and APP (chromosome 21). Presenilin is a catalytic subunit of γ-secretase, mutation in these PSEN-1/PSEN-2 can change the locations where gamma secretase cleaves APP, which increases the production of Aβ **(Esler & Wolfe, 2001)**.

6. Therapeutic effectiveness for Alzheimer's disease

Currently, there are no medications that can treat AD as it is complicated and caused by several different mechanisms. Moreover, drugs must cross the blood-brain barrier (BBB) before they can have any effect in the central nervous system. It is hard to find effective drugs **(Mogana et al., 2014; Paudel et al., 2018)**. However, there are medications that can treat symptoms of AD. These treatments include cholinesterase inhibitors and NMDA antagonists (table 3).

Table 3: **Table illustrates some symptomatic treatment of AD.**

Drugs	Mechanism of Action	Side effects	References
Tacrine	- Inhibited the action of acetylcholinesterase (ACHE), - Increased secretion and production of acetylcholine, - Stimulated glucose metabolism - Raised levels of monoamine metabolites and nicotine brain receptors.	Induced hepatotoxicity.	**(Wagstaff & McTavish, 1994; Watkins et al., 1994)**
Donepezil	- Inhibited AChE in erythrocyte more than tacrine (non-competitive inhibition), - Increased the level of acetylcholine, - Inhibited the excitotoxicity inducing by glutamate, - Reduced the level of inflammatory cytokine, etc.	Insomnia, diarrhoea, loss of appetite, muscle weakness, bradycardia, etc.	**(Bryson & Benfield, 1997; Sharma, 2019)**
Rivastigmine	- Inhibited AChE by binding in ionic and esteratic sites, and Butyrylcholinesterase (BChE). - Prevented belated neuronal death, - Could slow functional decline, - Activated the metabolism of global brain, etc.	Diarrhoea, vomiting, nausea, etc.	**(Desai & Grossberg, 2005; Potkin et al., 2001)**

Galantamine	- Inhibited AChE (competitive and reversible inhibition), - Boosted the cholinergic nicotinic neurotransmission.	Bronchospasm, nausea, vomiting, weakness, etc.	**(Nordgren et al., 2009; Olin & Schneider, 2002)**
Metrifonate	- Inhibited AChE (irreversible inhibition), - Boosted the cholinergic neurotransmission.	Anthelmintic, bradycardia, diarrhoea, rhinitis, and leg cramps…	**(López Arrieta & Schneider, 2006)**
Memantine	- Antagonist of NMDA receptors (non-competitive inhibitor), - It can be used with AChE inhibitor, - Had positive effect on neuropsychiatric symptoms, global functioning, and cognition.	Few side effects including hallucinations and aggression.	**(Reisberg et al., 2003; van Marum, 2009)**

Amyloid beta inhibition

Aβ inhibition by peptides and small molecules

The α5β1 integrin played a critical role in mediating cell adhesion to Aβ; the α5β1 integrin was also involved in the degradation and clearance of Aβ, and reduced Aβ deposition in cell culture **(Matter et al., 1998)**.

β-sheet breaker peptide (iAβ5p) was found to cross the blood-brain barrier at a higher rate. Before testing this peptide, it was first treated in the amino terminus with acetylation and in the carboxyl terminus with amidation to prevent its degradation. The results showed that iAβ5p was able to reduce amyloid disposition, brain inflammation, and cerebral damage induced by amyloid **(Permanne et al., 2002)**.

Chafekar et al. used dendritic KLVFF peptides (K_4: four KLVFF coupled with dendrimeric) and the monomeric KLVFF (K_1). They found that K_4 prevented the low molecular weight (LMW) $Aβ_{1–42}$ aggregation, disassembled Aβ fibrils (fAβ), disassembled protofibrillar $Aβ_{1–42}$, and reorganised it into amorphous aggregates. In short, K_4 was able to inhibit all stages of Aβ aggregation much better than K_1 and its inhibitor activity is due to the KLVFF sequence, not to the dendritic structure **(Chafekar et al., 2007)**.

The pentapeptide $G_{33}LMVG_{37}$ is anti-Aβ, it had the capacity to interact with the C-terminal region of Aβ; thus, preventing it from interacting with membranes, and reducing the synaptotoxicity **(Peters et al., 2013)**.

The BHdS structure is comprised of reverse β-turn and two opposite β-strands. The cyclic conformation of BHdS peptide was able to decrease in a dose-dependent manner the rate of $Aβ_{1-42}$ aggregation and reduce its toxicity against neuronal cells **(Jha et al., 2018)**.

Cyclohexanehexols were able to reduce $Aβ_{40/42}$ levels, Aβ oligomers, synaptic loss, plaque burden, and angiopathy. However, scyllo-cyclohexanehexol had no impact on the activity of β- and γ-secretase **(McLaurin et al., 2006)**.

Trehalose is a simple disaccharide, it was able to inhibit fibrillar and oligomeric of $Aβ_{40}$, fibrillar of $Aβ_{42}$, inhibit Aβ aggregation and reduce its toxicity **(R. Liu et al., 2005)**.

Vitamin K3 inhibited $A\beta_{42}$ aggregation, reduced its cytotoxicity, decreased the β-sheet structures **(Alam et al., 2016)**.

Vitamin B12 inhibited in a concentration dependent manner the aggregation of $A\beta_{42}$, prevented β-sheet generation by reducing the structural conversion in $A\beta_{42}$, and lowered the cytotoxicity of Aβ. In addition to that, Aβ fibrils in presence of vitamin B12 become less susceptible to hydrophobic patches **(Alam et al., 2017)**.

Aβ inhibition by plants

Owing to the side effects of the available medicines, studies started to think about the necessity of plant use because of their high flavonoid and phenol contents. In table 4 we have mentioned some plants that have inhibitor activity against Aβ.

Table 4: Examples of plants that induced the inhibition of amyloid beta and its toxicity.

Plants	Aims	Results	References
Tarenna obtusifolia	The purpose was to test the ability of vomifoliol, isolated from Tarenna obtusifolia, to inhibit beta amyloid aggregation using Thioflavin T (ThT) assay. Dichloromethane (CH_2Cl_2) is the solvent used for extraction. Three compounds have been isolated and identified after fractionation of CH_2Cl_2 extract: vomifoliol, stigmasterol, and p-coumaric acid.	CH_2Cl_2 extract was effective in inhibiting Aβ aggregation where percent inhibition was equal to 63.42 at 50µg/ml. However, the CH_2Cl_2 extract could also cause toxicity of neuroblastoma cells (SH-SY5Y): CH_2Cl2 extract at 50µg/ml inhibits 75% of cell growth. Among the 3 compounds (vomifoliol, stigmasterol, and p-coumaric acid), only the vomifoliol had a significant inhibition against Aβ aggregation (55.71% at 50µg/ml) and caused no toxicity of SH-SY5Y cells at 1 µM, 10 µM, and 20 µM concentrations. Additionally, vomifoliol at 20 µM protected SH-SY5Y cells when treating them with 1 µM Aβ, which demonstrated that this substance had a neuroprotective effect.	(Tan et al., 2020)
Withania somnifera (Ashwagandha)	The purpose of their research was to determine the inhibitory effects of four derivatives of Withania somnifera (Withanolide A,	After treating the amyloid samples with withanolides and withanosides derivatives and incubating for 6h, they noticed that the fluorescence intensity reduced considerably. The assumption was that there had been a reduction	(Dubey et al., 2021)

	B and Withanoside IV, V) on the formation of amyloid oligomers and fibrils, and to test their ability to protect the cell from the harmful effects of beta amyloid and their ability to inhibit ROS generation.	in the β-sheet structures. Briefly the use of ThT assay indicated that the derivatives were able to inhibit amyloid beta aggregation. The anti-amyloidogenic property of all four derivatives could be attributed to their similar nature. The result also showed that these derivatives could inhibit fibrillisation. MTT assay indicated that withanolide A, B and withanoside IV, V had a neuroprotective effect by reducing Aβ fibrillation toxicity. The use of TUNEL test showed that the derivatives of Ashwagandha could lead to a pronounced reduction in the apoptotic cell numbers. After treating the SH-SY5Y cells with Aβ there was a hyperproduction of ROS. However, when the cells were treated with the derivatives, there was a reduction in the production of ROS (Withanolide A and B are most effective against ROS). In silico studies were carried out to evaluate the molecular interaction between two molecules: Ashwagandha derivatives and β-amyloid. The Molecular docking studies were done using Autodock v.4.2.3. The study showed that the	

		withanolides and withanosides had the ability to interact with the hydrophobic core of Aβ ($Aβ_{17–21}$) consequently, the interaction of the monomers will not be developed, and the aggregation will decrease. The molecular simulation method indicated that the withanolides and withanosides attached in the LVFFA region, a region where several inhibitors of Aβ have proven to be effective.	
Soshiho-tang (SST) composed of: Bupleurum falcatum, Pinellia ternata, Zingiber officinale, Scutellaria baicalensis, Ziziphus jujube, Panax ginseng, Glycyrrhiza uralensis.	The objective of this study was to test the ability of this herb to inhibit amyloid beta and its toxicity.	Five compounds of SST have been isolated: liquiritin (a), baicalein (c), baicalin (b), glycyrrhizin (e), and wogonin (d). Male C57BL6 mice were injected by Aβ aggregates, and two tests were used, PAT (passive avoidance task) and MWM (Morris water maze). The PAT result showed that Aβ reduced the transfer latency in the retention trial. The MWM results showed that Aβ increased the escape latency to target and decreased the crossing number. Treatment with SST reverse the effects of Aβ: - Increased the transfer latency in the retention trial,	(Sohn et al., 2021)

		- Decreased the escape latency to target, - Increased the crossing number. They also found out that Aβ provoked the reduction of the surviving neurons number and increased the level of Iba-1 and AChE. While SST reduced neuronal loss, inhibited the microglial activity, and decreased the activity of AChE. Moreover, SST treatment boosted Aβ disaggregation.	
Salvia officinalis (Rosmarinic acid)	Examined the effect of Salvia officinalis compound, Rosmarinic acid on: - Cell viability, - ROS, - P38 MAP kinase and GSK-3β, - Tau phosphorylation, - Cell apoptosis.	When PC-12 cells assayed with $A\beta_{42}$, the latter: - Reduced cells viability, - Increased ROS production, - Increased p-p38 and p-GSK-3β expression, - Increased pp-tau (hyperphosphorylated tau), - Induced DNA fragmentation (the generation of oligonucleosomes and mononucleosomes) and reduced the ration of pro-caspase/total caspase-3, which induced apoptosis. Treatment of PC-12 by rosmarinic acid reverse the effect of $A\beta_{42}$: - Reduced cell death, - Deceased the production of ROS, - Reduced p-p38 expression, but it had no effect on GSK-3β,	(Iuvone et al., 2006)

		- Decreased pp-tau, - Decreased DNA fragmentation and increased the ration of pro-caspase/total caspase-3.	
Ecklonia radiata. Six fractions were prepared from this herb: Crude extract (CE), Phlorotannin (PT), Polysaccharide (PS), Free sugar (FS), Low molecular weight (LM), High molecular weight (HM).	Examined the neuroprotective activities of Ecklonia radiate extracts against $A\beta_{1-42}$.	- Cell viability: The fractions were tested to see if it had any effect on PC-12 cell viability. The data revealed that only HM, CE, and PS at 25µg/mL, 100 µg/mL, and 50 µg/mL respectively, induced cytotoxicity. When PC-12 cells assayed with $A\beta_{1-42}$, the latter reduced cell viability. The addition of these fractions showed neuroprotective activities and increased cell viability. The highest neuroprotective activity was found in the PS, CE, and PT fractions. - Anti-aggregative effects: All fractions were able to inhibit the aggregation of $A\beta_{1-42}$ The highest inhibitor activity was found in PT (90%) followed by FS, CE, LM, PS, and finally HM. - Anti- ROS (H_2O_2)	(Alghazwi et al., 2020)

		Incubation of PC-12 with H_2O_2 decreased cell viability. Treatment with fractions exhibited antioxidant activity (against H_2O_2) and increased cell viability. The heights antioxidants activity was found in CE fraction. The LM fraction was found to be least effective against H_2O_2. Whereas HM showed no activity against H_2O_2. - anti-apoptotic effects: $A\beta_{1-42}$ induced apoptosis in PC-12 cell. Treatment with fractions inhibited $A\beta_{1-42}$ induced apoptosis. The PT fraction was found to be most effective against apoptosis due to the hydroxylation. While HM was to be least effective against apoptosis. - Neurite outgrowth activity All fractions were able to enhance neurite outgrowth at the highest concentration. The PS was the most effective (> 19%) due to the fucose.	

Inhibition of tau pathologies

The majority of the approaches being investigated for the inhibition of tau pathologies are aimed at the inhibition of tau aggregation (table 5) and the inhibition of kinases including GSK-3β **(Boutajangout & Wisniewski, 2014)**.

Inhibition of GSK-3

Tau phosphorylation is a delicate balance between the kinases that phosphorylate tau and the phosphatases that remove the phosphate group from tau. However, a perturbation of this balance either by an increase of kinases or a decrease of phosphatases may be causative of abnormal tau phosphorylation and that abnormal tau phosphorylation in turn leads to the aggregation of tau **(Martin et al., 2013)**. In this review, we will shed a light on glycogen synthase kinase-3 (GSK-3).

GSK-3 is a serine-threonine kinase, and there are two forms of this kinase, GSK-3α and GSK-3β with masse value of 51 and 47 kDa, respectively **(Doble & Woodgett, 2003)**. GSK-3 can be phosphorylated on Tyr216 of GSK-3β and Tyr279 of GSK-3α. This phosphorylation enhances the activity of this kinase. The GSK-3 activity is inhibited when the Ser9 or Ser21 sites of GSK-3β and GSK-3α respectively, are phosphorylated **(Lei et al., 2011)**. It is implicated in various cellular processes including the regulation of glycogen metabolism, cell cycle progression, apoptosis, and neuronal development. GSK-3 is also a key regulator of the Wnt/β-catenin and insulin signalling pathways **(Beurel et al., 2015; Kim & Snider, 2011; C. Xu et al., 2009)**. GSK-3 is one of the kinases that is strongly associated with AD. Overexpression of GSK-3 is known to directly trigger Aβ peptide production by increasing the cleavage of APP by β and γ secretase, induces tau hyperphosphorylation, impairs the long-term potentiation (LTP), activates microglia to secrete the proinflammatory factors, and causes neurodegeneration **(Hooper et al., 2008)**.

By inhibiting GSK-3, the generation of Aβ can be reduced, and the phosphorylation of protein tau can be alleviated **(Kramer et al., 2012)**. The table 6 lists some GSK-3 inhibitors.

Table 5: Examples of some plants that induce the inhibition of tau aggregation.

Plants	Aims	Results	References
Salvia miltiorrhiza	For their study, Tanshinone IIA (Tan IIA), which is isolated from *Salvia miltiorrhiza*, is used to explore its effects on tau protein.	- Test viability As an introductory step, they tested the effects of Tan IIA on the viability of Neuro-2a (N2a) and Human embryonic kidney 293(HEK293)/Tau cells using the Cell Counting Kit-8 (CCK-8) assay. The results of the experiment indicated that the viability of the N2a and HEK293/Tau cells was not influenced by Tan IIA at 0, 0.5, 1, 2.5, 5, and 10 μM. - Inhibition of expression and phosphorylation of tau protein by Tan IIA After the N2a cells were treated with 0, 2.5, 5 μM Tan IIA for 24 h, western blot analysis showed that N2a cells expressed lower than normal levels of total tau and phospho-Tau (pS396-Tau) proteins. The same process was applied to HEK293/Tau cells in order to observe the effect of Tan IIA on total tau, pS404-Tau, and pS396-Tau protein levels. As a result, the data revealed a decrease in these. On the basis of the immunofluorescence staining results, Tan IIA was found to reduce the levels of total tau in HEK293/Tau cells. After treating the 3xTg-AD mice primary neuron cells with 5μM Tan IIA for 24 h, the western blot analysis revealed that Tan IIA significantly reduced the total tau, pS404-Tau, and pS396-Tau levels in 3×Tg-AD mouse neurons. - Degradation of Tau protein by Tan IIA	**(Cai et al., 2020)**

		In order to understand the role of Tan IIA in the degradation of tau, the researchers conducted experiments with two substances: MG132, an inhibitor of proteasome, and Baf-A1, an inhibitor of autophagy. In the presence of Tan IIA only, the level of total tau, pS404-Tau, and pS396-Tau are diminished in HEK293/Tau cells. Nevertheless, the treatment with MG132 can suppress the degradation of tau created by Tan IIA and as a result, the level of tau, pS404-Tau, and pS396-Tau are increased in HEK293/Tau cells. Contrary to what MG132 did, the Baf-A1 was unable to increase the levels of total Tau, pS404-Tau, and pS396-Tau. Based on the data provided, it appeared that Tau proteins are degraded by Tan IIA through the proteasome pathway; however, the autophagy pathway was not involved. Moreover, when the immunoprecipitation and western blot analysis was performed, it was revealed that the Tan IIA at 5μM was able to increase the ubiquitination of Tau. - The suppression effect of Tan IIA on Tau aggregation and fibril formation The ThT assay showed that the use of Tan IIA with assorted concentrations (0, 2.5, 5, 10 and 20 μM) inhibited the fibrillisation of Tau-R3 and resulted in a considerable reduction in the fluorescence intensity. Furthermore, the TEM analysis demonstrated the inhibitory effect of tan IIA on heparin-induced aggregation of Tau-R3. - In silico study (molecular docking) The interaction between Tan IIA and Tau protein was investigated using AutoDock Vina 1.1.2. The study revealed that Tan IIA forms	

		two hydrogen bonds with Tau protein: one of these is between Tan IIA and Ser-320, and the other is between Tan IIA and Lys-369. Other strong bonds were observed between the 1, 2, 3, 4 tetrahydronaphthalene of Tan IIA and the residues Cys-322, Lys-370, Val-363 and Pro-364, the hydrophobic binds. The strong fixation of Tan IIA with Tau-R3 prevents the assembly of tau protein.	
Azadirachta indica (Limonoids)	The aim of this study was to test the capacity of small molecule intermediate (nimbin) and final limonoids (salannin) isolated from *Azadirachta indica* to inhibit tau aggregation.	The aggregation of tau hTau40wt (expressed in *E. coli*) was characterised by the formation of hydrophobic patches and β- sheet structure. The results of ThS, ANS, and TEM assays showed that the treatment of hTau40wt with Limonoids (nimbin and salannin): - Blocked β-sheet formation, - Decreased hydrophobic patches formation. - Inhibited tau aggregation (nimbin inhibited 41.5% of tau aggregation, while salannin inhibited 27.6% of it) and formed short and fragile aggregates. The viability of HEK293T cells was not influenced by nimbin and salannin. Moreover, both limonoids reduced tau-mediated toxicity.	**(Gorantla et al., 2019)**
Cinnamomum zeylanicum (or Ceylon cinnamon)	The aim of the study was to test the capacity of cinnamon extract (CE) to inhibit tau aggregation	The incubation of Tau^{187} with heparin led to the formation of fibrils. The latter was under surveillance using turbidity, thioflavin-S fluorescence, centrifugation, and electron microscopy methods. The results showed that the treatment of Tau^{187} with CE: - Reduced 75% of turbidity and inhibited tau aggregation, - Inhibited bona fide fibres formation, - Reduced tau fibres formation.	**(Peterson et al., 2009)**

		Moreover, cinnamon extract promoted monomeric tau aggregation and polymeric tau fibres disassembly. The inhibitor activity of cinnamon extract against tau aggregation is probably due to cinnamaldehyde.	
Isobavachalcone (derived from *Psoralea corylifolia*)	For their study, isobavachalcone is used to explore its effects on tau protein.	The results of ThT fluorescence and TEM assays indicated that the treatment with isobavachalcone inhibited heparin-induced tau K18 aggregation and prevented tau K18 filaments formation. Moreover, tau K18 fibrils can be broken down by isobavachalcone. Isobavachalcone was able to prevent the occurrence of apoptosis by inhibiting phosphatidylserine-induced tau K18 oligomers and via the ER (endoplasmic reticulum) and mitochondria pathways. Isobavachalcone was also able to modulate the activity of GSK-3β and PP2A (decrease GSK-3β and increase PP2A), to reduce the phosphorylation of tau protein.	**(Xiao et al., 2021)**
Red Ginseng	Examined the effect of KRGE (Korean red ginseng extract) and KRGE fraction (SF, saponin fraction; NSF, nonsaponin fraction; and NFP, nonsaponin fraction with polysaccharide) on tau protein.	The data of ThT fluorescence and TEM assays indicated that the treatment with KRGE or KRGE fraction (SF, NSF, and NFP): - Inhibited heparin-induced tau K18 aggregation, - Induced tau aggregates dissociation.	**(Shin et al., 2020)**

Ramalina terebrata	The aim of the study was to test the capacity of *R. terebrata* compounds to inhibit the aggregation of tau protein.	22 compounds were identified in the methanolic extract of *R. terebrata* using UHPLC-PDA-Q/Orbitrap/MS/MS. The methanolic extract of *R. terebrata* inhibited almost all of the tau aggregation at 1000 μg/mL. Four compounds of *R. terebrata* were tested: parietin, usnic acid, atraric acid, and inositol. These compounds did not inhibit the aggregation of tau except the parietin (inhibited at 28 μg/mL 75% of tau aggregation). - Molecular docking The author of this article considered that parietin is one of the molecules that have a negative charge. The result of the molecular docking showed that parietin interacted with the lysine of tau VQIVYK motif within the microtubule binding domain.	**(Cornejo et al., 2016)**

Table 6: Example of some inhibitors of GSK-3

Inhibitors	Mains finding	References
Indirubins (Danggui Longhui Wan component).	GSK-3β was incubated with GS-1 peptide as substrate + ATP (15 μM) + indirubins (indirubin-3'-monoxime). Indirubins were found to be powerful inhibitors of GSK-3β. Recombinant human tau, expressed in bacteria, was treated with GSK-3β; the results showed that GSK-3 induced phosphorylation of tau. The addition of indirubins (indirubin-3'-monoxime) reduced in a dose dependent manner tau phosphorylation. Moreover, htau23 (exhibiting in Sf9 cells) was treated with or without indirubin-3'-monoxime. GSK-3β induced the phosphorylation of AT100, PHF-1, AT8, and AT180 sites. The addition of indirubin-3'-monoxime reduced the phosphorylation at PHF-1 and AT180 sites and completely	**(Leclerc et al., 2001)**

	inhibited the phosphorylation at AT100 and AT8 sites, which indicates that indirubin-3'-monoxime inhibits GSK-3β. CDK5 was also assayed using histone H1 as substrate + 15 μM ATP + indirubins. The results showed that indirubins were able to inhibit CDK5. Kinetic study was performed indicate that indirubins interacted with GSK-3β within the ATP-binding pocket, so the indirubins are ATP-competitive GSK-3β inhibitors.	
Lithium	After NT2N neurons were treated with various Lithium chloride (LiCl) concentrations (0, 0.5, 1, 5, 10, and 25 mM), the results showed that LiCl in a concentration-dependent manner decreased the PHF1 (phosphorylation-dependent) immunoreactivity and increased the T1 (non-phosphorylation dependent) immunoreactivity as well as the electrophoretic mobility of tau, which was detected by T14/46 (total tau), meaning lithium induced reduction of tau phosphorylation. - GSK-3 inhibition The increase in LiCl concentration (0, 1, 5, 10 mM) inhibited GSK-3 in a concentration-dependent manner. - GSK-3β WT/SFV and S9A/SFV (without lithium) When NT2N neurons were treated with GSK-3β WT/SFV and GSK-3β S9A/SFV, T1 immunoreactivity was found to be decreased and PHF1 immunoreactivity was found to be increased, meaning that GSK-3β S9A and GSK-3β WT increased phosphorylation of tau. - GSK-3β (WT and S9A) + Lithium The addition of lithium removed this increase in tau phosphorylation (decreased the PHF1 immunoreactivity and increased the T1 immunoreactivity). The results indicated that lithium was able to directly inhibit GSK-3 to reduce tau phosphorylation.	**(Hong et al., 1997; Kramer et al., 2012)**

	- Lithium has opposite effects to GSK-3 Lithium increased phosphorylation of tau on the T1 site and decreased phosphorylation of tau on the PHF1, PHF13, PHF6, T3P, AT8, and AT270 sites. Whereas GSK-3 decreased phosphorylation of tau on the T1 site and increased phosphorylation of tau on the PHF1, PHF13, PHF6, T3P, AT8, and AT270 sites (neither lithium nor GSK-3 altered 12E8 site). This confirms the previous results that lithium direct inhibits GSK-3. - NT2N neurons + Calyculin A (phosphatases inhibitor) The results showed that Calyculin A was able to inhibit phosphatases 1 and 2A and decrease T1 immunoreactivity. - NT2N neurons + Calyculin A + lithium The addition of lithium increased T1 immunoreactivity. Lithium's ability to reduce tau phosphorylation appears to be independent of the activation of phosphatase. The mechanism of lithium action on GSK-3β has been the subject of much speculation. Two hypotheses were put forth to explain how lithium inhibits GSK-3β: the first being that lithium (Li^{+}) is Mg^{2+}competitive inhibitor, it doesn't compete with substrate or ATP, and the second being that lithium inhibits potassium deficiency.	
Kangen-karyu (KK) made up of six herbs: *Paeoniae Radix*, *Cnidii Rhizoma*, *Carthami Flos*, *Cyperi Rhizoma*,	- GSK-3β inhibition by Kangen-karyu (KK) The results showed that the KK was able to inhibit GSK-3β with an IC_{50} of 17.05 ± 1.14 μg/ mL. - GSK-3β inhibition by the constituents of KK The smaller IC_{50} value (the higher inhibitory activity) was found in *Salviae Miltiorrhizae* (IC_{50}= 7.77 ± 1.38 μg/ mL), followed by *Cyperi Rhizoma* (20.68 ± 2.50 μg/ mL). The other constituents were not found to have remarkable GSK-3β inhibition.	**(Paudel et al., 2018)**

Aucklandiae Radix, and *Salviae Miltiorrhizae*. Polar compounds of *Salvia miltiorrhiza*: Salvianolic acid (A, B, and C), Magnesium lithospermate B, Rosmarinic acid, and Caffeic acid.	- GSK-3β inhibition by polar compounds of *Salvia miltiorrhiza* The higher inhibitory activity was found in Salvianolic acid B (Sal B; IC_{50}: 6.97 ± 0.96 μM), followed by Sal A, Sal C, and magnesium lithospermate B with IC_{50} values of 30.21 ± 3.14 μM, 31.82 ± 2.08 μM, 33.07 ± 3.88 μM, respectively. Rosmarinic acid exhibited moderate activity ((IC_{50}: 135.35 ± 4.69 μM). While caffeic acid exhibited IC_{50} values of more than 400 μM (mild inhibition). - Docking studies with AutoDock 4.2 (using AMP-PNP and Indirubine ATP-competitive as a reference) Sal B could bind to GSK-3β to the ATP binding site by forming H-Bond with Lys183, Gln185, and Cys199. Moreover, Sal B could bind to GSK-3β by forming H-bond with Thr138 (not present in the ATP-competitive reference). Sal B could bind to GSK-3β by forming a bond with Leu188 and Val70 by π-alkyl interaction and with Lys85 by π-cation interaction. Kinetic study indicated that Sal B is ATP-competitive GSK-3β inhibitor. - Docking studies using Andrographolide GSM (GSK3 substrate)-competitive as reference Within the GSM binding site, Sal B could bind to GSK-3β by forming a bond with Arg96 and Lys292 by H-bond interaction, Arg96 and Val263 by π-alkyl interaction, Phe293 by π–π T-shaped interaction, and with Lys292 by π–σ interaction.	
Salvia officinalis (SO), *Lavandula angustifolia* (LA), *Mentha piperita* (MP), *Melissa*	- GSK-3β inhibition All Lamiaceae extracts had GSK-3β inhibitory activity < 75 μg/mL. The highest inhibitory activity against GSK-3β was found in the OO, MP, OM, TV, OV, MO, and LA with IC_{50} values of 7.94 μg/ mL, 8.84 μg /mL, 12.75 μg /mL, 21.80 μg /mL, 24.20 μg /mL, 27.59 μg /mL, and 40.35 μg /mL, respectively. 14 chemicals were identified in the *O. onites*, of which apigenin 7-	**(Gürbüz et al., 2019)**

officinalis (MO), *Origanum onites* (OO), *Thymus vulgaris* (TV), *Origanum majorana* (OM), *Origanum vulgare* (OV), *Sideritis congesta* (SC), *Dorystoechas hastata* (DH).	O-glucuronide, rosmarinic acid, and luteolin 7-O-glucuronide were the major compounds of OO and also OM. Studies have shown that these compounds may be useful in AD prevention due to their neuroprotective and anti-inflammatory effects. For *M. piperita* eriocitrin, salvianolic acid E/B, and rosmarinic acid were the major compounds and may help to prevent the toxicity of amyloid beta. BACE-1 inhibition All extracts exhibited IC_{50} values of more than 200 μg/ mL and were therefore deemed to be ineffective in inhibiting BACE-1. - CK-1δ inhibition The extracts were not found to have remarkable CK-1δ inhibition.	
NP12: Thiadiazolidinone (TDZD) derivative.	TDZD is non-ATP competitive inhibitor. Ana Martinez et al. suggested that the TDZD was able to interact with GSK-3 within the oxyanion binding pocket. They also suggested that the rapprochement of Lys205, Arg96, and Arg180 was necessary and required the negative charge to allow the active conformation to be stabilised. NP12 treatment precluded the spatial memory decline observed in APP^{sw}- tau^{vlw} mice. It has been proven that the Ser9 phosphorylation inhibited GSK-3β. NP12 treatment increased GSK-3β phosphorylation at Ser9. Moreover, the treatment of NP12 reduced the phosphorylation (≈ 60%) at PHF1 and CP13 sites, which were the putative sites of GSK-3β on tau protein. Thus meaning that NP12 was capable to decrease phosphorylation of tau in APP^{sw}- tau^{vlw} mice.	**(Martinez et al., 2002; Serenó et al., 2009)**
Paullone (Alsterpaullone)	- GSK-3, CDK5, CDK3, CDK1 inhibition GSK-3 was incubated with GS-1 peptide (substrate) + ATP (15μm) + Paullone (alsterpaullone), CDKs were incubated with histone H1 (substrate) + ATP (15μm) + Paullone (alsterpaullone).	**(Leost et al., 2000)**

	The results showed that alsterpaullone was able to inhibit GSK-3α/GSK-3β, CDK2/cyclin A, CDK1/cyclin B, CDK5/p25 and CDK2/cyclin E with IC_{50} values of 0.004 μM, 0.015 μM, 0.035 μM, 0.040 μM, and 0.200 μM, respectively. The results of their research have demonstrated that paullone is one of the kinase inhibitors that could inhibit CDKs and GSK-3. Kinetic experiments showed that paullone inhibited CDKs within the ATP binding site, the same results found with GSK-3, thus the paullone was ATP competitive GSK-3β inhibitor. - *In vitro* Recombinant human tau (expressed in bacteria) was treated by GSK-3β, the latter induced tau phosphorylation. The addition of alsterpaullone inhibited this phosphorylation in a dose dependent manner ($IC_{50} \approx$ 33 nM). - *In vivo*: Human tau23 (exhibiting in Sf9 cells) was treated with or without 20 μM of alsterpaullone/ aminopurvalanol. The results showed that alsterpaullone inhibited the phosphorylation at PHF-1 and AT100 sites of GSK-3β. AT8 was the putative site of GSK-3β and CDK-like kinase; alsterpaullone also inhibited the phosphorylation at this site but either by inhibiting GSK-3β or CDK. Alsterpaullone at AT180 exhibited a weak inhibition. Concerning the aminopurvalanol (CDK inhibitors but not GSK-3β), it was able to inhibit the phosphorylation at AT8 and AT100 sites, to reduce the phosphorylation at AT180, but it showed a weak inhibition at PHF-1 site. This date indicated that alsterpaullone was capable to inhibit GSK3-β and reduce tau phosphorylation.	
Thienylhalomethyl-Ketones	- CSK-3β inhibition GSK-3β assayed using peptide GS-1 (substrate) + ATP and with or without compound (eight compounds were used, their structures are found in (Conde et al., 2003) article). The results showed that six of these compounds exhibited IC_{50} values of more than 100 μM, and one showed	**(Conde et al., 2003; Perez et al., 2009)**

an IC_{50}= 75 μM, thus ineffective in inhibiting GSK-3β. The highest inhibitory activity against GSK-3β was found in the 2-chloroacetyl-4,5- dichlorothiophene (**8**) with IC_{50} value of 2.5 μM.

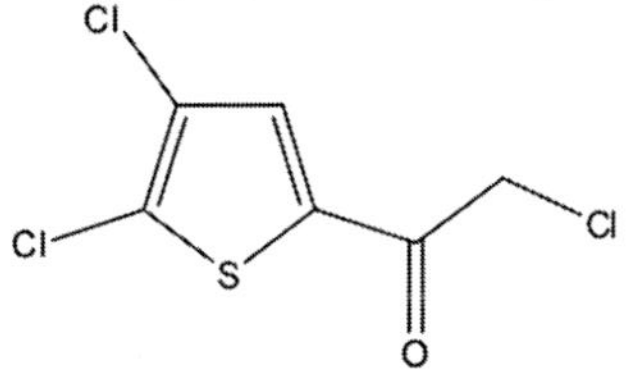

2-chloroacetyl-4,5- dichlorothiophene

A similar experiment was done but with other compounds. The results showed that chloromethylhalothienyl ketones (**20**, **19**, and **21**) had remarkable GSK-3β inhibition with IC_{50} value of 1 μM, 2 μM, and 3 μM, respectively.

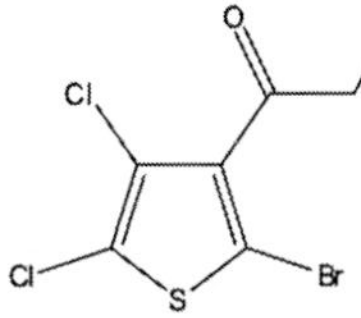

19

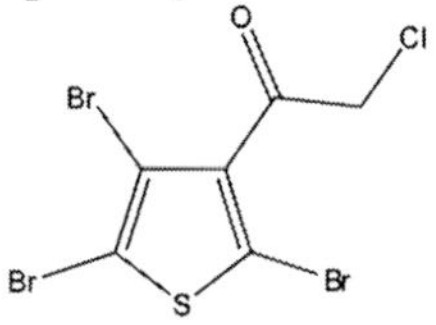

20

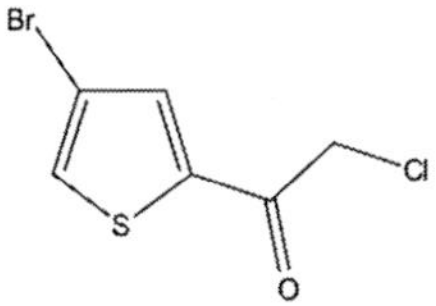

21

The results of kinetic experiments suggested that halomethylketones (HMKs) are non-ATP-competitive inhibitors. The authors of this paper suggested that HMKs modified the proper positioning of ATP within the ATP-binding pocket and induced a covalent modification of Cys199, which disrupts GSK-3β's phosphorylating activity. Therefore, HMKs can be considered as irreversible inhibitors.

	Granule cerebellar neuron (GCNs) was treated with HMKs (**18**, **19**, **23**, **28**, **29**, **30**, and **32**). The results showed that all compounds were able to decrease PHF-1 –immunoreactivity and increase Tau-1 –immunoreactivity. Thus, HMKs could reduce GSK-3β induced tau phosphorylation.	
Salvia fruticosa infusion (SFINF) and its predominant compounds: rosmarinic acid (RA), luteolin 7-O-glucuronide, and caffeic acid.	- GSK-3β, CK-1δ, and BACE-1 inhibition (using Kinase-Glo Kit assay SFINF was able to inhibit GSK-3β with an IC_{50} of 6.52 μg/mL. However, it was not found to have remarkable inhibitory activity against BACE-1 and CK-1δ (IC_{50}: 86 μg/mL and 121.57 μg/mL, respectively). - Molecular docking The docking score of rosmarinic acid was found to be the best (-14.62 kcal/mol: least binding energy), compared to luteolin 7-O-glucuronide (-13.98 kcal/mol), and caffeic acid (-11.43 kcal/mol). Moreover, RA and AR-A014418 (selective GSK-3 inhibitor) both orient similarly in the GSK-3β active site. However, rosmarinic acid (RA) exhibited IC_{50} values of more than 100 μM (ineffective in inhibiting GSK-3β), which means that the synergistic of SFINF compounds can inhibit GSK-3β. After treating the SH-SY5Y cells with amyloid beta (Aβ), the latter reduced cell proliferation. The addition of SFINF suppressed this reduction in cell proliferation and stimulated it in a non-dose dependent manner.	**(Gürbüz et al., 2021)**

4. Inhibition of ApoE4

Because of the side effects of ApoE4 that have been mentioned before, researchers discovered that the inhibition of ApoE4 may be considered as remedy for AD (table 7).

Table 7: Examples of some molecules induced ApoE4 inhibition.

Inhibitors	Main finding	References
Antisense oligonucleotides (ASOs)	After treating the P301S/ApoE4 mice with ASOs the results showed that ASOs: - Decreased ApoE4 expression, - Reduced the tau pathological forms, - Reduced levels of three cytokines IL6, TNFα, and IL1β to lessen the extent of neuroinflammation.	**(Litvinchuk et al., 2021)**
Budmunchiamine L5	Study in silico indicated that budmunchiamine L5: - Was less toxic, - Absorbed well, - Could cross the BBB, - Formed H-bond with Glu77, - Could stably bind to ApoE4 as shown the dynamics simulation. Budmunchiamine L5 could inhibit ApoE4.	**(H.-J. Huang et al., 2014)**
imipramine and olanzapine	The two compounds were found in the NCC drug library and tested by HTS (high-throughput screening) assay (the experiment was carried out on several compounds). The results showed that imipramine and olanzapine: - Could cross the BBB, - Inhibited the apoE4-Aβ interaction,	**(N. R. Johnson et al., 2021)**

	- Decreased the Aβ fibrillisation rate, After treating the 5xFAD mouse neurons with imipramine and olanzapine the data showed that these two compounds: - Had no effects on cell viability, - Decreased the level of Aβ and its neuropathology - Decreased the total tau and pTau.	
curcumin	11 cholinesterase inhibitors and 18 plant compounds were used in this experiment. The docking results showed that curcumin: - Had the best scoring function than the other compounds, - Had the best affinity toward the ApoE4 binding site: curcumin interacted with ApoE4 by forming an H-bond with Glu77 and with Glu27. Researchers proposed that curcumin could inhibit ApoE4. Another study was intended to look at the impacts of curcumin on ApoE4. After transfection, the SH-SY5Y cells with ApoE4, there has been an increase in proinflammatory factors, decrease in the expression of the peroxisome proliferator-activated receptor-γ (PPARγ), and activation of the NF-κB pathway. Treatment with curcumin: - Decreased the levels of inflammatory factors IL1β, TNF-α, nitric oxide, COX-2 and iNOS, - Inhibited the activation of nuclear factor kappa B (NF-κB) pathway by promoting the expression of PPARγ. According to this data curcumin was able to inhibit ApoE4 and its neurological damage.	**(Dhanachandra Singh et al., 2012; M. Wang et al., 2020)**
GIND25 and PH002	The data showed that both GIND25 and PH002: - Affected the domain interaction of ApoE4 in Neuro-2a cells, as a result decreased ApoE4 induced damaged intracellular trafficking.	**(Brodbeck et al., 2011; C. Wang et al., 2018)**

	GIND25 and PH002 are two small molecular compounds that can correct the structures of apoE4. Another research stated that apoE4-ACM treatment with PH002 decreased the ApoE4, reduced Aβ's$_{42/40}$ and pTau levels, and increased the number of GABAergic neurons.	
CS-6253	The addition of CS-6253 in apoE4-TR mice increased the level of ABCA1, which in turn increased the lipidation of ApoE4.	**(Boehm-Cagan et al., 2016)**

5. Acetylcholinesterase inhibition

Cholinesterase belongs to the family of serine hydrolase, it comes in two types: butyrylcholinesterase (BuChE) and acetylcholinesterase (AChE) (Talesa, 2001). AChE is an enzyme responsible for breaking down acetylcholine (ACh), a neurotransmitter that is sensitised by choline acetyltransferase. It is involved in the process of learning and memory **(Alvarez et al., 1997; Hasselmo, 2006)**. If the AChE is too high or the activity of choline acetyltransferase is below the usual level, the ACh levels become too low. Some issues may happen on the level of memory and concentration, and it will lead to a reduction in the cholinergic neurotransmission which will be a sign of AD **(Mukherjee et al., 2007)**. Aβ and P-tau promote the elevation of AChE in the case of illness. Moreover, AChE not only serves to hydrolyse ACh but also, it forms stable complexes with Aβ fibrils and boosts Aβ aggregation. On one hand, AChE influenced PS-1 to increase the production of Aβ, and on the other, GSK-3β also influenced by AChE induced tau hyperphosphorylation **(Alvarez et al., 1997; García-Ayllón et al., 2011)**. Researchers suggested that the inhibition of AChE is one of the possible treatments for AD. In this review, we will focus on the studies that used plants-based remedy to inhibit acetylcholinesterase (table 8).

Table 8: Examples of some plants exhibited anticholinesterase activity.

Plants	Aims	Results	References
Stephaniae Tetrandrae Radix (STR), *Coptidis Rhizoma* (CR), *Phellodendri Chinensis Cortex* (PCC).	The aim of the study was to test the combination of STR+CR and STR+PCC, as well as the combinations of their alkaloids, fangchinoline (isolated from STR), and coptisine (isolated from CR) /berberine (isolated from PCC) to inhibit acetylcholinesterase (AChE).	HPLC was used to identify the principal components in extracts of STR, CR, and PCC. The STR extract contains two major alkaloids: fangchinoline and tetrandrine. There are four major alkaloids found in the CR extract: berberine, coptisine, palmatine, and epiberberine. For PCC extract, the major alkaloid is berberine. - The Ellman method was used to determine the inhibition of AChE by extracts and their alkaloids For the herbal extract: The CR extract showed the strong inhibition of AChE with an IC_{50} of 4.11 ± 0.15 µg/mL, while the STR extract showed the moderate inhibition of AChE (IC_{50}= 570.11 ± 10.41 µg/mL). For their alkaloids: The smaller IC_{50} value, was found in fangchinoline (IC_{50}= 2.17 ± 0.05 µM), followed by berberine (2.33 ± 0.16 µM), palmatine (6.52 ± 0.84 µM), coptisine (13.50 ± 1.48 µM), and epiberberine (18.70 ± 0.83 µM), meaning that fangchinoline had the greatest inhibitory activity against AChE. Whereas the tetrandrine had no inhibitory activity against AChE. - The synergistic effect of herb extracts/alkaloids was calculated using the median-effect principle The combination of STR-CR (the combination index CI< 1 when Fa< 0.4), as well as the combination of STR-PCC (CI<	**(Kong et al., 2019)**

		1 when Fa< 0.8), showed better synergistic inhibition of AChE activity depending on the dose. When Fa=0.5 the CI of fangchinoline-coptisine and fangchinoline-berberine at various ratios was below 1, proposing a synergistic inhibitory effect on AChE when used together. - The molecular docking was employed using the MOE Dock module in order to assess the binding mechanisms of the active components on the AChE. Fangchinoline could bind to AChE by forming a bond with PHE_{288} (acyl active sites) by π-H interaction and with TYR_{334} (PAS active site) through an H-donor interaction. While berberine and coptisine could bind to AChE by forming a bond with PHE_{330} (gated flexible active site) by an H-π interaction and with TRP_{279} (PAS active site) by an H-π interaction. Berberine showed another interaction with PAS active site (TYR_{334}) of AChE by an H-π interaction. Molecular docking simulation revealed the feasibility of inhibiting AChE activity by these alkaloids.	
Juglans regia L	The extracts used: dichloromethane, methanol, acetone, ethyl acetate and distilled water. The purpose of study is to test antioxidant activity of these extracts (using DPPH, DMPD, SO, NO, H_2O_2,	The extracts were all effective against DPPH (the fruit acetone extract showed a higher scavenging activity at 2000 μg ml^{-1}). But they had no inhibitory effect on H_2O_2 and DMPD. SO and NO were scavenged by dichloromethane and water extracts respectively.	**(Orhan et al., 2011)**

	ferric ion-chelating capacity, FRAP and PRAP) and their anticholinesterase activity against acetylcholinesterase (AChE) and butyrylcholinesterase (BChE).	For the ferric ion-chelating capacity, water had the greatest activity, followed by dichloromethane, acetone, methanol, and ethyl acetate. The fruit acetone and the leaf dichloromethane inhibited FRAP and PRAP respectively. Concerning anticholinesterase activity, the leaf dichloromethane extract had a large capacity to inhibit BChE ($32.18 \pm 1.36\%$ at 200 $\mu g\ ml^{-1}$) compared to other extracts that have a no or low inhibitory capacity. However, no extracts were able to inhibit AChE.	
Juglans regia, Mentha piperita, Fragaria ananassa, Melissa officinalis, Salvia officinalis, Helichrysum arenarium.	The study examined the antioxidant activity (using the following methods: DPPH, LDL oxidation, β-carotene bleaching, Rancimat) and the anticholinesterase activity (against AChE) of the aqueous tea infusions of these plants.	The infusions were all effective against DPPH and β-carotene bleaching (they were able to inhibit the linoleic acid peroxidation and, therefore, block beta carotene oxidation). *Fragaria ananassa L.* and *Melissa officinalis L.* aqueous infusions showed a higher scavenging activity against LDL oxidation. The Rancimat method showed that the most effective at inhibiting lipid peroxide formation was *Salvia officinalis L.* and *Helichrysum arenarium L.* aqueous infusions. *Juglans regia L.* and *Fragaria ananassa L.* aqueous infusions (using Ellman´s method) were found to be the strongest inhibitors of AChE (with 45% and 42.5% inhibition) compared to other infusions.	**(Kulišić-Bilušić et al., 2008)**
Pulmonaria officinalis And	The study examined the anticholinesterase effect and antioxidant effect of *Pulmonaria*	Antioxidant activity (against DPPH and reducing power): - *C.umbellatum* ethanolic extract and *P.officinalis* ethanolic extract at 3 mg/ml were able to inhibit 84.9%,	**(Neagu et al., 2018)**

Centarium umbellatum	*officinalis* and *Centarium umbellatum* (aqueous and ethanolic extracts).	75.47%, respectively of DPPH more than the aqueous extracts. - The reason that ethanolic extracts of these two plants exhibited the higher antioxidant activity is the existence of flavone in large quantities. - The same results were found when using reducing power method. HPLC analysis: - Rosmarinic acid, rutin, and hyperoside were found in high concentration in *P. officinalis* ethanolic extract. - Caffeic acid was found in *P. officinalis* aqueous extract. - Caffeic acid and syringic acid were found in high concentration in *C. umbellatum* aqueous extract. - Hyperoside and rutin were found in high concentration in *C. umbellatum* ethanolic extract. Inhibition of acetylcholinesterase: - Ethanolic extracts were found to inhibit acetylcholinesterase more than aqueous extracts. - The *C.umbellatum* ethanolic extract inhibited 94.24% of AChE, followed by *C.umbellatum* aqueous extract, *P. officinalis* ethanolic extract, and *P. officinalis* aqueous extract with 92.28, 87.72, 72.24 percent inhibition, respectively.	
Citrullus colocynthis, *Emex spinosa*,	The aim of the study was to: - Test the ability of these plants to inhibit AChE,	- Activity antioxidant (against: DPPH) *Emex spinosa* (IC_{50} =10.89 µg/ml) > *Scrophularia hypericifolia* (IC_{50} =11.88 µg/ml) > *Caylusea hexagyna* (IC_{50}	**(Shadat et al., 2015)**

Rhazya stricta, *Scrophularia hypericifolia* and *Caylusea hexagyna*	- Examine their antioxidant effect.	=12.33 µg/ml) > *Rhazya stricta* (IC_{50} =12.80 µg/ml) > *Citrullus colocynthis* (IC_{50} =12.83 µg/ml). - Against Superoxide radical *Scrophularia hypericifolia* (IC_{50} =20.83 µg/ml) > *Rhazya stricta* (IC_{50} =37.51 µg/ml) > *Caylusea hexagyna* (IC_{50} =62.50 µg/ml) > *Citrullus colocynthis* (IC_{50} =62.51 µg/ml) > *Emex spinosa* (IC_{50} =68.18 µg/ml). - Against H_2O_2 *Scrophularia hypericifolia* (IC_{50} =8.66 µg/ml) > *Rhazya stricta* (IC_{50} =15.59 µg/ml) > *Caylusea hexagyna* (IC_{50} =24.53 µg/ml) > *Citrullus colocynthis* (IC_{50} =25.99 µg/ml) > *Emex spinosa* (IC_{50} =28.34 µg/ml). - Against Ferrous ions *Caylusea hexagyna* (IC_{50} =15.58 µg/ml) > *Emex spinosa* (IC_{50} =15.99 µg/ml) > *Citrullus colocynthis* (IC_{50} =16.67 µg/ml) > *Rhazya stricta* (IC_{50} =18.60 µg/ml) > *Scrophularia hypericifolia* (IC_{50} =20.51 µg/ml). - Activity anti acetylcholinesterase The height-inhibitor activity was found in *Citrullus colocynthis* (inhibited 83.54% of AChE), *Emex spinosa* (inhibited 81.92% of AChE), and *Rhazya stricta* (inhibited 76.36% of AChE). While the weak activity was found in *Caylusea hexagyna* (18.48%) and *Scrophularia hypericifolia* (15.79%).	
Curcuma longa (REVERC3)	The purpose of study is to test the anticholinesterase activity of	- AChE inhibition REVERC3 inhibited AChE with an IC_{50} of 29.08 µg/mL, which showed a higher inhibitor activity compared to the	**(Hv et al., 2020)**

	REVERC3 (turmeric extract) against AChE and BuChE.	regular turmeric extract (IC_{50}= 139.2 µg/ mL). Galantamine (used as reference) still had the higher inhibitor activity (IC_{50}= 0.31 µg/ mL). - BuChE inhibition REVERC3 inhibited BuChE with an IC_{50} of 33.59 µg/mL - Kinetic study Kinetic study showed that REVERC3 inhibited AChE activity competitively (Galantamine exhibited mixed inhibition). Inhibition of the BuChE by REVERC3 was by uncompetitive (Galantamine exhibited competitive inhibition). - Molecular docking The molecular docking was employed to assess the binding mechanisms of the bisdemethoxycurcumin (BDMC, REVERC3 constituent) on the cholinesterase. BDMC could strongly bind to AChE by forming an H-bond with PHE295 (acyl pocket). BDMC could bind to BuChE by forming a bond with Asp70 (PAS region), Ser198, and His438 (catalytic domain)	

Conclusion

Amyloid beta and tau protein are the main culprits in Alzheimer's disease (AD). Aβ is a protein that builds up in the brain and leads to the formation of plaques, whilst tau is a protein that forms tangles in the brain. When these proteins build up, the brain begins to deteriorate, and AD occurs. Today, there are no effective treatments for AD. However, scientists are still developing ways to slow the progression of the disease. Almost all researchers, whether old or new, have focused on the inhibition of amyloid beta formation, ROS production, cholinesterase, tau hyperphosphorylation, the toxic effects of apoE4, and kinases including GSK-3 as a solution to either cure or minimise the symptoms of AD. Moreover, therapies by medicinal plants are being pursued by researchers for the treatment of AD, due to many of their bioactive compounds that show a wide range of biological activities.

Acknowledgments: The authors acknowledge the facilities provided by the Algerian Ministry of Higher Education and Scientific Research.

References

Alam, P., Chaturvedi, S. K., Siddiqi, M. K., Rajpoot, R. K., Ajmal, M. R., Zaman, M., & Khan, R. H. (2016). Vitamin k3 inhibits protein aggregation: Implication in the treatment of amyloid diseases. *Scientific Reports*, *6*(1), 26759. https://doi.org/10.1038/srep26759

Alam, P., Siddiqi, M. K., Chaturvedi, S. K., Zaman, M., & Khan, R. H. (2017). Vitamin B12 offers neuronal cell protection by inhibiting Aβ-42 amyloid fibrillation. *International Journal of Biological Macromolecules*, *99*, 477-482. https://doi.org/10.1016/j.ijbiomac.2017.03.001

Alghazwi, M., Charoensiddhi, S., Smid, S., & Zhang, W. (2020). Impact of Ecklonia radiata extracts on the neuroprotective activities against amyloid beta (Aβ1-42) toxicity and aggregation. *Journal of Functional Foods*, *68*, 103893. https://doi.org/10.1016/j.jff.2020.103893

Alvarez, A., Opazo, C., Alarcón, R., Garrido, J., & Inestrosa, N. C. (1997). Acetylcholinesterase promotes the aggregation of amyloid-beta-peptide fragments by forming a complex with the growing fibrils. *Journal of Molecular Biology*, *272*(3), 348-361. https://doi.org/10.1006/jmbi.1997.1245

Baumkotter, F., Schmidt, N., Vargas, C., Schilling, S., Weber, R., Wagner, K., Fiedler, S., Klug, W., Radzimanowski, J., Nickolaus, S., Keller, S.,

Eggert, S., Wild, K., & Kins, S. (2014). Amyloid Precursor Protein Dimerization and Synaptogenic Function Depend on Copper Binding to the Growth Factor-Like Domain. *Journal of Neuroscience*, *34*(33), 11159-11172. https://doi.org/10.1523/JNEUROSCI.0180-14.2014

Beckman, J. S., Beckman, T. W., Chen, J., Marshall, P. A., & Freeman, B. A. (1990). Apparent hydroxyl radical production by peroxynitrite : Implications for endothelial injury from nitric oxide and superoxide. *Proceedings of the National Academy of Sciences of the United States of America*, *87*(4), 1620-1624. https://doi.org/10.1073/pnas.87.4.1620

Beurel, E., Grieco, S. F., & Jope, R. S. (2015). Glycogen synthase kinase-3 (GSK3) : Regulation, actions, and diseases. *Pharmacology & therapeutics*, *0*, 114-131. https://doi.org/10.1016/j.pharmthera.2014.11.016

Bird, T. D. (2008). Genetic Aspects of Alzheimer Disease. *Genetics in medicine: official journal of the American College of Medical Genetics*, *10*(4), 231-239. https://doi.org/10.1097/GIM.0b013e31816b64dc

Boehm-Cagan, A., Bar, R., Liraz, O., Bielicki, J. K., Johansson, J. O., & Michaelson, D. M. (2016). ABCA1 Agonist Reverses the ApoE4-Driven Cognitive and Brain Pathologies. *Journal of Alzheimer's Disease*, *54*(3), 1219-1233. https://doi.org/10.3233/JAD-160467

Boutajangout, A., & Wisniewski, T. (2014). Tau-Based Therapeutic Approaches for Alzheimer's Disease—A Mini-Review. *Gerontology*, *60*(5), 381-385. https://doi.org/10.1159/000358875

Boyles, J. K., Pitas, R. E., Wilson, E., Mahley, R. W., & Taylor, J. M. (1985). Apolipoprotein E associated with astrocytic glia of the central nervous system and with nonmyelinating glia of the peripheral nervous system. *The Journal of Clinical Investigation*, *76*(4), 1501-1513. https://doi.org/10.1172/JCI112130

Brodbeck, J., McGuire, J., Liu, Z., Meyer-Franke, A., Balestra, M. E., Jeong, D., Pleiss, M., McComas, C., Hess, F., Witter, D., Peterson, S., Childers, M., Goulet, M., Liverton, N., Hargreaves, R., Freedman, S., Weisgraber, K. H., Mahley, R. W., & Huang, Y. (2011). Structure-dependent Impairment of Intracellular Apolipoprotein E4 Trafficking and Its Detrimental Effects Are Rescued by Small-molecule Structure Correctors. *The Journal of Biological Chemistry*, *286*(19), 17217-17226. https://doi.org/10.1074/jbc.M110.217380

Broide, R. S., & Leslie, F. M. (1999). The α7 nicotinic acetylcholine receptor in neuronal plasticity. *Molecular Neurobiology*, *20*(1), 1-16. https://doi.org/10.1007/BF02741361

Bryson, H. M., & Benfield, P. (1997). Donepezil: *Drugs & Aging*, *10*(3), 234-239. https://doi.org/10.2165/00002512-199710030-00007

Buée, L., Bussière, T., Buée-Scherrer, V., Delacourte, A., & Hof, P. R. (2000). Tau protein isoforms, phosphorylation and role in neurodegenerative disorders11These authors contributed equally to this work. *Brain Research Reviews*, *33*(1), 95-130. https://doi.org/10.1016/S0165-0173(00)00019-9

Busciglio, J., Lorenzo, A., Yeh, J., & Yankner, B. A. (1995). β-Amyloid fibrils induce tau phosphorylation and loss of microtubule binding. *Neuron*, *14*(4), 879-888. https://doi.org/10.1016/0896-6273(95)90232-5

Cai, N., Chen, J., Bi, D., Gu, L., Yao, L., Li, X., Li, H., Xu, H., Hu, Z., Liu, Q., & Xu, X. (2020). Specific Degradation of Endogenous Tau Protein and Inhibition of Tau Fibrillation by Tanshinone IIA through the Ubiquitin–Proteasome Pathway. *Journal of Agricultural and Food Chemistry*, *68*(7), 2054-2062. https://doi.org/10.1021/acs.jafc.9b07022

Carrillo-Mora, P., Luna, R., & Colín-Barenque, L. (2014). Amyloid beta : Multiple mechanisms of toxicity and only some protective effects? *Oxidative medicine and cellular longevity*, *2014*.

Casley, C. S., Canevari, L., Land, J. M., Clark, J. B., & Sharpe, M. A. (2002). β-Amyloid inhibits integrated mitochondrial respiration and key enzyme activities. *Journal of Neurochemistry*, *80*(1), 91-100. https://doi.org/10.1046/j.0022-3042.2001.00681.x

Chafekar, S. M., Malda, H., Merkx, M., Meijer, E. W., Viertl, D., Lashuel, H. A., Baas, F., & Scheper, W. (2007). Branched KLVFF Tetramers Strongly Potentiate Inhibition of β-Amyloid Aggregation. *ChemBioChem*, *8*(15), 1857-1864. https://doi.org/10.1002/cbic.200700338

Chen, F., David, D., Ferrari, A., & Gotz, J. (2004). Posttranslational Modifications of Tau—Role in Human Tauopathies and Modeling in Transgenic Animals. *Current Drug Targets*, *5*(6), 503-515. https://doi.org/10.2174/1389450043345236

Chen, G., Xu, T., Yan, Y., Zhou, Y., Jiang, Y., Melcher, K., & Xu, H. E. (2017). Amyloid beta : Structure, biology and structure-based therapeutic development. *Acta Pharmacologica Sinica*, *38*(9), 1205-1235. https://doi.org/10.1038/aps.2017.28

Conde, S., Pérez, D. I., Martínez, A., Perez, C., & Moreno, F. J. (2003). Thienyl and Phenyl α-Halomethyl Ketones: New Inhibitors of Glycogen Synthase Kinase (GSK-3β) from a Library of Compound Searching. *Journal of Medicinal Chemistry*, *46*(22), 4631-4633. https://doi.org/10.1021/jm034108b

Cornejo, A., Salgado, F., Caballero, J., Vargas, R., Simirgiotis, M., & Areche, C. (2016). Secondary Metabolites in Ramalina terebrata Detected by UHPLC/ESI/MS/MS and Identification of Parietin as Tau

Protein Inhibitor. *International Journal of Molecular Sciences*, *17*(8), 1303. https://doi.org/10.3390/ijms17081303

Cox, K., Combs, B., Abdelmesih, B., Morfini, G., Brady, S. T., & Kanaan, N. M. (2016). Analysis of isoform-specific tau aggregates suggests a common toxic mechanism involving similar pathological conformations and axonal transport inhibition. *Neurobiology of Aging*, *47*, 113-126. https://doi.org/10.1016/j.neurobiolaging.2016.07.015

Desai, A. K., & Grossberg, G. T. (2005). Rivastigmine for Alzheimer's disease. *Expert Review of Neurotherapeutics*, *5*(5), 563-580. https://doi.org/10.1586/14737175.5.5.563

Dhanachandra Singh, Kh., Karthikeyan, M., Kirubakaran, P., Sathya, V., & Nagamani, S. (2012). Structure-based drug discovery of ApoE4 inhibitors from the plant compounds. *Medicinal Chemistry Research*, *21*(6), 825-833. https://doi.org/10.1007/s00044-011-9595-3

Doble, B. W., & Woodgett, J. R. (2003). GSK-3 : Tricks of the trade for a multi-tasking kinase. *Journal of Cell Science*, *116*(7), 1175-1186. https://doi.org/10.1242/jcs.00384

Dubey, S., Kallubai, M., & Subramanyam, R. (2021). Improving the inhibition of β-amyloid aggregation by withanolide and withanoside derivatives. *International Journal of Biological Macromolecules*, *173*, 56-65. https://doi.org/10.1016/j.ijbiomac.2021.01.094

Durand, D., Damon, M., & Gobert, M. (2013). Le stress oxydant chez les animaux de rente : Principes généraux. *Cahiers de Nutrition et de Diététique*, *48*(5), 218-224. https://doi.org/10.1016/j.cnd.2013.04.005

Esler, W. P., & Wolfe, M. S. (2001). A portrait of Alzheimer secretases–new features and familiar faces. *Science*, *293*(5534), 1449-1454.

García-Ayllón, M.-S., Small, D. H., Avila, J., & Sáez-Valero, J. (2011). Revisiting the Role of Acetylcholinesterase in Alzheimer's Disease : Cross-Talk with P-tau and β-Amyloid. *Frontiers in Molecular Neuroscience*, *4*, 22. https://doi.org/10.3389/fnmol.2011.00022

Gong, C.-X., Liu, F., Grundke-Iqbal, I., & Iqbal, K. (2005). Post-translational modifications of tau protein in Alzheimer's disease. *Journal of Neural Transmission*, *112*(6), 813-838. https://doi.org/10.1007/s00702-004-0221-0

Gorantla, N. V., Das, R., Mulani, F. A., Thulasiram, H. V., & Chinnathambi, S. (2019). Neem Derivatives Inhibits Tau Aggregation. *Journal of Alzheimer's Disease Reports*, *3*(1), 169-178. https://doi.org/10.3233/ADR-190118

Gosztyla, M. L., Brothers, H. M., & Robinson, S. R. (2018). Alzheimer's Amyloid-β is an Antimicrobial Peptide : A Review of the Evidence.

Journal of Alzheimer's Disease, *62*(4), 1495-1506. https://doi.org/10.3233/JAD-171133

Grøntvedt, G. R., Schröder, T. N., Sando, S. B., White, L., Bråthen, G., & Doeller, C. F. (2018). Alzheimer's disease. *Current Biology: CB*, *28*(11), R645-R649. https://doi.org/10.1016/j.cub.2018.04.080

Guix, F. X., Wahle, T., Vennekens, K., Snellinx, A., Chávez-Gutiérrez, L., Ill-Raga, G., Ramos-Fernandez, E., Guardia-Laguarta, C., Lleó, A., Arimon, M., Berezovska, O., Muñoz, F. J., Dotti, C. G., & De Strooper, B. (2012). Modification of γ-secretase by nitrosative stress links neuronal ageing to sporadic Alzheimer's disease. *EMBO Molecular Medicine*, *4*(7), 660-673. https://doi.org/10.1002/emmm.201200243

Guo, Y., Wang, Q., Chen, S., & Xu, C. (2021). Functions of amyloid precursor protein in metabolic diseases. *Metabolism: Clinical and Experimental*, *115*, 154454. https://doi.org/10.1016/j.metabol.2020.154454

Gürbüz, P., Dokumacı, A. H., Gündüz, M. G., Perez, C., Göger, F., Paksoy, M. Y., Yerer, M. B., & Ömür Demirezer, L. (2021). In vitro biological activity of Salvia fruticosa Mill. Infusion against amyloid β-peptide-induced toxicity and inhibition of GSK-3β, CK-1δ, and BACE-1 enzymes relevant to Alzheimer's disease. *Saudi Pharmaceutical Journal*, *29*(3), 236-243. https://doi.org/10.1016/j.jsps.2021.01.007

Gürbüz, P., Martinez, A., Pérez, C., Martínez-González, L., Göger, F., & Ayran, İ. (2019). Potential anti-Alzheimer effects of selected Lamiaceae plants through polypharmacology on glycogen synthase kinase-3β, β-secretase, and casein kinase 1δ. *Industrial Crops and Products*, *138*, 111431. https://doi.org/10.1016/j.indcrop.2019.05.080

Hasselmo, M. E. (2006). The role of acetylcholine in learning and memory. *Current Opinion in Neurobiology*, *16*(6), 710-715. https://doi.org/10.1016/j.conb.2006.09.002

Heinisch, J. J., & Brandt, R. (2016). Signaling pathways and posttranslational modifications of tau in Alzheimer's disease : The humanization of yeast cells. *Microbial Cell*, *3*(4), 135.

Hong, M., Chen, D. C. R., Klein, P. S., & Lee, V. M.-Y. (1997). Lithium Reduces Tau Phosphorylation by Inhibition of Glycogen Synthase Kinase-3. *Journal of Biological Chemistry*, *272*(40), 25326-25332. https://doi.org/10.1074/jbc.272.40.25326

Hooper, C., Killick, R., & Lovestone, S. (2008). The GSK3 hypothesis of Alzheimer's disease. *Journal of Neurochemistry*, *104*(6), 1433-1439. https://doi.org/10.1111/j.1471-4159.2007.05194.x

Hsieh, H., Boehm, J., Sato, C., Iwatsubo, T., Tomita, T., Sisodia, S., & Malinow, R. (2006). AMPAR Removal Underlies Aβ-Induced Synaptic

Depression and Dendritic Spine Loss. *Neuron*, *52*(5), 831-843. https://doi.org/10.1016/j.neuron.2006.10.035

Huang, D., Yu, M., Yang, S., Lou, D., Zhou, W., Zheng, L., Wang, Z., Cai, F., Zhou, W., Li, T., & Song, W. (2018). Ethanol Alters APP Processing and Aggravates Alzheimer-Associated Phenotypes. *Molecular Neurobiology*, *55*(6), 5006-5018. https://doi.org/10.1007/s12035-017-0703-3

Huang, H.-J., Chen, H.-Y., Lee, C.-C., & Chen, C. Y.-C. (2014). Computational Design of Apolipoprotein E4 Inhibitors for Alzheimer's Disease Therapy from Traditional Chinese Medicine. *BioMed Research International*, *2014*, e452625. https://doi.org/10.1155/2014/452625

Huang, Y., & Mahley, R. W. (2014). Apolipoprotein E : Structure and function in lipid metabolism, neurobiology, and Alzheimer's diseases. *Neurobiology of Disease*, *72*, 3-12. https://doi.org/10.1016/j.nbd.2014.08.025

Huang, Y.-W. A., Zhou, B., Wernig, M., & Südhof, T. C. (2017). ApoE2, ApoE3, and ApoE4 Differentially Stimulate APP Transcription and Aβ Secretion. *Cell*, *168*(3), 427-441.e21. https://doi.org/10.1016/j.cell.2016.12.044

Hv, S., Raj, A., K, G., S, C., & K, S. (2020). Kinetics and computational analysis of cholinesterase inhibition by REVERC3, a bisdemethoxycurcumin-rich *Curcuma longa* extract : Relevance to the treatment of Alzheimer's disease. *SAGE Open Medicine*, *8*, 205031212097349. https://doi.org/10.1177/2050312120973499

Ischiropoulos, H., & Al-Mehdi, A. B. (1995). Peroxynitrite-mediated oxidative protein modifications. *FEBS Letters*, *364*(3), 279-282. https://doi.org/10.1016/0014-5793(95)00307-U

Iuvone, T., De Filippis, D., Esposito, G., D'Amico, A., & Izzo, A. A. (2006). The Spice Sage and Its Active Ingredient Rosmarinic Acid Protect PC12 Cells from Amyloid-β Peptide-Induced Neurotoxicity. *Journal of Pharmacology and Experimental Therapeutics*, *317*(3), 1143-1149. https://doi.org/10.1124/jpet.105.099317

Iwatsubo, T., Odaka, A., Suzuki, N., Mizusawa, H., Nukina, N., & Ihara, Y. (1994). Visualization of Aβ42(43) and Aβ40 in senile plaques with end-specific Aβ monoclonals : Evidence that an initially deposited species is Aβ42(43). *Neuron*, *13*(1), 45-53. https://doi.org/10.1016/0896-6273(94)90458-8

Jha, A., Kumar, M. G., Gopi, H. N., & Paknikar, K. M. (2018). Inhibition of β-Amyloid Aggregation through a Designed β-Hairpin Peptide. *Langmuir*, *34*(4), 1591-1600. https://doi.org/10.1021/acs.langmuir.7b03617

Johnson, G. V. W., & Stoothoff, W. H. (2004). Tau phosphorylation in neuronal cell function and dysfunction. *Journal of Cell Science*, *117*(24), 5721-5729. https://doi.org/10.1242/jcs.01558

Johnson, N. R., Wang, A. C.-J., Coughlan, C., Sillau, S., Lucero, E., Viltz, L., Markham, N., Allen, C., Dhanasekaran, A. R., Chial, H. J., & Potter, H. (2021). *Imipramine and olanzapine block apoE4-catalyzed polymerization of Aβ and show evidence of improving Alzheimer's disease cognition* (p. 2021.03.28.437389). https://doi.org/10.1101/2021.03.28.437389

Kadavath, H., Hofele, R. V., Biernat, J., Kumar, S., Tepper, K., Urlaub, H., Mandelkow, E., & Zweckstetter, M. (2015). Tau stabilizes microtubules by binding at the interface between tubulin heterodimers. *Proceedings of the National Academy of Sciences*, *112*(24), 7501-7506. https://doi.org/10.1073/pnas.1504081112

Kessels, H. W., & Malinow, R. (2009). Synaptic AMPA Receptor Plasticity and Behavior. *Neuron*, *61*(3), 340-350. https://doi.org/10.1016/j.neuron.2009.01.015

Kienlen-Campard, P., Tasiaux, B., Hees, J. V., Li, M., Huysseune, S., Sato, T., Fei, J. Z., Aimoto, S., Courtoy, P. J., Smith, S. O., Constantinescu, S. N., & Octave, J.-N. (2008). Amyloidogenic Processing but Not Amyloid Precursor Protein (APP) Intracellular C-terminal Domain Production Requires a Precisely Oriented APP Dimer Assembled by Transmembrane GXXXG Motifs *. *Journal of Biological Chemistry*, *283*(12), 7733-7744. https://doi.org/10.1074/jbc.M707142200

Kim, W.-Y., & Snider, W. (2011). Functions of GSK-3 Signaling in Development of the Nervous System. *Frontiers in Molecular Neuroscience*, *4*, 44. https://doi.org/10.3389/fnmol.2011.00044

Koechlin, N. (2006). Santé mentale : Quelle place pour les fous? *Journal français de psychiatrie*, *4*, 35-37.

Kong, X.-P., Liu, E. Y. L., Chen, Z.-C., Xu, M. L., Yu, A. X. D., Wu, Q.-Y., Xia, Y.-J., Duan, R., Dong, T. T. X., & Tsim, K. W. K. (2019). Synergistic Inhibition of Acetylcholinesterase by Alkaloids Derived from Stephaniae Tetrandrae Radix, Coptidis Rhizoma and Phellodendri Chinensis Cortex. *Molecules*, *24*(24), 4567. https://doi.org/10.3390/molecules24244567

Kramer, T., Schmidt, B., & Lo Monte, F. (2012). Small-Molecule Inhibitors of GSK-3 : Structural Insights and Their Application to Alzheimer's Disease Models. *International Journal of Alzheimer’s Disease*, *2012*, e381029. https://doi.org/10.1155/2012/381029

Kulišić-Bilušić, T., Katalinić, V., Dragović-Uzelac, V., Ljubenkov, I., Kriško, A., Dejanović, B., Jukić, M., Politeo, O., Pifat, G., & Miloš, M.

(2008). Antioxidant and Acetylcholinesterase Inhibiting Activity of Several Aqueous Tea Infusions in vitro. *Food Technology and Biotechnology*, *46*(4), 368-375.

Leclerc, S., Garnier, M., Hoessel, R., Marko, D., Bibb, J. A., Snyder, G. L., Greengard, P., Biernat, J., Wu, Y.-Z., Mandelkow, E.-M., Eisenbrand, G., & Meijer, L. (2001). Indirubins Inhibit Glycogen Synthase Kinase-3β and CDK5/P25, Two Protein Kinases Involved in Abnormal Tau Phosphorylation in Alzheimer's Disease. *Journal of Biological Chemistry*, *276*(1), 251-260. https://doi.org/10.1074/jbc.M002466200

Lee, H. J., Seo, H. I., Cha, H. Y., Yang, Y. J., Kwon, S. H., & Yang, S. J. (2018). Diabetes and Alzheimer's Disease : Mechanisms and Nutritional Aspects. *Clinical Nutrition Research*, *7*(4), 229. https://doi.org/10.7762/cnr.2018.7.4.229

Lee, S. J. C., Nam, E., Lee, H. J., Savelieff, M. G., & Lim, M. H. (2017). Towards an understanding of amyloid-β oligomers : Characterization, toxicity mechanisms, and inhibitors. *Chemical Society Reviews*, *46*(2), 310-323. https://doi.org/10.1039/C6CS00731G

Lei, P., Ayton, S., Bush, A. I., & Adlard, P. A. (2011). GSK-3 in Neurodegenerative Diseases. *International Journal of Alzheimer & #x2019; s Disease*, *2011*, e189246. https://doi.org/10.4061/2011/189246

Leost, M., Schultz, C., Link, A., Wu, Y.-Z., Biernat, J., Mandelkow, E.-M., Bibb, J. A., Snyder, G. L., Greengard, P., Zaharevitz, D. W., Gussio, R., Senderowicz, A. M., Sausville, E. A., Kunick, C., & Meijer, L. (2000). Paullones are potent inhibitors of glycogen synthase kinase-3β and cyclin-dependent kinase 5/p25 : Paullones inhibit GSK-3β and CDK5/p25. *European Journal of Biochemistry*, *267*(19), 5983-5994. https://doi.org/10.1046/j.1432-1327.2000.01673.x

Li, C., Chai, S., Ju, Y., Hou, L., Zhao, H., Ma, W., Li, T., Sheng, J., & Shi, W. (2017). Pu-erh Tea Protects the Nervous System by Inhibiting the Expression of Metabotropic Glutamate Receptor 5. *Molecular Neurobiology*, *54*(7), 5286-5299. https://doi.org/10.1007/s12035-016-0064-3

Litvinchuk, A., Huynh, T. V., Shi, Y., Jackson, R. J., Finn, M. B., Manis, M., Francis, C. M., Tran, A. C., Sullivan, P. M., Ulrich, J. D., Hyman, B. T., Cole, T., & Holtzman, D. M. (2021). Apolipoprotein E4 Reduction with Antisense Oligonucleotides Decreases Neurodegeneration in a Tauopathy Model. *Annals of Neurology*, *89*(5), 952-966. https://doi.org/10.1002/ana.26043

Liu, F., Grundke-Iqbal, I., Iqbal, K., & Gong, C.-X. (2005). Contributions of protein phosphatases PP1, PP2A, PP2B and PP5 to the regulation of tau phosphorylation. *European Journal of Neuroscience*, *22*(8), 1942-1950. https://doi.org/10.1111/j.1460-9568.2005.04391.x

Liu, F., Iqbal, K., Grundke-Iqbal, I., Hart, G. W., & Gong, C.-X. (2004). O-GlcNAcylation regulates phosphorylation of tau : A mechanism involved in Alzheimer's disease. *Proceedings of the National Academy of Sciences*, *101*(29), 10804-10809. https://doi.org/10.1073/pnas.0400348101

Liu, R., Barkhordarian, H., Emadi, S., Park, C., & Sierks, M. (2005). Trehalose differentially inhibits aggregation and neurotoxicity of beta-amyloid 40 and 42. *Neurobiology of Disease*, *20*(1), 74-81. https://doi.org/10.1016/j.nbd.2005.02.003

López Arrieta, J., & Schneider, L. (2006). Metrifonate for Alzheimer's disease. *Cochrane Database of Systematic Reviews*, *2*. https://doi.org/10.1002/14651858.CD003155.pub3

Lovinger, D. M. (2008). Communication Networks in the Brain. *Alcohol Research & Health*, *31*(3), 196-214.

Lyketsos, C. G., Colenda, C. C., Beck, C., Blank, K., Doraiswamy, M. P., Kalunian, D. A., Yaffe, K., & Task Force of American Association for Geriatric Psychiatry. (2006). Position statement of the American Association for Geriatric Psychiatry regarding principles of care for patients with dementia resulting from Alzheimer disease. *The American Journal of Geriatric Psychiatry: Official Journal of the American Association for Geriatric Psychiatry*, *14*(7), 561-572. https://doi.org/10.1097/01.JGP.0000221334.65330.55

Ma, K.-G., & Qian, Y.-H. (2019). Alpha 7 nicotinic acetylcholine receptor and its effects on Alzheimer's disease. *Neuropeptides*, *73*, 96-106. https://doi.org/10.1016/j.npep.2018.12.003

Mahley, R. (1988). Apolipoprotein E : Cholesterol transport protein with expanding role in cell biology. *Science*, *240*(4852), 622-630. https://doi.org/10.1126/science.3283935

Mahley, R. W., & Rall, S. C. (2000). Apolipoprotein E : Far More Than a Lipid Transport Protein. *Annual Review of Genomics and Human Genetics*, *1*(1), 507-537. https://doi.org/10.1146/annurev.genom.1.1.507

Mamun, A., Uddin, Md. S., Mathew, B., & Ashraf, G. (2020). Toxic Tau : Structural Origins of Tau Aggregation in Alzheimer's Disease. *Neural Regeneration Research*, *15*, 1417-1420. https://doi.org/10.4103/1673-5374.274329

Martin, L., Latypova, X., & Terro, F. (2011). Post-translational modifications of tau protein : Implications for Alzheimer's disease. *Neurochemistry International*, *58*(4), 458-471.

https://doi.org/10.1016/j.neuint.2010.12.023
Martin, L., Latypova, X., Wilson, C. M., Magnaudeix, A., Perrin, M.-L., Yardin, C., & Terro, F. (2013). Tau protein kinases : Involvement in Alzheimer's disease. *Ageing Research Reviews*, *12*(1), 289-309. https://doi.org/10.1016/j.arr.2012.06.003
Martinez, A., Alonso, M., Castro, A., Pérez, C., & Moreno, F. J. (2002). First non-ATP competitive glycogen synthase kinase 3 beta (GSK-3beta) inhibitors : Thiadiazolidinones (TDZD) as potential drugs for the treatment of Alzheimer's disease. *Journal of Medicinal Chemistry*, *45*(6), 1292-1299. https://doi.org/10.1021/jm011020u
Mathew, R., Srinivas, G., & Mathuranath, P. S. (2011). Tau and Tauopathies. In J. P. Blass (Éd.), *Neurochemical Mechanisms in Disease* (p. 633-667). Springer. https://doi.org/10.1007/978-1-4419-7104-3_19
Matter, M. L., Zhang, Z., Nordstedt, C., & Ruoslahti, E. (1998). The α5β1 Integrin Mediates Elimination of Amyloid-β Peptide and Protects Against Apoptosis. *Journal of Cell Biology*, *141*(4), 1019-1030. https://doi.org/10.1083/jcb.141.4.1019
McLaurin, J., Kierstead, M. E., Brown, M. E., Hawkes, C. A., Lambermon, M. H. L., Phinney, A. L., Darabie, A. A., Cousins, J. E., French, J. E., Lan, M. F., Chen, F., Wong, S. S. N., Mount, H. T. J., Fraser, P. E., Westaway, D., & George-Hyslop, P. S. (2006). Cyclohexanehexol inhibitors of Aβ aggregation prevent and reverse Alzheimer phenotype in a mouse model. *Nature Medicine*, *12*(7), 801-808. https://doi.org/10.1038/nm1423
Mietelska-Porowska, A., Wasik, U., Goras, M., Filipek, A., & Niewiadomska, G. (2014). Tau Protein Modifications and Interactions : Their Role in Function and Dysfunction. *International Journal of Molecular Sciences*, *15*(3), 4671-4713. https://doi.org/10.3390/ijms15034671
Mogana, R., Adhikari, A., Debnath, S., Hazra, S., Hazra, B., Teng-Jin, K., & Wiart, C. (2014). The Antiacetylcholinesterase and Antileishmanial Activities of Canarium patentinervium Miq. *BioMed Research International*, *2014*, 1-7. https://doi.org/10.1155/2014/903529
Möller, H. J., & Graeber, M. B. (1998). The case described by Alois Alzheimer in 1911. Historical and conceptual perspectives based on the clinical record and neurohistological sections. *European Archives of Psychiatry and Clinical Neuroscience*, *248*(3), 111-122. https://doi.org/10.1007/s004060050027
Monyer, H., Sprengel, R., Schoepfer, R., Herb, A., Higuchi, M., Lomeli, H., Burnashev, N., Sakmann, B., & Seeburg, P. H. (1992). Heteromeric

NMDA Receptors : Molecular and Functional Distinction of Subtypes. *Science*, *256*(5060), 1217-1221. https://doi.org/10.1126/science.256.5060.1217

Mukherjee, P. K., Kumar, V., Mal, M., & Houghton, P. J. (2007). Acetylcholinesterase inhibitors from plants. *Phytomedicine*, *14*(4), 289-300. https://doi.org/10.1016/j.phymed.2007.02.002

Neagu, E., Radu, G. L., Albu, C., & Paun, G. (2018). Antioxidant activity, acetylcholinesterase and tyrosinase inhibitory potential of Pulmonaria officinalis and Centarium umbellatum extracts. *Saudi Journal of Biological Sciences*, *25*(3), 578-585. https://doi.org/10.1016/j.sjbs.2016.02.016

Nguyen, K. V. (2015). The human β-amyloid precursor protein : Biomolecular and epigenetic aspects. *Biomolecular Concepts*, *6*(1), 11-32. https://doi.org/10.1515/bmc-2014-0041

Nordgren, I., Bengtsson, E., Holmstedt, B., & Pettersson, B.-M. (2009). Levels of Metrifonate and Dichlorvos in Plasma and Erythrocytes during Treatment of Schistosomiasis with Bilarcil®. *Acta Pharmacologica et Toxicologica*, *49*, 79-86. https://doi.org/10.1111/j.1600-0773.1981.tb03256.x

Olin, J. T., & Schneider, L. (2002). Galantamine for Alzheimer's disease. *Cochrane Database of Systematic Reviews*, *3*. https://doi.org/10.1002/14651858.CD001747

Orhan, I. E., Suntar, I. P., & Akkol, E. K. (2011). In vitro neuroprotective effects of the leaf and fruit extracts of Juglans regia L. (walnut) through enzymes linked to Alzheimer's disease and antioxidant activity. *International Journal of Food Sciences and Nutrition*, *62*(8), 781-786. https://doi.org/10.3109/09637486.2011.585964

PACHER, P., BECKMAN, J. S., & LIAUDET, L. (2007). Nitric Oxide and Peroxynitrite in Health and Disease. *Physiological reviews*, *87*(1), 315-424. https://doi.org/10.1152/physrev.00029.2006

Pagano, K., Tomaselli, S., Molinari, H., & Ragona, L. (2020). Natural Compounds as Inhibitors of Aβ Peptide Aggregation : Chemical Requirements and Molecular Mechanisms. *Frontiers in Neuroscience*, *0*. https://doi.org/10.3389/fnins.2020.619667

Paglini, G., Peris, L., Mascotti, F., Quiroga, S., & Caceres, A. (2000). Tau Protein Function in Axonal Formation. *Neurochemical Research*, *25*(1), 37-42. https://doi.org/10.1023/A:1007531230651

Pallas-Bazarra, N., Jurado-Arjona, J., Navarrete, M., Esteban, J. A., Hernández, F., Ávila, J., & Llorens-Martín, M. (2016). Novel function of Tau in regulating the effects of external stimuli on adult hippocampal neurogenesis. *The EMBO Journal*, *35*(13), 1417-1436.

https://doi.org/10.15252/embj.201593518

Paudel, P., Seong, S., Zhou, Y., Park, C., Yokozawa, T., Jung, H., & Choi, J. (2018). Rosmarinic Acid Derivatives' Inhibition of Glycogen Synthase Kinase-3β Is the Pharmacological Basis of Kangen-Karyu in Alzheimer's Disease. *Molecules*, *23*(11), 2919. https://doi.org/10.3390/molecules23112919

Perez, D. I., Conde, S., Pérez, C., Gil, C., Simon, D., Wandosell, F., Moreno, F. J., Gelpí, J. L., Luque, F. J., & Martínez, A. (2009). Thienylhalomethylketones : Irreversible glycogen synthase kinase 3 inhibitors as useful pharmacological tools. *Bioorganic & Medicinal Chemistry*, *17*(19), 6914-6925. https://doi.org/10.1016/j.bmc.2009.08.042

Permanne, B., Adessi, C., Saborio, G. P., Fraga, S., Frossard, M., Van Dorpe, J., Dewachter, I., Banks, W. A., Van Leuven, F., & Soto, C. (2002). Reduction of amyloid load and cerebral damage in transgenic mouse model of Alzheimer's disease by treatment with a β-sheet breaker peptide. *The FASEB Journal*, *16*(8), 860-862. https://doi.org/10.1096/fj.01-0841fje

Peters, C., Fernandez-Perez, E. J., Burgos, C. F., Espinoza, M. P., Castillo, C., Urrutia, J. C., Streltsov, V. A., Opazo, C., & Aguayo, L. G. (2013). Inhibition of amyloid beta-induced synaptotoxicity by a pentapeptide derived from the glycine zipper region of the neurotoxic peptide. *Neurobiology of Aging*, *34*(12), 2805-2814. https://doi.org/10.1016/j.neurobiolaging.2013.06.001

Peterson, D. W., George, R. C., Scaramozzino, F., LaPointe, N. E., Anderson, R. A., Graves, D. J., & Lew, J. (2009). Cinnamon Extract Inhibits Tau Aggregation Associated with Alzheimer's Disease In Vitro. *Journal of Alzheimer's Disease*, *17*(3), 585-597. https://doi.org/10.3233/JAD-2009-1083

Plum, L., Schubert, M., & Brüning, J. C. (2005). The role of insulin receptor signaling in the brain. *Trends in Endocrinology & Metabolism*, *16*(2), 59-65. https://doi.org/10.1016/j.tem.2005.01.008

Potkin, S. G., Anand, R., Fleming, K., Alva, G., Keator, D., Carreon, D., Messina, J., Wu, J. C., Hartman, R., & Fallon, J. H. (2001). Brain metabolic and clinical effects of rivastigmine in Alzheimer's disease. *The International Journal of Neuropsychopharmacology*, *4*(03). https://doi.org/10.1017/S1461145701002528

Rajmohan, R., & Reddy, P. H. (2017). Amyloid Beta and Phosphorylated Tau Accumulations Cause Abnormalities at Synapses of Alzheimer's disease Neurons. *Journal of Alzheimer's disease : JAD*, *57*(4), 975-999. https://doi.org/10.3233/JAD-160612

Reisberg, B., Doody, R., Stöffler, A., Schmitt, F., Ferris, S., & Möbius, H. J. (2003). Memantine in Moderate-to-Severe Alzheimer's Disease. *New England Journal of Medicine*, *348*(14), 1333-1341. https://doi.org/10.1056/NEJMoa013128

Renner, M., Lacor, P. N., Velasco, P. T., Xu, J., Contractor, A., Klein, W. L., & Triller, A. (2010). Deleterious Effects of Amyloid β Oligomers Acting as an Extracellular Scaffold for mGluR5. *Neuron*, *66*(5), 739. https://doi.org/10.1016/j.neuron.2010.04.029

Robert D. Terry & Peter Davies. (1980). *Dementia of the Alzheimer Type | Annual Review of Neuroscience.* https://www.annualreviews.org/doi/pdf/10.1146/annurev.ne.03.030180.000453

Rodrigues, C. M. P., Solá, S., Brito, M. A., Brondino, C. D., Brites, D., & Moura, J. J. G. (2001). Amyloid β-Peptide Disrupts Mitochondrial Membrane Lipid and Protein Structure : Protective Role of Tauroursodeoxycholate. *Biochemical and Biophysical Research Communications*, *281*(2), 468-474. https://doi.org/10.1006/bbrc.2001.4370

Rossi, F., & Bianchini, E. (1996). Synergistic Induction of Nitric Oxide by β-Amyloid and Cytokines in Astrocytes. *Biochemical and Biophysical Research Communications*, *225*(2), 474-478. https://doi.org/10.1006/bbrc.1996.1197

Sadigh-Eteghad, S., Sabermarouf, B., Majdi, A., Talebi, M., Farhoudi, M., & Mahmoudi, J. (2015). Amyloid-Beta : A Crucial Factor in Alzheimer's Disease. *Medical Principles and Practice*, *24*(1), 1-10. https://doi.org/10.1159/000369101

Saha, R. N., & Pahan, K. (2006). Regulation of Inducible Nitric Oxide Synthase Gene in Glial Cells. *Antioxidants & redox signaling*, *8*(5-6), 929-947. https://doi.org/10.1089/ars.2006.8.929

Schedin-Weiss, S., Winblad, B., & Tjernberg, L. O. (2014). The role of protein glycosylation in Alzheimer disease. *FEBS Journal*, *281*(1), 46-62. https://doi.org/10.1111/febs.12590

Serenó, L., Coma, M., Rodríguez, M., Sánchez-Ferrer, P., Sánchez, M. B., Gich, I., Agulló, J. M., Pérez, M., Avila, J., Guardia-Laguarta, C., Clarimón, J., Lleó, A., & Gómez-Isla, T. (2009). A novel GSK-3β inhibitor reduces Alzheimer's pathology and rescues neuronal loss in vivo. *Neurobiology of Disease*, *35*(3), 359-367. https://doi.org/10.1016/j.nbd.2009.05.025

Shadat, A., Ibrahim, A., Ezzeldin, E., & Alsaid, M. (2015). Acetylcholinesterase inhibition and antioxidant activity of some medicinal plants for treating neuro degenarative disease. *African*

Journal of Traditional, Complementary and Alternative Medicines, *12*(3), 97. https://doi.org/10.4314/ajtcam.v12i3.12

Shankar, G. M., Li, S., Mehta, T. H., Garcia-Munoz, A., Shepardson, N. E., Smith, I., Brett, F. M., Farrell, M. A., Rowan, M. J., Lemere, C. A., Regan, C. M., Walsh, D. M., Sabatini, B. L., & Selkoe, D. J. (2008). Amyloid-β protein dimers isolated directly from Alzheimer's brains impair synaptic plasticity and memory. *Nature Medicine*, *14*(8), 837-842. https://doi.org/10.1038/nm1782

Sharma, K. (2019). Cholinesterase inhibitors as Alzheimer's therapeutics (Review). *Molecular Medicine Reports*, *20*(2), 1479-1487. https://doi.org/10.3892/mmr.2019.10374

Shelat, P. B., Chalimoniuk, M., Wang, J.-H., Strosznajder, J. B., Lee, J. C., Sun, A. Y., Simonyi, A., & Sun, G. Y. (2008). Amyloid beta peptide and NMDA induce ROS from NADPH oxidase and AA release from cytosolic phospholipase A2 in cortical neurons. *Journal of Neurochemistry*, *106*(1), 45-55. https://doi.org/10.1111/j.1471-4159.2008.05347.x

Shin, S. J., Park, Y. H., Jeon, S. G., Kim, S., Nam, Y., Oh, S.-M., Lee, Y. Y., & Moon, M. (2020). Red Ginseng Inhibits Tau Aggregation and Promotes Tau Dissociation *In Vitro*. *Oxidative Medicine and Cellular Longevity*, *2020*, 1-12. https://doi.org/10.1155/2020/7829842

Skoog, I., & Gustafson, D. (2006). Update on hypertension and Alzheimer's disease. *Neurological Research*, *28*(6), 605-611. https://doi.org/10.1179/016164106X130506

Smith, D. G., Cappai, R., & Barnham, K. J. (2007). The redox chemistry of the Alzheimer's disease amyloid β peptide. *Biochimica et Biophysica Acta (BBA) - Biomembranes*, *1768*(8), 1976-1990. https://doi.org/10.1016/j.bbamem.2007.02.002

Snyder, E. M., Nong, Y., Almeida, C. G., Paul, S., Moran, T., Choi, E. Y., Nairn, A. C., Salter, M. W., Lombroso, P. J., Gouras, G. K., & Greengard, P. (2005). Regulation of NMDA receptor trafficking by amyloid-β. *Nature Neuroscience*, *8*(8), 1051-1058. https://doi.org/10.1038/nn1503

Sohn, E., Kim, Y. J., & Jeong, S.-J. (2021). Korean traditional herbal formula Soshiho-tang attenuates memory impairment and neuronal damage in mice with amyloid-beta-induced Alzheimer's disease. *Integrative Medicine Research*, *10*(3), 100723. https://doi.org/10.1016/j.imr.2021.100723

Stanley, P., Schachter, H., & Taniguchi, N. (2009). N-Glycans. In A. Varki, R. D. Cummings, J. D. Esko, H. H. Freeze, P. Stanley, C. R. Bertozzi,

G. W. Hart, & M. E. Etzler (Éds.), *Essentials of Glycobiology* (2nd éd.). Cold Spring Harbor Laboratory Press. http://www.ncbi.nlm.nih.gov/books/NBK1917/

Stoothoff, W. H., & Johnson, G. V. W. (2005). Tau phosphorylation : Physiological and pathological consequences. *Biochimica et Biophysica Acta (BBA) - Molecular Basis of Disease*, *1739*(2), 280-297. https://doi.org/10.1016/j.bbadis.2004.06.017

Strittmatter, W. J., Saunders, A. M., Schmechel, D., Pericak-Vance, M., Enghild, J., Salvesen, G. S., & Roses, A. D. (1993). Apolipoprotein E : High-avidity binding to beta-amyloid and increased frequency of type 4 allele in late-onset familial Alzheimer disease. *Proceedings of the National Academy of Sciences*, *90*(5), 1977-1981. https://doi.org/10.1073/pnas.90.5.1977

Swerdlow, R. H., Burns, J. M., & Khan, S. M. (2014). The Alzheimer's Disease Mitochondrial Cascade Hypothesis : Progress and Perspectives. *Biochimica et biophysica acta*, *1842*(8), 1219-1231. https://doi.org/10.1016/j.bbadis.2013.09.010

Szabó, C. (2003). Multiple pathways of peroxynitrite cytotoxicity. *Toxicology Letters*, *140-141*, 105-112. https://doi.org/10.1016/S0378-4274(02)00507-6

Tabaton, M., & Tamagno, E. (2007). The molecular link between β- and γ-secretase activity on the amyloid β precursor protein. *Cellular and Molecular Life Sciences*, *64*(17), 2211-2218. https://doi.org/10.1007/s00018-007-7219-3

Talesa, V. N. (2001). Acetylcholinesterase in Alzheimer's disease. *Mechanisms of Ageing and Development*, *122*(16), 1961-1969. https://doi.org/10.1016/S0047-6374(01)00309-8

Tan, M. A., Gonzalez, S. J. B., Alejandro, G. J. D., & An, S. S. A. (2020). Neuroprotective effects of vomifoliol, isolated from Tarenna obtusifolia Merr. (Rubiaceae), against amyloid-beta1-42-treated neuroblastoma SH-SY5Y cells. *3 Biotech*, *10*(10), 424. https://doi.org/10.1007/s13205-020-02421-z

Tesseur, I., Van Dorpe, J., Spittaels, K., Van den Haute, C., Moechars, D., & Van Leuven, F. (2000). Expression of Human Apolipoprotein E4 in Neurons Causes Hyperphosphorylation of Protein Tau in the Brains of Transgenic Mice. *The American Journal of Pathology*, *156*(3), 951-964. https://doi.org/10.1016/S0002-9440(10)64963-2

Theendakara, V., Peters-Libeu, C. A., Bredesen, D. E., & Rao, R. V. (2018). Transcriptional Effects of ApoE4 : Relevance to Alzheimer's Disease. *Molecular Neurobiology*, *55*(6), 5243-5254. https://doi.org/10.1007/s12035-017-0757-2

Vamecq, J., Vallée, L., Storme, L., Gelé, P., & Bordet, R. (2004). Les acteurs immédiats du stress oxydatif. *P HARMACOLOGIE*, *18*, 8.

Van Nostrand, W. E. (2016). The influence of the amyloid β-protein and its precursor in modulating cerebral hemostasis. *Biochimica et biophysica acta*, *1862*(5), 1018-1026. https://doi.org/10.1016/j.bbadis.2015.10.020

van Marum, R. J. (2009). Update on the use of memantine in Alzheimer's disease. *Neuropsychiatric Disease and Treatment*, *5*, 237-247.

Wagstaff, A. J., & McTavish, D. (1994). Tacrine. *Drugs & aging*, *4*(6), 510-540.

Walsh, D. M., Minogue, A. M., Sala Frigerio, C., Fadeeva, J. V., Wasco, W., & Selkoe, D. J. (2007). The APP family of proteins : Similarities and differences. *Biochemical Society Transactions*, *35*(2), 416-420. https://doi.org/10.1042/BST0350416

Wang, C., Najm, R., Xu, Q., Jeong, D., Walker, D., Balestra, M. E., Yoon, S. Y., Yuan, H., Li, G., Miller, Z. A., Miller, B. L., Malloy, M. J., & Huang, Y. (2018). Gain of toxic Apolipoprotein E4 effects in Human iPSC-Derived Neurons Is Ameliorated by a Small-Molecule Structure Corrector. *Nature medicine*, *24*(5), 647-657. https://doi.org/10.1038/s41591-018-0004-z

Wang, H.-Y., Li, W., Benedetti, N. J., & Lee, D. H. S. (2003). A7 Nicotinic Acetylcholine Receptors Mediate β-Amyloid Peptide-induced Tau Protein Phosphorylation *. *Journal of Biological Chemistry*, *278*(34), 31547-31553. https://doi.org/10.1074/jbc.M212532200

Wang, M., Kou, J., Wang, C., Yu, X., Xie, X., & Pang, X. (2020). Curcumin inhibits APOE4-induced injury by activating peroxisome proliferator-activated receptor-γ (PPARγ) in SH-SY5Y cells. *Iranian Journal of Basic Medical Sciences*, *23*(12), 1576-1583. https://doi.org/10.22038/ijbms.2020.47184.10858

Watkins, P. B., Zimmerman, H. J., Knapp, M. J., Gracon, S. I., & Lewis, K. W. (1994). Hepatotoxic Effects of Tacrine Administration in Patients with Alzheimer's Disease. *JAMA*, *271*(13), 992-998. https://doi.org/10.1001/jama.1994.03510370044030

Weber, S. A., Patel, R. K., & Lutsep, H. L. (2018). Cerebral amyloid angiopathy : Diagnosis and potential therapies. *Expert Review of Neurotherapeutics*, *18*(6), 503-513. https://doi.org/10.1080/14737175.2018.1480938

White, M. R., Kandel, R., Tripathi, S., Condon, D., Qi, L., Taubenberger, J., & Hartshorn, K. L. (2014). Alzheimer's Associated β-Amyloid Protein Inhibits Influenza A Virus and Modulates Viral Interactions with Phagocytes. *PLoS ONE*, *9*(7), e101364. https://doi.org/10.1371/journal.pone.0101364

Xiao, S., Wu, Q., Yao, X., Zhang, J., Zhong, W., Zhao, J., Liu, Q., & Zhang, M. (2021). Inhibitory Effects of Isobavachalcone on Tau Protein Aggregation, Tau Phosphorylation, and Oligomeric Tau-Induced Apoptosis. *ACS Chemical Neuroscience*, *12*(1), 123-132. https://doi.org/10.1021/acschemneuro.0c00617

Xu, C., Kim, N.-G., & Gumbiner, B. M. (2009). Regulation of protein stability by GSK3 mediated phosphorylation. *Cell cycle (Georgetown, Tex.)*, *8*(24), 4032-4039.

Xu, Q. (2006). Profile and Regulation of Apolipoprotein E (ApoE) Expression in the CNS in Mice with Targeting of Green Fluorescent Protein Gene to the ApoE Locus. *Journal of Neuroscience*, *26*(19), 4985-4994. https://doi.org/10.1523/JNEUROSCI.5476-05.2006

Yan, D., Zhang, Y., Liu, L., & Yan, H. (2016). Pesticide exposure and risk of Alzheimer's disease : A systematic review and meta-analysis. *Scientific Reports*, *6*, 32222. https://doi.org/10.1038/srep32222

Zhao, N., Liu, C.-C., Van Ingelgom, A. J., Martens, Y. A., Linares, C., Knight, J. A., Painter, M. M., Sullivan, P. M., & Bu, G. (2017). Apolipoprotein E4 Impairs Neuronal Insulin Signaling by Trapping Insulin Receptor in the Endosomes. *Neuron*, *96*(1), 115-129.e5. https://doi.org/10.1016/j.neuron.2017.09.003

Zhao, W.-Q., Felice, F. G. D., Fernandez, S., Chen, H., Lambert, M. P., Quon, M. J., Krafft, G. A., & Klein, W. L. (2008). Amyloid beta oligomers induce impairment of neuronal insulin receptors. *The FASEB Journal*, *22*(1), 246-260. https://doi.org/10.1096/fj.06-7703com